Allergy and the Nervous System

Chemical Immunology and Allergy

Vol. 98

Allergy and the Nervous System

Volume Editor

John Bienenstock Hamilton, Ont.

51 figures, and 4 tables, 2012

KARGER Basel · Freiburg · Paris · London · New York · New Delhi · Bangkok · Beijing · Tokyo · Kuala Lumpur · Singapore · Sydney

Chemical Immunology and Allergy
Formerly published as 'Progress in Allergy' (Founded 1939),
continued 1990–2002 as 'Chemical Immunology'
Edited by Paul Kallós 1939–1988, Byron H. Waksman 1962–2002

Dr. John Bienenstock
Departments of Pathology and
Molecular Medicine
McMaster University
Brain-Body Institute, St. Joseph's Healthcare
50 Charlton Avenue East, T3304
Hamilton, Ontario L8N 4A6 (Canada)
E-Mail bienens@mcmaster.ca

Bibliographic Indices. This publication is listed in bibliographic services, including Current Contents® and PubMed/MEDLINE.

Disclaimer. The statements, opinions and data contained in this publication are solely those of the individual authors and contributors and not of the publisher and the editor(s). The appearance of advertisements in the book is not a warranty, endorsement, or approval of the products or services advertised or of their effectiveness, quality or safety. The publisher and the editor(s) disclaim responsibility for any injury to persons or property resulting from any ideas, methods, instructions or products referred to in the content or advertisements.

Drug Dosage. The authors and the publisher have exerted every effort to ensure that drug selection and dosage set forth in this text are in accord with current recommendations and practice at the time of publication. However, in view of ongoing research, changes in government regulations, and the constant flow of information relating to drug therapy and drug reactions, the reader is urged to check the package insert for each drug for any change in indications and dosage and for added warnings and precautions. This is particularly important when the recommended agent is a new and/or infrequently employed drug.

www.karger.com
Printed in Germany on acid-free and non-aging paper (ISO 9706) by Kraft Druck GmbH, Ettlingen
ISSN 1660–2242
e-ISSN 1662–2898
ISBN 978–3–8055–9984–9
e-ISBN 978–3–8055–9985–6

Contents

Preface

Until a few decades ago, many allergic manifestations were largely regarded as being psychosomatic in origin. This was particularly thought to apply to asthma even though it had been demonstrated that skin allergic reactions could be adoptively transferred from one patient to another with serum in the famous Prausnitz-Kustner reaction [1]. The identification of the role of mast cells in allergy and their content of histamine helped to emphasize the biological nature of allergic reactions [2], and this was finally resolved with the identification of IgE as the key antibody responsible in mice by Ishizaka and Ishizaka [3]. The final confirmation that this not only applied to rodents but also humans in the clinical setting, came with the discovery of a human IgE equivalent by Johansson and Bennich [4].

The subsequent identification that asthma was an inflammatory disease [5], as with many discoveries in medicine, really engendered a paradigm shift away from a consideration of the role of the brain and nervous system in allergy and especially in asthma. In recent times it has become increasingly clear that the immune and nervous systems are integrated and that constant bidirectional communication is occurring between them, and the term psychoneuroimmunology has been used to describe this [6]. Most immune cells possess receptors for neurotransmitters and neurotrophic factors, and indeed also have the capacity to synthesize many of them. That the brain is often involved in modulating inflammation and immune activity has now been well described in the literature, and we showed some time ago that it was possible to condition mast cells to degranulate using a Pavlovian conditioning model [7]. More recently, the potential role of chronic stress in allergic disease has been identified and raises the important question of the role of psychosocial circumstances as determinants of various allergic conditions.

The mechanisms and pathways whereby the nervous system may be involved in beneficial or detrimental outcomes in allergy are still somewhat obscure, but new light is being shed on this complex biology through technological and conceptual advances. These include magnetic resonance imaging of the brain and epigenetics. The chapters in this book cover many but not all aspects of the potential and actual role of the nervous system in the modulation of allergy, and our hope is that they may help restore some balance in our thinking about allergic disease and offer a more holistic approach to its understanding and treatment.

John Bienenstock

References

1 Prausnitz C, Küstner H: Studien über die Ueberempfindlichkeit. Zentralbl Bakteriol 1921;86:160–169.

2 Selye H: The Mast Cells. Washington, Butterworth, 1965.

3 Ishizaka K, Ishizaka T: Identification of gamma E antibody as a carrier of reaginic activity. J Immunol 1967;99:1187–1198.

4 Johansson SGO, Bennich H: Immunological studies of an atypical (myeloma) immunoglobulin. Immunology 1967;13:381–394.

5 Chung KF, Durham SR: Asthma as an inflammatory disease: clinical perspectives. Br Med Bull 1992;48:179–189.

6 Ader R, Felten D, Cohen N (eds): Psychoneuroimmunology, ed 4. New York, Academic Press, 2006.

7 MacQueen G, Marshall J, Perdue M, Siegel S, Bienenstock J: Pavlovian conditioning of rat mucosal mast cells to secrete rat mast cell protease II. Science 1989;243:83–85.

Bienenstock J (ed): Allergy and the Nervous System.
Chem Immunol Allergy. Basel, Karger, 2012, vol 98, pp 1–13

Relations between Asthma and Psychological Distress: An Old Idea Revisited

Ryan J. Van Lieshout[a] · Glenda M. MacQueen[b]

[a]Department of Psychiatry and Behavioral Neurosciences, McMaster University, Hamilton, Ont., and
[b]Department of Psychiatry, University of Calgary, Calgary, Alta., Canada

Abstract
Asthma has long been considered a condition in which psychological distress exerts a negative impact. Epidemiological studies confirm that depression and anxiety disorders, amongst the most common psychiatric disorders, occur in higher rates in people with asthma than in the general population. Alterations in the stress axis, immune and autonomic nervous systems appear to be involved in the pathogenesis of each disorder and may contribute to the observed associations between these conditions. Although there is increasing recognition of the importance of treating psychological distress to optimize symptom control in people with asthma, there are few studies examining whether specific treatments for depression or anxiety can improve symptom control in asthma and result in better overall function and outcome.

Links between psychological factors and allergic disorders have been observed in clinical practice for centuries [1]. More formalized hypotheses regarding the link between asthma and psychological factors were put forward in the 1930s by French and Alexander [2], who described asthma as one of the seven classic psychosomatic disorders caused by specific psychological conflicts. There has been a dramatic shift in the conceptualization and treatment of asthma in the last 50 years or so, but Douwes et al. [3] recently suggested that the original conceptualization of asthma being importantly influenced by psychological factors is experiencing something of a renaissance.

Depression and the anxiety disorders have diagnostic overlap and probably shared pathophysiological processes and are two of the most common psychiatric illnesses. Below, we focus prominently on the association between asthma and either depression or anxiety (depression/anxiety). Mood and anxiety disorders are associated with both a high burden of suffering and immense health care costs. Individuals with asthma and depression/anxiety may be disproportionately affected than those with either condition alone. In youth with depression, asthma severity is increased relative to those with asthma alone [4]. In adults with asthma, mental health problems are also associated with poor asthma control [5]. Pulmonary function tends to be lower in people with asthma and depression or anxiety [6].

Why asthma and certain mental disorders commonly co-occur is not understood. It has been suggested that asthma increases the risk of developing anxiety and depression. Less frequently, it is proposed that mental disorders increase one's risk of developing asthma, but as over half of people with asthma become symptomatic within the first decade of life, this is unlikely to account for the majority of cases. The most provocative explanation is that asthma, depression and anxiety share common pathophysiological pathways. Given that all these conditions are complex chronic illnesses that result from interacting genetic and environmental factors, it is conceivable that they share common susceptibility genes [7] and/or environmental risk factors which account for their high rates of comorbidity.

In this chapter, we examine the clinical and epidemiological evidence supporting the links between asthma and mental disorders and examine data that suggest that the high rate of co-occurrence between these illnesses may arise at least in part via common risk factors and pathways. We then review the evidence that outcome in asthma may be improved through psychiatric interventions that may act in part to decrease features of depression, anxiety and somatization.

Epidemiologic Evidence of the Association between Asthma and Mood and Anxiety Disorders

Individuals with asthma appear to have about a twofold higher risk of having one or more anxiety or depressive disorders [8]. To date, the most methodologically rigorous and generalizable study of the comorbidity of asthma and mental disorders suggests that adults with asthma are at increased risk of manifesting major depressive disorder or dysthymia (OR = 1.6, 95% CI = 1.4–1.8), anxiety disorders including generalized anxiety disorder, panic disorder, posttraumatic stress disorder and social phobia (OR = 1.5, 95% CI = 1.4–1.7) [9]. In this synthesis of studies from 17 different countries, individuals with asthma had rates of major depressive disorder that ranged from 5 to 25.5%, and generalized anxiety disorder from 0 to 6.7%. Despite significant variability in the populations assessed, the sampling methods utilized and means of defining both asthma and mental disorders in studies done to date, the findings of this work generally support the majority of those in the published literature to date [10, 11]. In general, population-based studies have not reported rates of co-morbidity as high as studies that evaluated depression in clinical cohorts of patients with asthma, for whom lifetime rates of depression have been recorded to be as high as 41% [12]. This may represent an accurate reflection of variation in rates of depression occurring as a function of severity of asthma; as it is possible that the overall rates of psychiatric illness in those with mild and well-controlled asthma are low, with elevated rates observed in patients surveyed in tertiary care clinical settings who are likely to have more severe and chronic asthma.

Asthma may be more deleterious to emotional well-being than other chronic illnesses. Children with asthma appeared to be at higher risk for depression than children with other illnesses including cancer and cystic fibrosis [13] and asthmatic children seem to have more problems with affective adjustment and functional impairment than children with a cancer diagnosis [14]. In adults, particularly older adults [11], asthma is associated with higher rates of depression than other chronic illnesses, even after adjusting for psychosocial factors, physical comorbidity and the use of medications linked to depression. The study of Ortega et al. [15] of 2,554 American Latinos showed that of cardiovascular disease, diabetes and asthma, only persons with asthma had an increased risk of a depressive disorder. Ng et al. [11], compared rates of depression in older adults with doctor-diagnosed asthma to nonasthmatic controls including those with chronic illness. They found an increased risk of depressive disorders relative to controls (OR = 2.45, 1.06–5.69) and controls with chronic illnesses even after adjusting for potential confounders (OR = 2.42, 1.04–5.64). Finally, Niti and colleagues compared the rates of depression among older Asian adults with chronic medical illnesses to controls and between the types of illness. In addition to finding that depressive symptoms were higher in those with chronic illness overall, crude odds ratios were elevated for only certain chronic illnesses after adjustment for a number of relevant variables, of which asthma/COPD was the one with the highest risk (OR = 2.85, 1.36–5.98) [16]. Interestingly, though subjective health and functional status explained most of the link between depression and chronic illness, in those with asthma/COPD, these variables did not completely explain depression rates. As a result, the authors concluded that chronic respiratory illness might have a direct psychobiological link to depression.

Mechanisms Underlying the Association between Asthma and Mood and Anxiety Disorders

Why asthma and depression/anxiety are frequently comorbid is not well understood. One cognitive theory posits that asthma produces mental disorders because the repeated experience of asthma produces fearful or catastrophic thoughts about respiratory symptoms that produces anxiety problems over time [17]. It has also been suggested that the experience of unpredictable asthma attacks can lead to a state of learned helplessness that can produce depression [18]. Finally, others believe that the family's exposure to asthma can produce a depressogenic environment, overwhelming parents with excessive care and financial demands [19]. One biological theory that supports the asthma→mental disorder hypothesis suggests that repeated episodes of hypoxia and hypercapnia leads brain circuits that modulate responses to fear including those in the locus ceruleus and amygdala to become hyperreactive in response to asthma attacks or the experience of shortness of breath [17]. Over time this is thought to result in states of anxiety that can become clinical in severity.

Few studies have examined the possibility that asthma and mental disorders share common pathophysiologic pathways. The potential environmental and molecular pathways that might underlie this finding are myriad and could include diverse environmental and genetic influences potentially mediated by dysregulation of a plethora of biological pathways. We have previously reviewed these [20] and here only briefly discuss the range of genetic, familial and environmental factors that may link asthma and depression.

Familial and Genetic Associations between Asthma and Depression

It has been hypothesized that individual genes or even multiple genes in close proximity to one another (and under the control of similar regulatory elements) may be involved in the causal pathways of asthma and depression. However, while heritability estimates for asthma and depression vary from 60 to 80% [21], there is little extant evidence to support the existence of shared polymorphisms between these conditions. Indirect proof of a link between asthma and depression comes from family studies that suggest that the prevalence of one disorder is increased in the family members of index cases with the other [22]. Wamboldt et al. [23] reported that mood but not anxiety disorders were increased in the relatives of adolescents with severe asthma and that the onset of these problems was equally likely to have occurred before as after the proband's asthma diagnosis. More recent studies provide further proof that the prevalence of mood disorders is increased in the parents of children with asthma [24] even when childhood mental illness is considered [25].

More direct evidence supporting a genetic link between asthma and depression comes from the study of Wamboldt et al. [26] of Finnish twin pairs in which they assessed the prevalence of atopic disease and depressive symptomatology. They found a within-person correlation between atopic and depressive symptoms of 0.103 and, using a best-fit model, estimated that 64% of this association was due to shared familial vulnerability, mainly additive genetic factors.

Hypothalamic Pituitary Adrenal Axis

Exposure to highly and/or chronically psychologically stressful environments in early life may also contribute to the increased risk of comorbid asthma and depression or anxiety. Indeed, research in both animals and humans suggests that chronic stress disrupts a series of physiological systems that may actually increase the risk of both asthma and mental disorders. Some have proposed that perinatal exposure to stress in youth at risk of asthma results in alterations of the hypothalamic pituitary adrenal (HPA) axis that is at first hyperresponsive but that becomes hyporesponsive over time. This downregulation of stress hormones and their effects on their receptors may lead to reduced regulation of inflammatory responses in response to asthma triggers [27].

Maternal experience of stress in pregnancy can affect the development of central nervous, immune and respiratory systems. Indeed, the fetus is particularly sensitive to stressful environmental stimuli in utero since DNA synthesis rates are highest at that time. A recent study in humans demonstrated that prenatal psycholgocial stress can induce alterations in both innate and adaptive immune responses as measured in cord blood [28]. Additional physiologic stresses encountered in pregnancy could also confer risk for depression or asthma to offspring. Maternal smoking in pregnancy appears to increase the risk of mental disorders [29], and asthma [30]. Given obesity's association with a systemic inflammatory milieu [31] and since exposure to maternal obesity in pregnancy may increase the risk of psychiatric illness in offspring [32] and the likelihood that they will develop asthma later in life [33], obesity in pregnancy might also be a shared risk factor for asthma and psychiatric illness.

Postnatal stress also appears to play a role in the genesis of asthma. Childhood stress exposure is associated with an increased risk of developing asthma [34] and it is well known that stresses experienced in childhood increase the risk of a variety of psychiatric disorders. Stresses relevant to the pathogenesis of asthma and mental disorders are not merely limited to those experienced in or as a result of the child's proximal physical environment, however. Stress exposure often occurs in multiple contexts in those chronically exposed to it. Children who grow up poor not only experience more family violence, separation, and chaos but have parents who are more authoritarian and less responsive. They are also exposed to higher levels of air and water pollution, more dangerous neighborhoods and attend poorer schools and day cares [35]. The prevalence of asthma also appears to be inversely related to levels of social support [11]. In light of this evidence, it is not difficult to extrapolate this to the conclusion that early life stress may trigger genetic predispositions to asthma as well as to mental disorders.

The Immune System

Given the multiple, complex and reciprocal links between stress response systems and the immune system and the importance of both to the pathogenesis of asthma and certain mental disorders, it would not be surprising if the immune system mediated some of the effects of environmental stresses on asthma and depression. While the immune alterations in asthma, including a predilection for Th2-based immune responses are well known, immune dysregulation is also present in people with depression [36]. Sickness behavior, the emotional and behavioral symptoms that develop as a consequence of acute infection or cytokine therapy, can result from increased levels of interleukin-1 and tumor necrosis factor, and is a frequently cited link between cytokine activation and major depressive disorder (MDD) [37].

A bidirectional relationship seems to exist between cytokine and glucocorticoid (GC) signaling pathways that might explain how stress links asthma and mental illness via the immune system. Cytokine effects on GC signaling are complex as proinflammatory cytokines seem to increase expression of the β-isoform of human GC receptor relative to the α-isoform. This imbalance contributes to GC resistance in a number of disorders, including asthma and may also be important to the development of depression. Certainly, numerous cytokines and their signaling pathways can inhibit glucocorticoid receptor signaling by downregulating the translocation and function of these receptors [20].

Stress-elicited changes in the immune and central nervous systems may occur as early as fetal life. Indeed, maternal stress responses involving the HPA axis in pregnancy and leading to cortisol release affect fetal immunomodulation and induce a Th2 cell predominance by directly affecting cytokine production [38] and preventing the development of regulatory T cells [39]. Postnatal stresses can affect immune development just as prenatal exposures can [40].

The Autonomic Nervous System

The ANS is comprised of the sympathetic (adrenergic, noradrenergic) and parasympathetic (cholinergic) systems. Depression is associated with parasympathetic, vagal or cholinergic bias [41] and people with asthma may also manifest dysregulation of cholinergic systems. As stress can affect the development of the ANS, its dysregulation could be another mechanism by which stress increases the risk of developing both asthma and emotional problems. In addition to being affected by stress, the balance between parasympathetic and sympathetic nervous system activity occurring in response to emotions may be also be germane to immune system alterations that result in airway inflammation and hyperreactivity [42]. Both GC and sympathovagal balances play a role in the development of the immune system as well as intrauterine and postnatal lung maturation [43]. Stress in utero as well as postnatally can also alter sympthovagal balance [44] and affect immunoregulation [45]. In one study, children without asthma and exposed to maternal distress showed an elevation of cortisol in response to acute stressors while asthmatic children had lower cortisol levels. The results of this work suggest that changes in the HPA axis and potentially also the ANS alter inflammatory responses to asthma triggers and may contribute to the association [46] between asthma and certain mental disorders.

While stress generally decreases parasympathetic nervous system activity in healthy persons, Lehrer et al. [47] proposed that in those with asthma, stress may lead to an increased response of both parasympathetic and sympathetic nervous systems. Miller [48] has suggested that depression is accompanied by a pattern of autonomic dysregulation that entails a cholinergic or vagal bias (i.e. vagal over sympathetic reactivity) that amplifies airway instability in asthma. He proposes that depression alters the extent of the vagal or cholinergically mediated response of airways to asthma triggers. Indeed, his group has recently demonstrated that children with asthma and depression demonstrate vagal bias when stressed, as well as increased airway resistance. While this model was not designed to assess the etiologies of asthma or depression, it may provide a framework by which stress increases the risk of this comorbidity via the ANS.

It is apparent that the pathways linking asthma and mental disorders are complex. This is illustrated in a study by Chen et al. [49] in which low family support was associated with worse asthma symptoms via allergic inflammation and worse neighborhood conditions led to worsened morbidity via smoking. As Shalowitz [50] has noted, the studies required to understand these associations require the collection of a wide variety of variables at the individual, family, neighborhood and societal level.

Examining Psychological Influences on Asthma Using Neuroimaging

In addition to the impact psychosocial stress can have on the immune and autonomic nervous systems, it is possible that stress can modulate asthma symptoms [51] via direct effects on the brain [52]. There is anecdotal and empirical evidence that the stable variable of nonhypnotic suggestibility can determine the susceptibility of asthmatic patients to suggestion of bronchoconstriction, providing a construct for understanding how some, but not all, patients with asthma might be influenced by asthma-related cues [53]. Until recently, however, there were no studies that directly imaged the brain during exposure to asthma-related stimuli.

In a seminal study, Rosenkranz et al. [54] used functional magnetic resonance imaging (fMRI) to examine activity in the anterior cingulate cortex (ACC) and insula during exposure to asthma-related words when patients with asthma were exposed to allergen. The results provide provocative evidence that these brain regions were hyperresponsive to asthma related emotional cues and afferent physiologic signals. As Rosenkrantz and Davidson [55] subsequently noted, the relative interoceptive ability of asthmatics is unknown. Asthma is characterized by hypersensitive airways, including the sensory nerves that innervate the airway; it is unknown whether this sensitization to noxious stimuli extends to the cortex. Other chronic inflammatory conditions, such as irritable bowel syndrome, show this form of sensitization [56]. The ACC receives input regarding key physical symptoms (e.g. shortness of breath) of relevance to asthma (for an extensive review of the ACC, see Devinsky et al. [57]). Along with the insula, the ACC is also crucial for the processing of emotional stimuli and is implicated in the pathophysiology of MDD. Rosenkranz et al. [54] contextualized their study by stating that 'despite the compelling support for a model integrating psychological and physiological factors in asthma, the brain has been largely absent from any discussion of its mechanistic underpinnings'.

Capuron et al. [58] also used fMRI to examine patients receiving interferon (IFN) therapy, finding that IFN-treated patients had activation of the dorsal ACC during a visuospatial task that was not present in control subjects. Interestingly, IFN-treated patients performed well on the task but appeared to require more extensive involvement of the ACC than was necessary from control subjects. Although indirect, this study supports the hypothesis that the ACC may be important for understanding the interface of cognition, emotion, and peripheral inflammation. Studies such as these, which integrate brain imaging with physiologic symptoms or inflammatory markers, are complex to undertake but represent extraordinary opportunities to reveal the role of the brain in modulating various components of the asthmatic response.

Treatment of Psychiatric Symptoms to Improve Asthma and Health-Related Quality of Life

Katon et al. [59] examined depression and anxiety in adolescents with asthma, reporting that only about one-third of youth with anxiety had the condition recognized within the last year, and only about one in five youth with depression had adequate treatment. A commentary accompanying this article concluded that the methods used by Katon et al. [59] were probably conservative in the estimates of rates receiving treatment, so the actual rates of treatment of depression or anxiety in youth with asthma may be even lower than 20% [60]. Thus, there appears to be a significant dissociation between studies that, despite limitations, suggest that anxiety and MDD occur frequently in asthma and studies that suggest that in routine clinical practice comorbid psychiatric conditions are infrequently recognized in patients with asthma and even less frequently treated.

There does, however, appear to be increasing recognition of the importance of attending to psychological function in order to optimize outcome in patients with asthma, particularly children and youth. In general, such treatment could involve the direct treatment of symptoms of depression or anxiety in patients with asthma, or it may involve the use of psychological therapies targeted directly at the management of symptoms of asthma [61].

Pharmacologic Treatment

There is a notable paucity of data examining whether treating depression in people with asthma will improve asthma outcome. Brown et al. [62] randomized 90 patients with asthma and an episode of depression to citalopram, a commonly used antidepressant, or placebo. The impact of this intervention on asthma symptoms was difficult to evaluate between antidepressant- and placebo-treated patients because at end point there was no difference in depression scores between antidepressant- and placebo-treated patients. Nonetheless, antidepressant-treated patients required fewer oral corticosteroids and there was a correlation between asthma symptom severity and depression symptoms. Patients who had substantial improvement in depressive symptoms (regardless of whether they were medication or placebo treated) had greater improvement in a variety of asthma-related scales than patients whose depressive symptoms did not improve significantly. These results do, therefore, support the notion that improvement in depressive symptoms may improve outcome in patients with asthma.

Another trial, conducted several decades ago, evaluated the impact of antidepressant treatment on asthma outcome. Completed in 1969, investigators examined whether the antidepressants amitriptyline and doxepin improved depressive and anxiety symptoms in patients with allergic diseases, including some patients with asthma [63]. Doxepin appeared to have a more pronounced benefit than amitriptyline but the particularly potent antihistaminergic properties of doxepin may have mediated the observed effect.

There is some evidence that tianeptine, a selective 5HT reuptake enhancer, reduces respiratory symptoms in those with asthma [64]. A small study that treated depressed people with asthma [65] found that bupropion treatment improved depressive and anxiety symptoms, but this did not translate into significant impact on FEV1 or self-reported asthma control.

In contrast to improved asthma control following treatment of depression, therapeutic agents used for asthma may worsen symptoms of depression and anxiety. Exogenous steroid administration commonly induce mood shifts and experience with immune-based therapies for other conditions highlights the fact that profound changes in mood can occur with immunotherapy, making CNS side effects, including depressive symptoms, a leading reason for treatment discontinuation. More recently, concerns were raised that the leukotriene receptor antagonist montelukast could produce suicidal thinking though thorough reviews of the evidence leading to this assertion suggest that this finding may have been spurious [66]. Studies that consider the pathophysiological points of convergence between MDD and asthma may result at a minimum in the development of new therapies that do not worsen symptoms of the other condition, increasing the likelihood that novel therapeutics will be acceptable to clinicians, patients and regulatory bodies.

Behavioral Treatment

A number of studies have examined the efficacy of psychological therapies at improving various aspects of asthma control or quality of life. These studies have been reviewed for both adults [67] and children [68] and are briefly reviewed here.

Cognitive behavior therapy (CBT) incorporates the key elements of both behavioral and cognitive models. Two studies measuring asthma knowledge as an outcome reported benefits of CBT [69], and CBT has been reported to have a positive effect on self-efficacy measures. The cognitive element of therapy tends to focus on identification and constructive management of incorrect and damaging thoughts, such as perceptions of helplessness or inappropriate fear of asthma attack that can trigger episodes. Information (e.g. about the relations between anxiety and bronchoconstriction) also targets cognitions. Behavioral elements of therapy focus on identifying the processes by which behavior has been learned and modifying behavior using methods such as systematic desensitization, selective reinforcement, and positive modeling.

Dahl found positive results following behavioral therapy when school absenteeism and use of as-needed medications were the outcome measures in young people with asthma [70].

Relaxation techniques are generally conducted with or without biofeedback and were the focus of several earlier studies of psychological interventions in asthma. Such programs generally include progressive relaxation, autogenic training, which focuses on attending to bodily feelings and mentally controlling them, and hypnosis or deep relaxation, which may be induced using mental imagery. This is often accompanied by autosuggestion to create positive thoughts and feedback of biologic indicators, which the subject must control via relaxation. Alexander et al. [71] measured the effect of relaxation therapy on peak expiratory flow and found effects favoring the treatment group compared with the control group. In addition, self-hypnosis assisted relaxation reduced emergency room visits, again in a single study that also found that self-reports of asthma improved in the self-hypnosis group [72]. In contrast, hospital admission rates were not decreased following biofeedback [73], nor were self-hypnosis rates or use of as-needed medications [74], but emergency room visits were in a single study [75]. The results from these studies highlight the variability in outcome measures employed and the difficulty of understanding these studies in a systematic manner given this variability. Breathing retraining exercises include a range of techniques for improving breathing control in asthma. These are not regarded as standard psychotherapics, although aspects of breathing retraining may be included in behavioural therapy or CBT. A Cochrane review [76] has previously examined the effectiveness of breathing retraining exercises, suggesting that conclusions must be viewed with caution.

Despite the trials of various psychological approaches in asthma, there are no sufficiently powered studies of any single therapy to draw conclusions regarding the utility of these approaches for improving asthma-related outcome. In addition to adequate power, a key issue limiting the interpretation of these studies is how to select patients with asthma for psychological intervention. It may be that a randomized controlled trial that includes patients with very mild or well-controlled asthma or only minimal psychological distress may not yield much evidence of improvement in asthma symptoms following intervention.

Conclusions

Psychiatric illnesses, particularly depression and anxiety, occur at higher rates in individuals with asthma than in the general population and perhaps at elevated levels compared to those with other chronic illnesses. Alterations in the HPA axis, immune system and ANS may confer risk of both disorders and account for a major component of the co-occurrence of the conditions. Work is required to understand the environmental and genetic factors relevant to the development of asthma and depression/

anxiety and the molecular pathways that underlie this. Given the high rates of depression and anxiety in people with asthma, the detection and management of psychiatric symptoms should be an integral component of medical care for people with asthma, perhaps children and youth in particular. Pharmacological and nonpharmacological treatments for depression may translate into better control of asthma, but trials are needed to determine the optimal approach to managing depression and anxiety in people with asthma.

References

1 Di Marco F, Santus P, Centanni S: Anxiety and depression in asthma. Curr Opin Pulm Med 2011; 17:39–44.

2 French T, Alexander F: Psychogenic factors in bronchial asthma. Psychosomatic Medicine Monographs, vol 4. National Research Council, 1941.

3 Douwes J, Brooks C, Pearce N: Asthma nervosa: old concept, new insights. Eur Respir J 2011;37: 986–990.

4 Waxmonsky J, Wood BL, Stern T, Ballow M, Lillis K, Cramer-Benjamin D, Mador J, Miller BD: Association of depressive symptoms and disease activity in children with asthma: methodological and clinical implications. J Am Acad Child Adolesc Psychiatry 2006;45:945–954.

5 Laforest L, Van Ganse E, Devouassoux G, Bousquet J, Chretin S, Bauguil G, Pacheco Y, Chamba G: Influence of patients' characteristics and disease management on asthma control. J Allergy Clin Immunol 2006;117:1404–1410.

6 Krommydas GC, Gourgoulianis KI, Angelopoulos NV, Kotrotsiou E, Raftopoulos V, Molyvdas P-A: Depression and pulmonary function in outpatients with asthma. Resp Med 2004;98:220–224.

7 Mrazek DA: Psychiatric symptoms in patients with asthma causality, comorbidity, or shared genetic etiology. Child Adolesc Psychiatr Clin North Am 2003; 12:459–471.

8 Kuehn B: Asthma linked to psychiatric disorders. JAMA 2008;299:158–160.

9 Scott KM, Von Korff M, Ormel J, Zhang M-y, Bruffaerts R, Alonso J, Kessler RC, Tachimori H, Karam E, Levinson D, Bromet EJ, Posada-Villa J, Gasquet I, Angermeyer MC, Borges G, de Girolamo G, Herman A, Haro JM: Mental disorders among adults with asthma: results from the World Mental Health Survey. Gen Hosp Psychiatry 2007;29: 129–133.

10 Goodwin RD, Jacobi F, Thefeld W: Mental disorders and asthma in the community. Arch Gen Psychiatry 2003;60:1125–1130.

11 Ng TP, Chiam PC, Kua EH: Mental disorders and asthma in the elderly: a population-based study. Int J Geriatr Psychiatry 2007;22:668–674.

12 Nejtek VA, Brown ES, Khan DA, Moore JJ, Van Wagner J, Perantie DC: Prevalence of mood disorders and relationship to asthma severity in patients at an inner-city asthma clinic. Ann Allergy Asthma Immunol 2001;87:129–133.

13 Bennett DS: Depression among children with chronic medical problems: a meta-analysis. J Pediatr Psychol 1994;19:149–169.

14 Padur JS, Rpoff MA, Houston BK, Barnard M, Daovsky M, Olson NY, Moore WV, Vats TS, Lieberman B: Psychosocial adjustment and the role of functional status for children with asthma. J Asthma 1995;32:345–353.

15 Ortega AN, Feldman JM, Canino G, Steinman K, Alegria M: Co-occurrence of mental and physical illness in US Latinos. Soc Psychiatry Psychiatr Epidemiol. 2006;41:927–934.

16 Niti M, Ng TP, Kua EH, Ho RC, Tan CH: Depression and chronic medical illnesses in Asian older adults: the role of subjective health and functional status. Int J Geriatr Psychiatry 2007;22:1087–1094.

17 Katon WJ, Richardson L, Lozano P, McCauley E: The relationship of asthma and anxiety disorders. Psychosom Med 2004;66:349–355.

18 Chaney JM, Mullins LL, Uretsky DL, Pace TM, Werden D, Hartman VL: An experimental examination of learned helplessness in older adolescents and young adults with longstanding asthma. J Pediatr Psychol 1999;24:259–270.

19 Galil N: Depression and asthma in children. Curr Opin Pediatrics 2000;12:331–335.

20 Van Lieshout RJ, Bienenstock J, MacQueen GM: A review of candidate pathways underlying the association between asthma and major depressive disorder. Psychosom Med 2009;71:187–195.

21 Rutter ML: The interplay of nature, nurture, and developmental influences: the challenge ahead for mental health. Arch Gen Psychiatry 2002;59: 996–1000.

22 Davis JB: Neurotic illness in the families of children with asthma and wheezy bronchitis: a general practice population study. Psychol Med 1977;7:305–310.
23 Wamboldt MZ, Weintraub P, Krafchick D, Wamboldt FS: Psychiatric family history in adolescents with severe asthma. J Am Acad Child Adolesc Psychiatry 1996;35:1042–1049.
24 Brown ES, Gan V, Jeffress J: Psychiatric symptomatology and disorders in caregivers of children with asthma. Pediatrics 2006;118:e1715–e1720.
25 Ortega AN, Goodwin RD, McQuaid EL, Canino G: Parental mental health, childhood psychiatric disorders, and asthma attacks in island Puerto Rican youth. Ambul Pediatr 2004;4:308–315.
26 Wamboldt MZ, Hewitt JK, Schmitz S: Familial association between allergic disorders and depression in adult Finnish twins. Am J Med Genet 2000;96: 146–153.
27 Segerstrom SC, Miller GE: Psychological stress and the human immune system: a meta-analytic study of 30 years of inquiry. Psychol Bull 2004;130: 601–630.
28 Wright RJ, Visness CM, Calatroni A, Grayson MH, Gold DR, Sandel MT, Lee-Paritz A, Wood RA, Kattan M, Bloomberg GR, Burger M, Toglas A, Witter FR, Sperling RS, Sadovsky Y, Gern JE: Prenatal maternal stress and cord blook innate and adaptive cytokine responses in an inner-city cohort. Am J Resp Crit Care Med 2010;182:25–33.
29 Langley K, Rice F, van den Bree MB, Thapar A: Maternal smoking during pregnancy as an environmental risk factor for attention deficit hyperactivity disorder behavior. A review. Minerva Pediatr 2005; 57:359–371.
30 Ng SP, Zelikoff JT: Smoking during pregnancy: subsequent effects on offspring immune competence and disease vulnerability in later life. Reprod Toxicol 2007;23:428–437.
31 Fantuzzi G: Adipose tissue, adipokines, and inflammation. J Allergy Clin Immunol 2005;115:911–919.
32 Van Lieshout RJ, Taylor VH, Boyle MH: Pregnancy and pre-pregnancy obesity and neurodevelopmental outcomes in offspring: a systematic review. Obes Rev 2011;12:e548–e559.
33 Scholtens S, Wijga AH, Brunekreef B Kerkhof M, Postma DS, Oldenwening M, de Jongste JC, Smit HA: Maternal overweight before pregnancy and asthma in offspring followed for 8 years. Int J Obes 2010;34:606–613.
34 Wright RJ, Finn P, Contreras JP, Cohen S, Wright RO, Staudenmayer J, Wand M, Perkins D, Weiss ST, Gold DR: Chronic caregiver stress and IgE expression, allergen-induced proliferation, and cytokine profiles in a birth cohort predisposed to atopy. J Allergy Clin Immunol 2004;113:1051–1057.
35 Evans GW: The environment of childhood poverty. Am Psychol 2004;59:77–92.
36 Raison CL, Capuron L, Miller AH: Cytokines sing the blues: inflammation and the pathogenesis of depression. Trends Immunol 2006;27:24–31.
37 Wichers MC, Maes M: The role of indoleamine 2,3-dioxygenase (IDO) in the pathophysiology of interferon-alpha-induced depression. J Psychiatry Neurosci 2004;29:11–17.
38 von Hertzen LC: Maternal stress and T-cell differentiation of the developing immune system: possible implications for the development of asthma and atopy. J Allergy Clin Immunol 2002;109:923–928.
39 Stock P, Akbari O, Berry G, Freeman GJ, Dekruyff RH, Umetsu DT: Induction of T helper type 1-like regulatory cells that express foxp3 and protect against airway hyper-reactivity. Nat Immunol 2004; 5:1149–1156.
40 Taussig LM, Wright AL, Holberg CJ, Halonen M, Morgan WJ, Martinez FD: Tucson children's respiratory study: 1980 to present. J Allergy Clin Immunol 2003;111:661–675.
41 Janowsky D, Risch C, Parker D, HueyL, Judd L: Increased vulnerability to cholinergic stimulation in affective disorder patients. Psychopharmacol Bull 1980;16:29–31.
42 Wright RJ: Epidemiology of stress and asthma: from constricting communities and fragile families to epigenetics. Immunol Allergy Clin N Am 2011;31: 19–39.
43 Wright RJ: Perinatal stress and early life programming of lung structure and function. Biol Psychol 2010;84:46–56.
44 Card JP, Levitt P, Gluhovsky M, Rinaman L: Early experience modifies the postnatal assembly of autonomic emotional motor circuits in rats. J Neurosci 2005;25:9102–9111.
45 Tracey KJ: Physiology and immunology of the cholinergic anti-inflammatory pathway. J Clin Invest 2007;117:289–296.
46 Chen E, Miller GE: Stress and inflammation in exacerbations of asthma. Brain Behav Immun 2007; 21:993–999.
47 Lehrer PM, Isenberg S, Hochron SM: Asthma and emotion: a review. J Asthma 1993;30:5–21.
48 Miller BD: Depression and asthma: a potentially lethal mixture. J Allergy Clin Immunol 1987;80: 481–486.
49 Chen E, Chim L, Strunk R, Miller G: The role of the social environment in children and adolescents with asthma. Am J Respir Crit Care Med 2007;176: 644–649.
50 Shalowitz MU: Advancing analytic methods to understand asthma control and disease morbidity. J Allergy and Clin Immunol 2008;122:496–499.

51 Liu LY, Coe CL, Swenson CA: School examinations enhance airway inflammation to antigen challenge. Am J Respir Crit Care Med 2002;165:1062–1067.
52 Charil A, LaPlante DP, Vaillancourt C, King S: Prenatal stress and brain development. Brain Res Rev 2010;65:56–79.
53 Leigh R, MacQueen G, Tougas G: Change in forced expiratory volume in 1 second after sham bronchoconstrictor in suggestible but not suggestion-resistant asthmatic subjects: a pilot study. Psychosom Med 2003;65:791–795.
54 Rosenkranz MA, Busse WW, Johnstone T: Neural circuitry underlying the interaction between emotion and asthma symptom exacerbation. Proc Natl Acad Sci USA 2005;102:13319–13324.
55 Rosenkranz MA, Davidson RJ: Afftective neural circuitry and mind-bind influences in asthma. Neuroimage 2009;47:972–980.
56 Mayer EA, Berman S, Suyenobu B, Labus J, Mandelkern MA, Naliboff BD, Chang L: Differences in brain responses to visceral pain between patients with irritable bowel syndrome and ulcerative colitis. Pain 2005;115:398–409.
57 Devinsky O, Morrell MJ, Vogt BA: Contributions of anterior cingulate cortex to behaviour. Brain 1995; 118:279–306.
58 Capuron L, Pagnoni G, Demetrashvili M: Anterior cingulate activation and error processing during interferon-alpha treatment. Biol Psychiatry 2005;58: 190–196.
59 Katon WJ, Richardson L, Russo J: Quality of mental health care for youth with asthma and comorbid anxiety and depression. Med Care 2006;44: 1064–1072.
60 Kelleher KJ, Horwitz SM: Quality of mental health care for children: a familiar storyline. Med Care 2006;44:1061–1063.
61 Peters TE, Fritz GK: Psychological considerations of the child with asthma Pediatr Clin North Am 2011; 58:921–935.
62 Brown ES, Vigil L, Khan DA: A randomized trial of citalopram versus placebo in outpatients with asthma and major depressive disorder: a proof of concept study. Biol Psychiatry 2005;58:865–870.
63 Sanger MD: Depression and allergic dermatologic disease. Psychosomatics. 1969;10:25–27.
64 Lechin F, van der Dijs B, Orozco B, Jara H, Rada I, Lechin ME, Lechin AE: Neuropharmacologic treatment of bronchial asthma with the antidepressant tianeptine: a double-blind, crossover placebo-controlled study. Clin Pharmacol Ther 1998;64: 223–232.
65 Brown ES, Vornik LA, Khan DA, Rush AJ: Bupropion in the treatment of outpatients with asthma and major depressive disorder. Int J Psychiatry Med 2007;37:23–28.
66 Philip G, Hustad CM, Malice M-P, Noonan G, Ezekowitz A, Reiss TF, Knorr B: Analysis of behaviour-related adverse experiences in clinical trials of montelukast. J Allergy Clin Immunol 2009; 124:699–706.
67 Yorke J, Fleming SL, Shuldham CM: Psychological interventions for adults with asthma. Cochrane Database Syst Rev 2006;1; CD002982.
68 Yorke J, Fleming SL, Shuldham C: A systematic review of psychological interventions for children with asthma. Pediatr Pulmonol 2007;42:114–124.
69 Colland VT: Learning to cope with asthma: a behavioural self-management program for children. Patient Educ Couns 1993;22:141–152.
70 Dahl J, Gustafsson D, Melin L: Effects of a behavioral treatment program on children with asthma. J Asthma 1990;27:41–46.
71 Alexander AB, Miklich DR, Hershkoff H: The immediate effects of systematic relaxation training on peak expiratory flow rates in asthmatic children. Psychosom Med 1972;34:388–394.
72 Kohen DP: Hypnotherapeutic management of pediatric and adolescent trichotillomania. J Dev Behav Pediatr 1996;17:328–334.
73 Khan AU: Effectiveness of biofeedback and counter-conditioning in the treatment of bronchial asthma. J Psychosom Res 1977;21:97–104.
74 Kotses H, Harver A, Segreto J: Long-term effects of biofeedback-induced facial relaxation on measures of asthma severity in children. Biofeedback Self Regul 1991;16:1–21.
75 Khan AU, Staerk M, Bonk C: Role of counter-conditioning in the treatment of asthma. J Psychosom Res 1973;17:389–392.
76 Holloway E, Ram FSF: Breathing exercises for asthma. Cochrane Database Syst Rev 2004; CD001277

Dr. Glenda M. MacQueen
Department of Psychiatry, University of Calgary
1403 29th St
Calgary, AB, T2N 2T9 (Canada)
Tel. +1 403 944 1296, E-Mail gmmacque@ucalgary.ca

Bienenstock J (ed): Allergy and the Nervous System.
Chem Immunol Allergy. Basel, Karger, 2012, vol 98, pp 14–31

The Brain and Asthma: What Are the Linkages?

William W. Busse

Division of Allergy, Pulmonary and Critical Care, Department of Medicine, University of Wisconsin School of Medicine and Public Health, Madison, Wisc., USA

Abstract

Stress has been associated as an important contributor to asthma in some patients. The mechanisms, however, which underlie this relationship remain unclear. In this review, the role of stress will be examined in relationship to the development of airway inflammation. As will be discussed, stress may not cause inflammation but enhances its expression when it develops to a second signal. In addition, recent studies using function magnetic resonance imaging (fMRI) have shown that specific circuits in the brain, i.e., anterior cingulate cortex and insula, are activated in relationship and intensity to the development of a late-phase response (LPR) to inhaled antigen, and that these brain signals are predictive and associated with the development of airway inflammation as measured by sputum eosinophils. Finally, in studies with mice, chronic stress enhances airway inflammation to an inhaled antigen, and these effects are associated with the development of corticosteroid unresponsiveness. Collectively, these data suggest that chronic stress enhances asthma severity through a number of novel mechanisms and the resulting increase in severity of asthma may not be responsiveness to standardly used treatments.

Asthma is characterized by reversible airflow obstruction, bronchial hyperresponsiveness, and airway inflammation [1]. Of these characteristics, airway inflammation is central to the pathogenesis and pathophysiology of asthma, as well as being a principal target for treatment. In addition, it is well demonstrated that environmental factors interact with the at-risk host to initiate immune responses that lead to airway inflammation [2–4]. These factors include allergens, respiratory infections, microbes, dietary factors, and stress [5]. Understanding how these factors may affect asthma and its underlying features has provided insight into the pathophysiology of airway dysfunction seen in this disease. Following on this concept, considerable insight has been gained into the pathophysiology of asthma through the study of the influence of respiratory infections and allergic sensitization [6]. In contrast, the role and contribution of stress to asthma has turned out to be a more complex, and at times, confusing story [7–10] with limited information on how stress affects or interacts with airway inflammation and thus influence asthma.

For many years, the focus on stress in asthma was largely limited to acute events and exploring the interaction of these stimuli on the autonomic nervous system regulation of airway smooth muscle responses, i.e. bronchospasm. These observations were helpful in providing insight into acute dysregulation of airway smooth muscle tone and an 'attack' of asthma, but did not fully advance our thinking or provide information on how stress could relate to the persistence and severity of asthma, and, in particular, how airway inflammation would fit into this process. In the past decade, there has been a shift in our thinking and the study of stress, or psychological factors, on asthma from acute responses towards how stress-related events influence airway inflammation and serve to influence the persistence and severity of disease.

This shift in focus has occurred, from my perspective, for a number of reasons. First, a recognition and realization that airway inflammation is a central and critical feature of asthma both at a pathogenetic and pathophysiologic level [2–4]. Second, there has been clarification of differential and distinct effects to acute versus chronic stress on the immune response, and the greater importance of chronic stress to asthma and underlying inflammation. Third, it has become apparent that stress, like other inciters or triggers of asthma, may be primarily a cofactor in the expression of asthma or its severity, and stress by itself may have limited effects on asthma. Fourth, technologic advances now provide tools to identify and measure the myriad of mediators and cells involved in the inflammatory processes; in addition, these products can now be detected and quantitated in relationship to airway dysfunction. Fifth, tools are available to identify the regulatory genetic signals involved in these reactions. Finally, imaging techniques were previously not available to detect central nervous system activation or the pathways activated in association with peripheral responses, in the case of asthma, the airflow obstruction and inflammation, and to link these neurocircuits to the resulting immune function, inflammation, and clinical characteristics. Given these advances, there has emerged significantly greater insight and appreciation of the involvement and integration of emotions, stress, and the nervous system in the pathophysiology of asthma. These advances will be the focus of the following discussion.

Differences in Acute versus Chronic Stress and Their Potential Role in Asthma (fig. 1)

Acute stress, or the 'fight-or-flight' response, is provoked by the appearance of a sudden, single event and the immediate response of the host to this event; a response which is largely designed for host preservation. Immediately following an acute stressful event, there is the activation of the adrenal gland with a rapid outpouring of catecholamines and corticosteroids. Both of these adrenal mediators are important to host protection and can have profound effects on features of asthma, which include

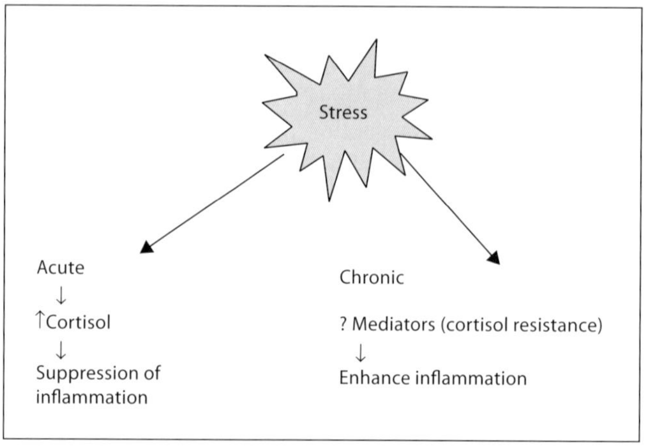

Fig. 1. Comparison of acute vs. chronic stress. Acute stress leads to increases in cortisol which can suppress inflammation. In contrast, during chronic stress, regulation by cortisol is attenuated and the normal suppression of cortisol is diminished.

a relaxation of airway smooth muscle tone by catecholamines and anti-inflammatory actions on phylogenetic cell function by corticosteroids.

Using allergic-sensitized mice, Forsythe et al. [11] compared the effects of acute vs. chronic stress on the airway inflammatory response to an inhaled allergen. In naïve, allergen-sensitized, nonstressed mice, inhalation of ovalbumin caused the mouse to have a significant increase in bronchial alveolar leukocytes in their lavage fluid. In the presence of an acute stress, however, this allergen-provoked increase in leukocytes was significantly suppressed. Using adrenal-cortical blocking agents, the investigators were able to show that cortisol secretion in response to an acute stress prior to the allergen challenge was responsible for suppression of resulting allergic inflammation.

In contrast, when mice were subjected to chronic stress and then challenged with ovalbumin, the increase in airway leukocytes to inhaled allergen was enhanced. Furthermore, with the use of pharmacological probes, the investigators were able to show that cortisol generation did not play a role in regulating this enhanced response to an allergen challenge or was ineffective. They proposed that during chronic stress, the inflammatory response was 'corticosteroid resistant'. Using chronic stress, Forsythe et al. [11] were able to show that the normal suppression of inflammation found with acute stress was lost because the regulatory effects of corticosteroids were altered from chronic stress.

These animal studies help set the stage for our subsequent discussion and point out how stress, and what kinds of stress, may interact with inflammation in asthma. First, these studies indicate that the type of stress that influences allergic inflammation is important and evidence points to chronic rather than acute events as being most important. Second, chronic stress enhances, but possibly does not cause, inflammation, and its action on inflammation may be more of an 'adjuvant' or 'primer' than an initiator. Third, the effects of stress can be reflected in respiratory response of the

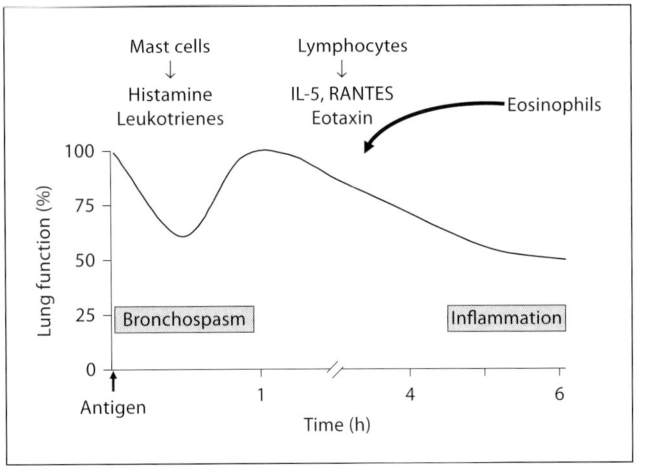

Fig. 2. Biology of the airway response to antigen. In some patients with asthma, there is a response to inhaled allergen. The immediate reaction with an acute fall in the FEV_1 is secondary to mast cell activation and its mediators leading to a bronchospastic response. Following this immediate reaction, there is the development of an inflammatory response, reflected by the recruitment of eosinophils, which produces a late-phase reaction with pulmonary obstruction.

airway to an allergen challenge with the bronchial recruitment and presence of leukocytes serving as a marker for inflammatory activity. As will be discussed below, this approach can serve as a model for study. Finally, the effects of chronic stress that lead to enhanced allergic inflammation may relate to a loss of a normal corticosteroid-regulating action on leukocytes such that, under chronic stress, these cells become resistant to the anti-inflammatory actions of corticosteroids.

Models in Asthma to Study the Effect of Stress on Airway Inflammation

In patients with asthma, the inhalation of allergen to which they are sensitive can initiate an allergic reaction in the airways and can serve as a model to describe key features of the airway responses which include bronchospasms (immediate reaction) and inflammation (late-phase reaction) (fig. 2) [12]. These pulmonary reactions to inhaled allergen can be divided into immediate and late phase responses. The late-phase response also has airflow obstruction, but the late phase effects on airflow obstruction are secondary to inflammation.

In these reactions, inhaled allergen is first recognized by mast cell-bound, antigen-specific IgE which serves to signal this airway cell to release its preformed mediators, like histamine, and generate the production of other mediators, like leukotrienes, to cause acute airflow obstruction [13]. In addition to this immediate bronchospastic response to antigen, many patients will recover from the acute or immediate reaction and go on to have a late phase reaction 4–8 h later [12]. The late phase reaction is also characterized by bronchial obstruction, but, in contrast to the immediate event, is more persistent, less responsive to bronchodilation, and associated with the recruitment of inflammatory cells, the principle of which are eosinophils. The airway response to allergen can, therefore, provide a model to study events central to asthma:

bronchospasm and airway inflammation. This model also allows the investigators to examine the effect of a co-factor, i.e. stress, on aspects of the allergic airway response: acute bronchospasm, cellular inflammation, and late phase airflow obstruction. Collectively, this model allows the investigator to parse the effects of a reaction to inhaled allergens on these individual aspects of an allergic response, bronchospasm and inflammation, and determine how co-factors, in our case, stress, affects various aspects of this response.

Using the airway response to an inhaled antigen, we evaluated the effects of chronic stress on allergic inflammation [14]. In initial efforts, we used models of acute stress in relationship to an allergen provocation and did not note enhancement of the underlying inflammatory response (data not shown) or the reaction to the antigen challenge. As a consequence, we shifted our attention to the use of chronic stress and under these conditions to begin to determine and define the effects of stress on airway inflammation in asthma. For study, we used the final examination period of college as a chronic stress stimulus [14]. Final examination time at the University of Wisconsin occurs at the end of each semester and lasts for at least a week. For most undergraduate classes, the final examination is a, if not the, major determinant of a student's final grade in a class, making this exercise highly important to the semester grade and potentially a source of considerable stress. Furthermore, most students have 4–5 final examinations during this week interval adding to the overall stress load of the individual during this time. As these examinations take place over at least a week, we considered them to be representative of chronic stress.

In this study [14], 20 University of Wisconsin undergraduate students volunteered to participate in our research project where we hypothesized that chronic stress associated with a final examination period would enhance allergic inflammation, and this enhancement could be demonstrated by using an allergen bronchoprovocation challenge as a model to elicit airway inflammation. All participants had asthma, did not take any asthma medications on a regular basis other than an as-needed short-acting bronchodilator, had an allergy to one of three test antigens used for an inhalation challenge (ragweed, cat or house dust mite), had an immediate response to an allergen inhalation challenge (fall in FEV_1 of at least 20%), and were able to produce sputum following saline induction and, in the sputum, demonstrate an increase in eosinophils following allergen challenge. The students underwent two allergen challenges: one during mid-semester (which we referred to as low stress) and one immediately following their last final examination (our stress phase). The order of these challenges was randomized such that one-half of the students had their initial study in the final examination stress phase and the other one-half with an initial study in the low-stress phase at mid-semester.

To determine if there were psychological effects of the final examination, stress-phase, students were asked to evaluate their levels of anxiety and depression. Scores for both anxiety (STAI) and depression (BDI score) showed small, but significant, increases during the stress phase of final examinations. Antigen challenge during

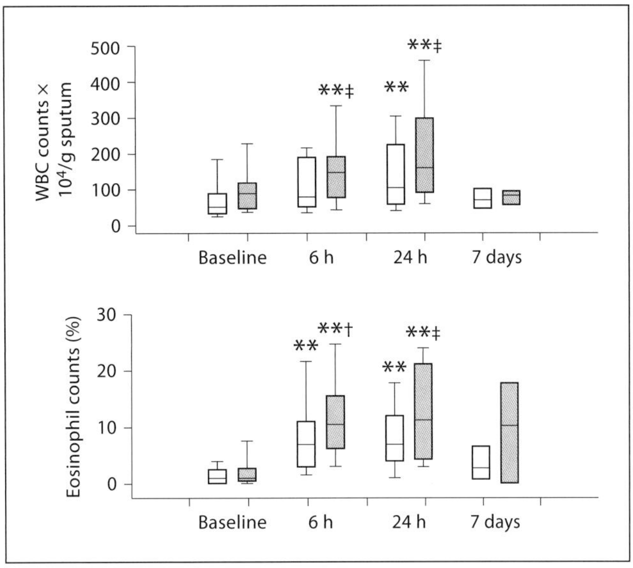

Fig. 3. The effect of stress from final examinations on sputum markers of inflammation. Sputum was obtained at baseline prior to antigen challenge and then again at 6 and 24 h postprovocation and 7 days later (n = 20). Reprinted with permission from Liu et al. [14]. □ = Low stress phase; ■ = high stress phase; ** = $p < 0.01$, vs. baseline; † = $p < 0.05$; ‡ = $p < 0.01$, stress vs. low-stress.

the stress-phase was associated with a significantly greater recruitment of leukocyte recruitment to the airway as measured in the induced sputum sample (fig. 3). The increase in leukocytes recruited to the airway during the stress phase was reflective of a greater proportion of these cells being eosinophils. Prior to the antigen challenge, the number of leukocytes and eosinophils were the same as the pre-stress-phase values suggesting that the effects of chronic stress on underlying airway inflammation in these students were largely on recruitment of cells at the time of the allergen challenge and stress, by itself, had not changed baseline levels of inflammation.

Blood samples had also been obtained in relationship to levels of stress. Interestingly, we found an increase in circulating eosinophils during the stress-phase and prior to challenge. Although not proven, these observations suggest that stress, by itself, had led to an increase in circulating eosinophils. Whether this was a result of stress stimulating the bone marrow to selectively release more eosinophils was not established but compatible with current information [15]. When a provocation of the airway in allergic subjects occurred with an antigen challenge, there were more eosinophils available in circulation to be recruited to the airway, and this was reflected by an increase in sputum eosinophils. It was almost like stress 'primed the pump,' in this case an increase in circulating eosinophils, for a greater response to a subsequent stimulus of asthma. Coinciding with this observation and, as a speculation to the cause of the increase in circulating eosinophils, was the finding that the ratio of interferon (IFN)-γ to interleukin (IL)-5 had shifted more towards a Th2 pattern. Collectively, these data suggest that chronic stress may affect asthma, and allergic inflammation, by causing a shift towards a greater Th2-like status, thus allowing for a greater inflammatory response with activation of asthma. The signals associated with stress that increased

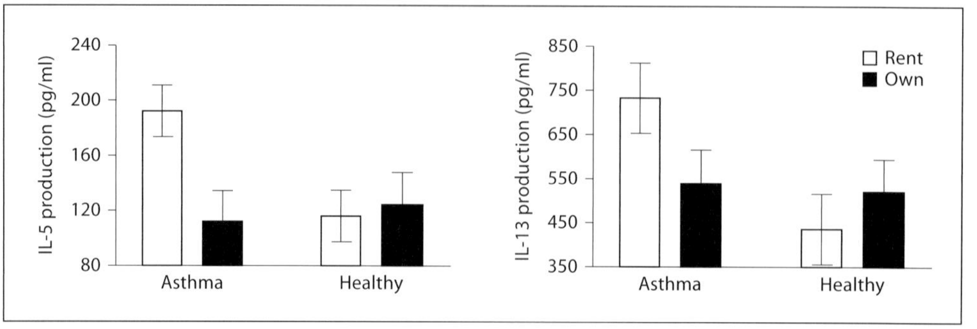

Fig. 4. A comparison of differences in production of IL-5 and IL-13 from PBMC for families who rent their homes versus families who own their own home by medical group status. PBMC were incubated with phorbol myristate acetate and calcium ionophore. The supernatants were analyzed for Th2 cytokines, IL-5 and IL-13. Reprinted with permission from Chen et al. [17].

circulating eosinophils were not identified, but the shift in Th1/Th2 ratio toward a greater Th2 response may have contributed to these changes.

Socioeconomic Status, Stress and Th2 Expression

Children living in the inner cities with asthma or born to a lower socioeconomic status are at risk for more severe asthma [16]. To define the mechanisms of this relationship, Chen et al. [17] recruited children with asthma who were being raised in a lower socioeconomic status (SES) and healthy children without this economic burden. Blood samples were obtained from both groups of children, and peripheral blood mononuclear cells (PBMC) were isolated and then activated by a combination of phorbol myristate acetate and calcium ionophore to generate cytokines. Supernatants were collected after a 48-hour incubation to measure a cytokine profile, IL-4, IL-5, IL-13 (Th2) and INF-γ (Th1) (fig. 4). The investigators used home ownership as a marker for socioeconomic status. Those patients with asthma who lived in a home which was owned by their parents, likely reflecting a higher SES, had less IL-5 generated when compared to children not living in a home owned by their parents. Moreover, IL-13 production from PBMC was inversely related to the family's SES and directly to levels of chronic home stress.

These data add further support to the argument that stress, in this case reflected by a low SES, was more likely to be associated with a Th2, or allergic, profile, and when activated, cells from these subjects were able to generate more Th2-associated cytokines. Although not directly stated by the investigators, their findings suggest that allergic sensitization and stress, or, in this case, SES, are associated with a greater Th2 expression and thus a greater tendency to allergic diseases and likelihood to create an allergic inflammatory response when activated.

In another study, Miller and Chen [18] evaluated molecular mechanisms which might explain how stress may further enhance features relevant to asthma: airflow obstruction and allergic inflammation. Using the same sample of children as described above, Miller and Chen [18] measured mRNA to the β_2-adrenergic receptor (β_2AR) and the glucocorticoid receptor (GR) in leukocytes and evaluated these patterns of expression in relationship to asthma and a recent major life event in the life of the subject. In patients with asthma, decreased mRNA to β_2AR and GR were found in asthma patients when a major life event had occurred recently and chronic stress was present. One of these molecules affects the regulation of airway tone (β_2AR), and the other, the regulator of inflammation (GR). Collectively, a decrease in the presence of these molecules could relate to a decrease in bronchodilating regulation of airway smooth muscle tone and inflammation, respectively. This effect on these two molecules during a major life event and chronic stress was not seen in healthy volunteers.

The observations of Chen and Miller and colleagues [17, 18] raise a number of factors to consider in how and under what circumstances stress affects allergic inflammation in asthma. First, patients with asthma and life-stress conditions appear to be more susceptible to changes in the regulation of beta adrenergic and glucocorticoid responsiveness because of a deficiency of these two systems. Second, changes in expression of these two regulating molecules can translate into a diminished bronchodilating response and diminished inflammation regulation by corticosteroids. Collectively, these findings imply that stress can enhance inflammation and airflow obstruction, and in addition, decrease the effectiveness of medications, i.e. bronchodilators and corticosteroids, used to regulate these two responses.

Use of Animal Models to Gain Insight to the Effects of Stress on Allergic Inflammation

For the past decades, the laboratory of John Sheridan [15] at Ohio State has been interested in the effects of stress on immune responses and immune responsiveness. To evaluate these aspects of interest, Dr. Sheridan's laboratory has developed an animal model in which he can induce and quantitate stress and examine its effects on a number of aspects of airway inflammation and factors associated with its regulation (see below). In his experimental design, mice are housed under different conditions. To create stress in animals, mice are placed in a cage with another mouse that is a predator who is allowed to create significant social disruption (SDR) stress over 6 consecutive days. Under these conditions, the mice display signs of stress with SDR. To evaluate the effects of this modeled stress on immune function, spleens were collected from the animals, both normal, nonstressed mice, and those who had undergone 6 days of SDR. A number of key observations were made in these experiments. First, the regulation of splenocyte cellular proliferation by corticosteroids was significantly decreased in mice that had undergone 6 days of SDR stress. Moreover, the

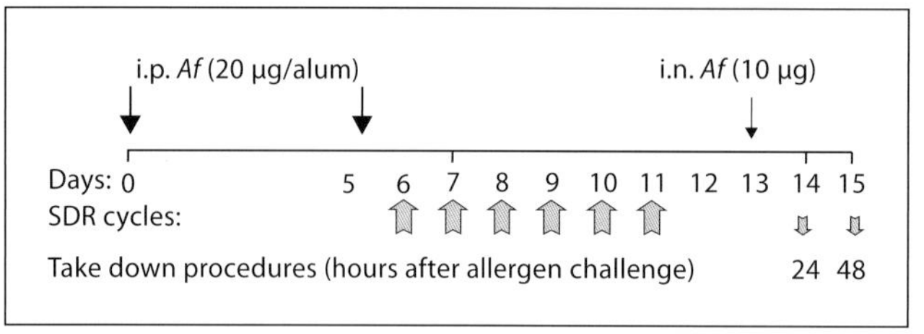

Fig. 5. In a combined protocol for allergic sensitization and SDR stress, mice received i.p. *Af* in alum on days 0 and 5, followed by repeated SDR for 2 h on days 6–11. Mice received intranasal (i.n.) allergen challenge on day 13 and were sacrificed either 24 or 48 h later. Control naive and SDR mice were sacrificed on day 15. Reprinted with permission from Bailey et al. [15].

suppression of IL-6 release to LPS by corticosteroids was decreased when cells were obtained from stressed animals. These observations support the findings by Miller and Chen [18] and suggest that one effect of stress on immune or allergic responses is a decrease in the anti-inflammatory effects of corticosteroids. It is possible that this effect may relate to in vivo events as seen during activation of asthma as well as in the response to treatment. Thus, a mechanistic action of stress is to compromise the effectiveness of corticosteroids in the regulation of inflammation.

To expand on these findings, Bailey et al. [15] used the same social disruption mouse model of stress. In addition, the mice underwent allergen sensitization prior to the social disruptive experience and then received an airway antigen challenge to explore the effects of stress on allergic inflammation (fig. 5). Four conditions were part of the study design: (1) naïve; (2) SDR (social disruptive response); (3) Af (*Aspergillus fumigatus* sensitized), and (4) Af + SDR. A number of key findings emerged. First, as expected, allergic sensitization and allergen challenge elicited a predictable inflammatory response in which eosinophils were the predominant cell recruited to the lung (fig. 6). In the presence of SDR and allergic sensitization, the eosinophilic lung response to allergen challenge was significantly increased as reflected by a greater eosinophil recruitment to the lung. SDR, in the absence of allergic sensitization, had no effect on underlying features of allergic inflammation. These data suggest, as noted in our studies of stress associated with final examinations in college students, that stress enhanced the allergic response and demonstrated that for the effects of stress to be apparent, it was necessary to have a second stimulus present, in this case, an allergen provocation. The investigators also found that the increase of airway hyperresponsiveness to methacholine following an allergen challenge was enhanced by SDR (fig. 7). Allergen challenge increases the airway response to methacholine, and this reaction to methacholine is further enhanced by the addition of SDR. This enhancing effect on the methacholine response associated with stress likely reflects a heightened degree of airway inflammation reflected by a greater eosinophil recruitment to the airway.

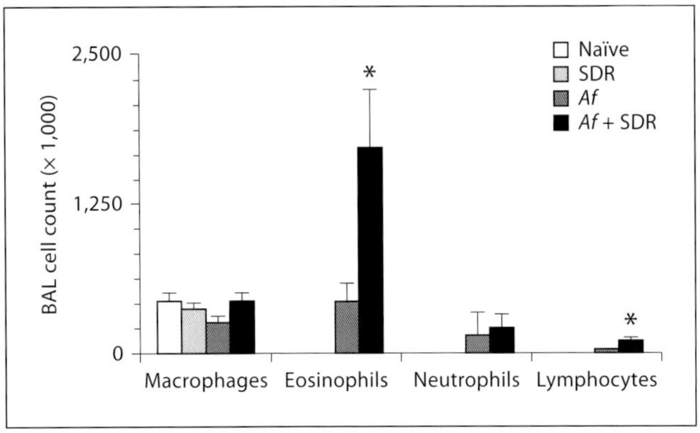

Fig. 6. BAL differential cell count was evaluated in Giemsa preparations. Stress (*Af* SDR) and allergic sensitization *(Af)* enhanced numbers of eosinophils and lymphocytes, but not neutrophils and macrophages in the BAL fluid. There was no difference between naive and SDR mice. Reprinted with permission from Bailey et al. [15].

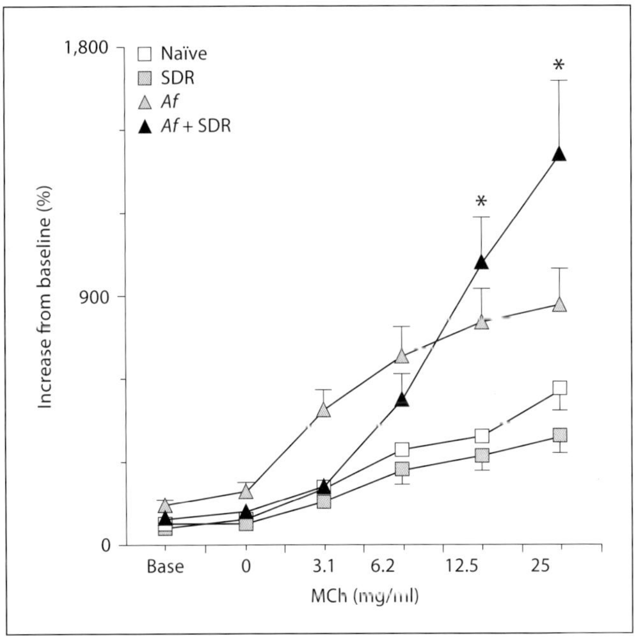

Fig. 7. MCh dose response at day 15. Exposure to allergen and stress enhanced airway hyperresponsiveness at high MCh concentrations. Mice were studied 48 h after a single *Af* challenge. Mice received increasing doses of inhaled MCh. Lung function was assessed using noninvasive plethysmography and Penh. There was no difference between naïve and SDR mice. Reprinted with permission from Bailey et al. [15].

In earlier work, the Sheridan investigative group had also found that corticosteroid responsiveness was diminished by stress [19]. In these experiments with mice, which combined stress and allergic sensitization, the investigators pursued two avenues of study to address the effects of these variables on corticosteroid responsiveness. First, corticosteroids suppress leukocyte generation of cytokines, IL-4, IL-5, and granulocyte-macrophage colony-stimulating factor. In the presence of stress, corticosteroids did not suppress the release of these mediators as effectively as under the non-stress and allergen sensitized conditions (fig. 8). In addition, the expression of the mRNA for the GR on splenocytes was significantly reduced in cells from Af-SDR mice (fig. 9).

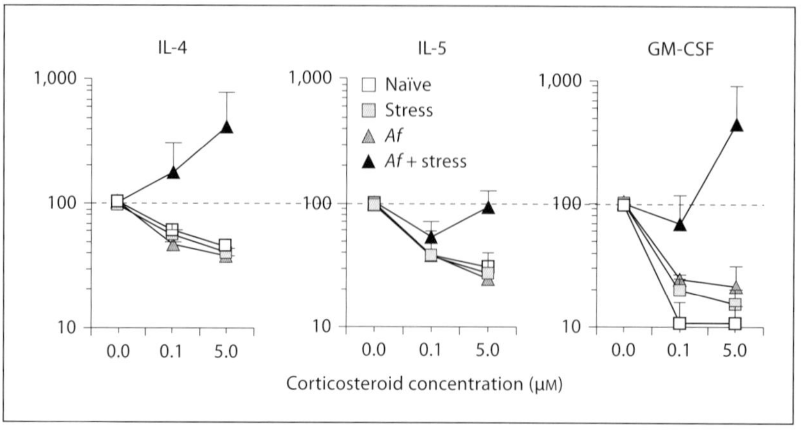

Fig. 8. Inhibition of CpG generation of cytokines. Combination of stress and allergen challenge abolished the dose-dependent inhibitory effects of corticosterone on LPS-stimulated splenocytes. Spleens were harvested from naive or SDR controls, and from *Af*-sensitized mice 24 h after *Af* challenge (*Af*, gray triangles; *Af* plus SDR, (d)). Splenocytes were cultured in the presence of LPS (1 μg/ml) and 0, 0.01, 0.05, 0.1, 0.5 or 5 μM corticosterone for 48 h. Cell viability (top left panel) was determined using a colorimetric assay. Cytokine, chemokine, and Ig levels in the supernatant were measured by SearchLight technology in each group. Data are presented as the percentage of cell viability or cytokine, chemokine, and Ig concentration of control values measured in the absence of corticosterone, marked by dashed lines (mean ± SEM of 5–8 per group). Reprinted with permission from Bailey et al. [15].

Fig. 9. GR protein levels in splenocytes. To study the effects of stress and asthma on function and expression of the GR, splenocytes and whole lung tissue were investigated. Naive mice and mice subjected to stress (SDR), allergen (*Af*), or allergen and stress (*Af* + SDR, gray hatched bars) were studied. On day 15 (48 h after *Af* challenge), spleens for GR nuclear translocation and lungs for GR mRNA and protein expression were harvested. Western blot analysis was performed using an anti-mouse GRα mAb. Expression was assessed using densitometric analysis and GAPDH as control. Mean ± SEM of 6 (duplicate experiment). Data were analyzed using the ΔΔCt method. Mean ± SEM of 4–6 (duplicate experiments). * $p < 0.05$, *Af* vs. *Af* plus SDR. Reprinted with permission from Bailey et al. [15].

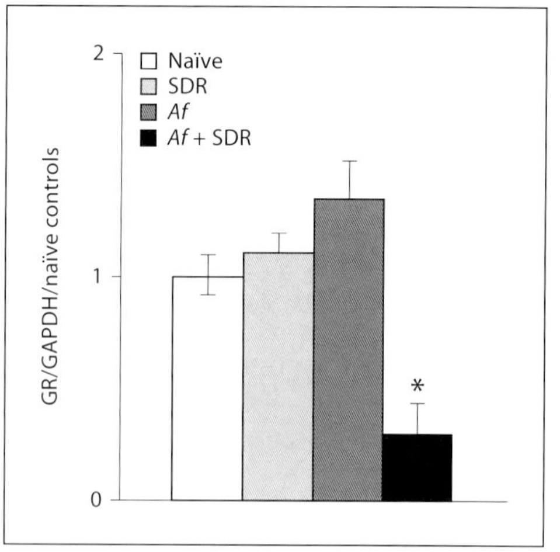

A number of conclusions can be made from these observations. First, the effects of stress on allergic inflammation were enhanced by conditions of chronic stress. Second, stress by itself did not appear to induce changes in the underlying features of allergic inflammation. Third, the effects of stress were found in the face of a second signal, i.e. allergen challenge. Fourth, these data suggest that stress primes the host's response to a second challenge. Lastly, at least in part, a mechanism by which chronic stress enhances allergic inflammation may relate to a diminished corticosteroid-regulating effect. Thus, from the assessment of stress in allergic sensitized animals, it was possible to corroborate findings we noted in humans [14] and to identify a potential underlying mechanism, i.e. diminished corticosteroid responsiveness, for the enhanced allergic inflammatory response associated with stress.

How Is the Central Nervous System, or Brain, Involved in the Allergic Airway Response in Asthma and How May this Relate to Stress?

Functional magnetic response imaging (fMRI) provides a technique to detect and quantitate sites of activation in the brain and to map circuits that might be associated with or involved in the response to peripheral signals such as from the lung. Applying this technology to the study of asthma, we conducted a series of experiments to determine whether an inhaled antigen challenge that provoked airway inflammation was associated with activation of specific areas, or circuits, of the brain [20]. We were primarily interested in two predetermined areas of the brain, the insula and anterior cingulate cortex. Both of these areas receive afferent input from the periphery, which carries information on physiological activity. Second, these areas of the brain have strong connections with neural structures that are essential in the processing of emotional information from the host. Finally, both centers are capable of modulating autonomic and motor activity to maintain homeostasis. Although these specific regions were of greatest interest to us, all areas of the brain were evaluated for possible associations with the allergic reactions in the lung.

Six subjects with mild asthma were selected for study. All subjects had a positive response to a methacholine provocation, an immediate fall in FEV_1 of at least 20%, and were allergic to environmental allergens by skin testing. In addition, each of the subjects underwent an allergen bronchoprovocation challenge and demonstrated: (1) an immediate response as indicated by a fall in FEV_1 >20% within 1 h of challenge, and (2) a late-phase response as reflected by fall in FEV_1 >15% at 4–8 h post-allergen challenge. The study design is shown in figure 10.

Each subject underwent three bronchoprovocation challenges. First, with saline to determine effects of a nonbronchoconstricting agent, methacholine, and allergen on airway function and sputum markers of inflammation as well as to provide experience and comfort with the scanning procedures. Then, in a double-blinded fashion, the subjects were given either methacholine or antigen. Following each challenge, the subjects had an fMRI scan one and 4 h post-challenge. These times were selected for the following reasons. By 1 h, the airflow obstruction to either methacholine or allergen had resolved and returned to baseline values. A second fMRI was conducted four hours post-challenge. At four hours, the late phase reaction to allergen had yet to fully manifest itself. The 4-hour timing allowed us to retain a blinding during the fMRI

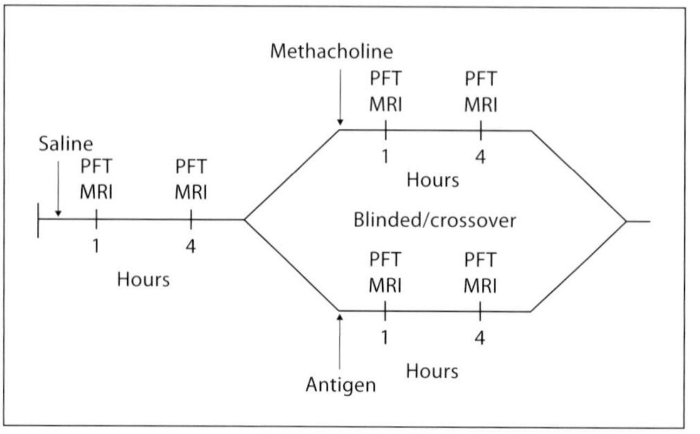

Fig. 10. Experimental design (brain): timing of experimental challenges and measures collected. Participants underwent both Ag and Meth challenges separated by at least 4 weeks in a complete within-subjects crossover design. Challenge order was counterbalanced.

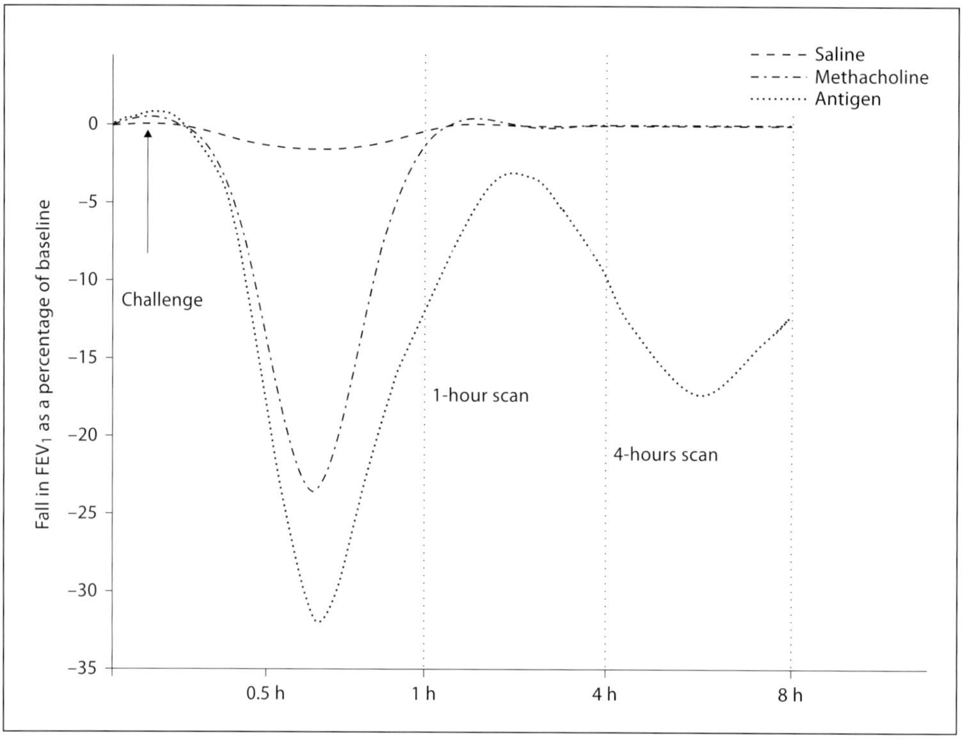

Fig. 11. Pulmonary response to bronchoprovocation with saline, methacholine and antigen.

as neither the subject nor investigator could tell if the challenge had been antigen or methacholine and the late-phase reaction, as reflected in a fall in the FEV_1, had not fully developed. Twenty-four hours after the challenge sputum was collected.

Figure 11 shows the effect of the bronchoprovocation on lung function. Saline had no effect on lung functions (FEV_1) over 8 h of observation and served as a negative

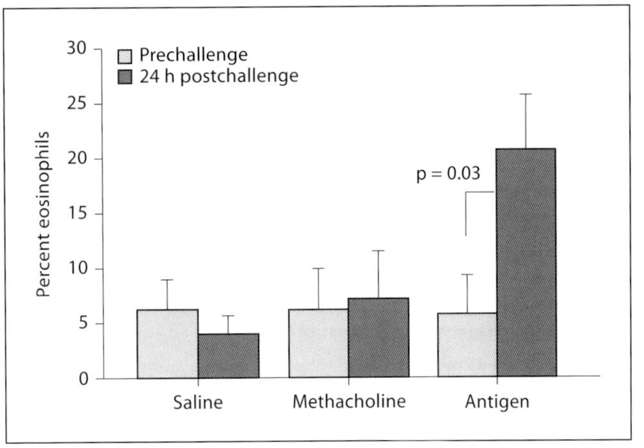

Fig. 12. Sputum eosinophils before and 24 h after bronchoprovocation (n = 6).

response control. Methacholine caused a predictable immediate fall in FEV_1 within 15 min of administration, and the FEV_1 returned to baseline values by 1 h post-challenge. Antigen, in contrast, caused not only an immediate fall in FEV_1 but also a late-phase response as indicated by a decrease in FEV_1 values beginning at 4 h postantigen challenge with maximal effects noted at 6–8 h postchallenge. fMRI studies were, as noted above, conducted at 1 and 4 h postbronchoprovocation. As noted, these times were selected to be at a point when the immediate response had resolved and preceded the full development of the late-phase reaction to antigen. These times were also selected for design and safety reasons. We did not want patients in the brain scan at the time of significant airflow obstruction. In addition, we wished to maintain a blinded aspect to the study for the 4-hour scan and to be representative of brain activation prior to the development of airway obstruction and inflammation. Pulmonary functions served as a marker of one of the peripheral responses of asthma – airflow obstruction; sputum analysis provided an assessment of inflammation.

Sputum samples were obtained prior to the bronchoprovocation studies and 24 h post-challenge; sputum analysis allowed us to measure airway inflammation with the percentage of eosinophils used as a representative marker of this reaction (fig. 12). At baseline, e.g. pre-challenge, sputum eosinophils were detected in the induced sputum samples and were similar at each of the study phases – saline, methacholine, and antigen. Following either saline or methacholine, there was no increase in sputum eosinophils. This lack of an increase in eosinophils was expected as inflammation is not a component of the reaction to methacholine or saline. With antigen, in contrast, there was a 3-fold, significant increase in sputum eosinophils and reflected the development of allergic inflammation associated with the fall in FEV_1.

These endpoints of changes in lung function and sputum eosinophils provided a clear distinction between the responses to methacholine and antigen. Methacholine's action was limited to an immediate bronchospastic response with no evidence of

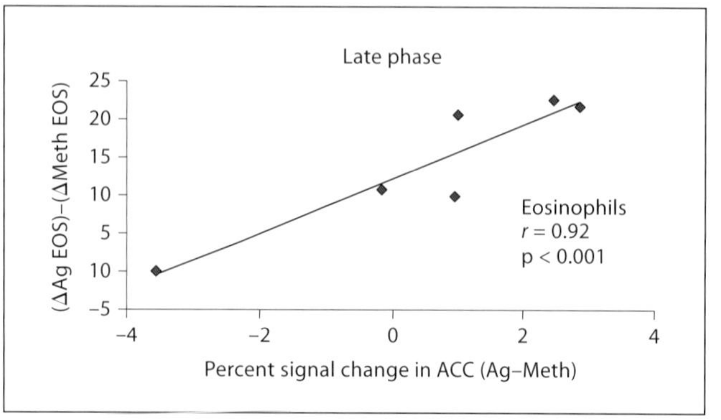

Fig. 13. Relationship of sputum eosinophils and anterior cingulate cortex (ACC) activation to antigen as compared to methacholine challenge. Reprinted with permission from Rosenkranz et al. [20].

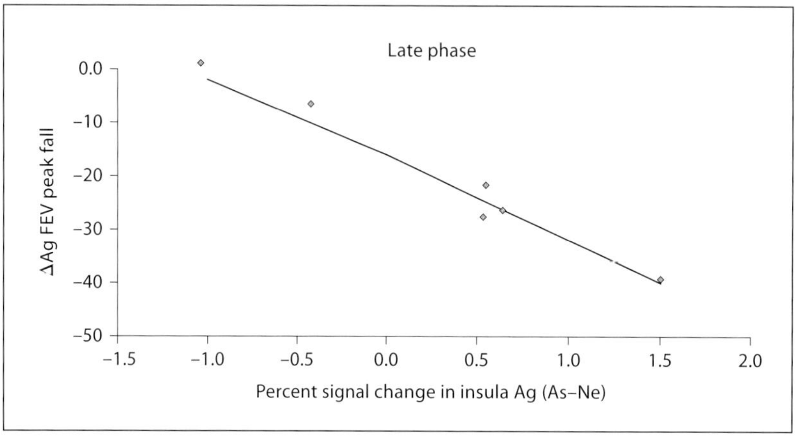

Fig. 14. Insula activity predicts peripheral measures of lung function. Percent signal change in the left insula in response to As compared with Ne words [As–Ne] and peak fall FEV_1 during late phase antigen [Ag] challenge *(b)* ($r = 0.97$, $p = 0.01$). Reprinted with permission from Rosenkranz et al. [20].

inflammation, at least as represented by sputum eosinophils. Antigen, in contrast, caused an immediate and late-phase fall in lung function; the development of the late-phase response was associated with an increase in this marker of inflammation. These measurements also allowed us to compare and contrast the effects of bronchospasm with methacholine and no inflammation on neural circuitry activation to the response to antigen, which caused both airflow obstruction and inflammation.

Given these differences between the responses to antigen and methacholine, we compared brain circuitry activation to pulmonary inflammation and airflow obstruction. There was a direct relationship between the degree of inflammation to an antigen challenge and brain circuitry activation, in this case, the anterior cingulate cortex (ACC) and insula (fig. 13). Conversely, activation of the insula was inversely related to the late-phase fall in FEV_1 postantigen challenge (fig. 14). In both cases the intensity of the allergic reaction related to the size of either the ACC or insula signals found on fMRI images. Although other areas of the brain were similarly evaluated, significant signals of activation were not found.

We feel that there are a number of features of our findings that are of interest to mechanisms of asthma and its control. First, activation of the ACC and insula preceded the appearance of late-phase pulmonary inflammation and airflow obstruction. This finding raises the possibility that neural circuitry activation following inhaled antigen occurs in advance of the late-phase events in the lung and may be either a reflection of the onset of these events or predictive of the responses, thus suggesting an involvement of brain activation that contributes to the intensity of this reaction. Second, it is possible that the principal response to neural circuitry activation is a lung-derived signal associated with the development of airway inflammation. This possibly remains speculative and is based on the observation that the airflow obstruction from methacholine did not elicit a neurosignal. Finally, we do not have information as to whether the neuroactivation is generated to enhance or downregulate the pulmonary responses to antigen (fig. 13). It is our speculation at present that the brain signal is a contributor to allergic inflammation.

At the present, it is difficult to fully put these observations into either a clinical context or pathophysiology relationship. Nonetheless, our findings indicate that the activation of the neurocircuits occurs in relationship to responses important in asthma: airflow obstruction and airway inflammation. Our observations also raise a realistic possibility that the brain is potentially an important and contributing component of the asthma response, or, at least in some individuals. To extend and expand on these data, we have the following speculations. Neurocircuits can contribute to clinical aspects of asthma, and their activation occurs primarily in response to stress, thus priming the patient for a greater inflammatory reaction when challenged with an asthma provoker, such as allergen.

We also noted in these experiments that cells isolated from the peripheral circulation at the time of the LPR were less responsive to anti-inflammatory actions of corticosteroids. These preliminary data also suggest that neuroactivated events may be associated with the appearance, or recruitment, of inflammatory cells to the lung that are less likely to be regulated by corticosteroids, thus making the resulting inflammatory response more severe.

If, indeed, these possibilities exist, we speculate that patients with asthma who experience a greater activation of the central nervous system will have a greater inflammatory response, or, at least, the events leading to airway inflammation are less well regulated, with the consequence being heightened airway injury and more severe disease. Therefore, we also propose that the environmental factors that generate chronic stress will activate specific brain circuits to create a situation which makes these affected individuals more susceptible to a more severe asthmatic reaction if a second stimulus is encountered. For example, the 'neurophenotype' asthmatic subject will be 'primed' by activation of these neurocircuits by stress. If they are subsequently exposed to antigen, or develop a respiratory infection, for example, the reaction is likely to be

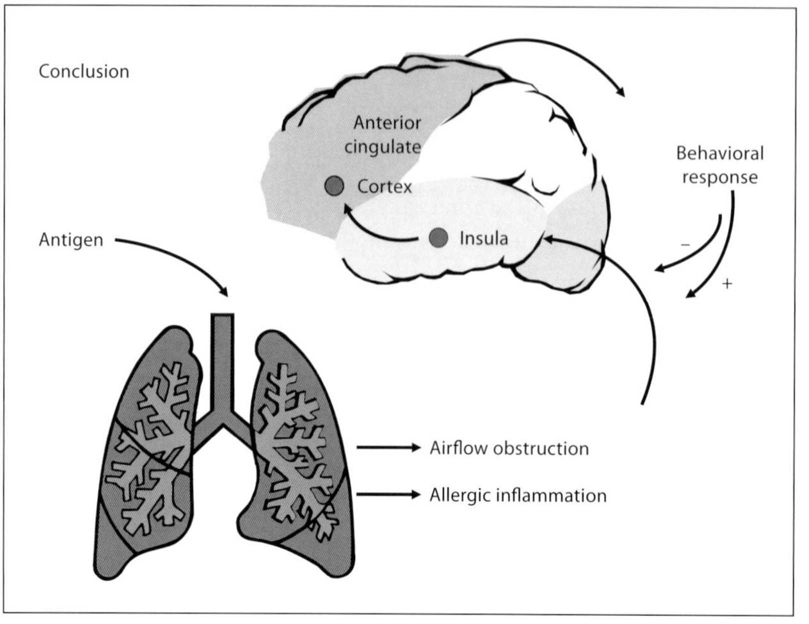

Fig. 15. Inhalation of antigen activates a pulmonary response which is characterized by airflow obstruction and inflammation, as reflected by sputum eosinophils. These lung responses are associated with an activation of brain circuits; the insula and anterior cingulate cortex. We propose that these same neurocircuits can be activated by behavior responses, such as stress. What needs to be determined is whether the activation of these brain regions upregulate or modulate the response in the lung.

more severe because selective neurocircuits have undergone activation and prime the asthmatic host for a greater inflammatory reaction to a second challenge. Moreover, because of an associated reduction in response to corticosteroids, regulation with this class of medications will be less with the end result being greater inflammation. Overall, this group of patients will be likely to have more severe disease.

Conclusions

Psychological stress can influence the severity of many diseases including asthma. The mechanisms by which stress affects asthma are not clearly defined nor are the patients at risk for its actions fully identified. We, and others, have shown that chronic stress enhances allergic airway inflammation and may shift Th cell responses more to a Th2 pattern. In addition, we have evidence that neurocircuits of the brain are activated in relationship and intensity to airway inflammation following an allergen challenge. Collectively, these data raise the possibility that areas of the brain participate in the pathophysiology of asthma and may have this effect by upregulating the inflammatory response (fig. 15). These observations are the beginning of work which will integrate more fully and comprehensively how the brain is involved in asthma and whether these brain-related areas can become new targets for asthma treatment.

References

1 Busse WW: The relationship of airway hyperresponsiveness and airway inflammation. Airway hyperresponsiveness in asthma: its measurement and clinical significance. Chest 2010;138:4S–10S.

2 Barnes PJ: Pathophysiology of allergic inflammation. Immunol Rev 2011;242:31–50.

3 Agrawal DK, Shao Z: Pathogenesis of allergic airway inflammation. Curr Allergy Asthma Rep 2010; 10:39–48.

4 Hamid Q, Tulic M: Immunobiology of asthma. Annu Rev Physiol 2009;71:489–507.

5 Holgate ST: Has the time come to rethink the pathogenesis of asthma? Curr Opin Allergy Clin Immunol 2010;10:48–53.

6 Busse WW, Lemanske RF Jr, Gern JE: Role of viral respiratory infections in asthma and asthma exacerbations. Lancet 2010;376:826–834.

7 Chen E, Miller GE: Stress and inflammation in exacerbations of asthma. Brain Behav Immun 2007; 21:993–999.

8 Miller GE, Cohen S, Ritchey AK: Chronic psychological stress and the regulation of pro-inflammatory cytokines: a glucocorticoid-resistance model. Health Psychol 2002;21:531–541.

9 Dave ND, Xiang L, Rehm KE, Marshall GD Jr: Stress and allergic diseases. Immunol Allergy Clin North Am 2011;31:55–68.

10 Rosenkranz MA, Davidson RJ: Affective neural circuitry and mind-body influences in asthma. Neuroimage 2009;47:972–980.

11 Forsythe P, Ebeling C, Gordon JR, Befus AD, Vliagoftis H: Opposing effects of short and long term stress on airway inflammation. Am J Resp Crit Care Med 2004:169:220–226.

12 O'Byrne PM, Gauvreau GM, Brannan JD: Provoked models of asthma: what have we learnt? Clin Exp Allergy 2009;39:181–192.

13 Boyce JA: Mast cells and eicosanoid mediators: a system of reciprocal paracrine and autocrine regulation. Immunol Rev 2007;217:168–185.

14 Liu LY, Coe CL, Swenson CA, Kelly EA, Kita H, Busse WW: School examinations enhance airway inflammation to antigen challenge. Am J Respir Crit Care Med 2002;165:1062–1067.

15 Bailey MT, Kierstein S, Sharma S, Spaits M, Kinsey SG, Tliba O, Amrani Y, Sheridan JF, Panettieri RA, Haczku A: Social stress enhances allergen-induced airway inflammation in mice and inhibits corticosteroid responsiveness of cytokine production. J Immunol 2009;182:7888–7896.

16 Busse WW, Mitchell H: Addressing issues of asthma in inner-city children. J Allergy Clin Immunol 2007; 119:43–49.

17 Chen E, Hanson MD, Paterson LQ, Griffin MJ, Walker HA, Miller GE: Socioeconomic status and inflammatory processes in childhood asthma: the role of psychological stress. J Allergy Clin Immunol 2006;117:1014–1020.

18 Miller GE, Chen E, Fok AK, Walker H, Lim A, Nicholls EF, Cole S, Kobor MS: Low early-life social class leaves a biological residue manifested by decreased glucocorticoid and increased proinflammatory signaling. Proc Natl Acad Sci USA 2009;106: 14716–14721.

19 Stark JL, Avitsur R, Padgett DA, Campbell KA, Beck FM, Sheridan JF: Social stress induces glucocorticoid resistance in macrophages. Am J Physiol Regul Integr Comp Physiol 2001;280:R1799–R1805.

20 Rosenkranz MA, Busse WW, Johnstone T, Swenson CA, Crisafi GM, Jackson MM, Bosch JA, Sheridan JF, Davidson RJ: Neural circuitry underlying the interaction between emotion and asthma symptom exacerbation. Proc Natl Acad Sci USA 2005;102: 13319–13324.

Prof. William W. Busse
Division of Allergy, Pulmonary and Critical Care, Department of Medicine
University of Wisconsin School of Medicine and Public Health
K4/910 CSC, MC 9988, 600 Highland Ave.
Madison, WI 53792 (USA)
Tel. +1 608 263 6183, E-Mail wwb@medicine.wisc.edu

Bienenstock J (ed): Allergy and the Nervous System.
Chem Immunol Allergy. Basel, Karger, 2012, vol 98, pp 32–47

Stress-Related Programming of Autonomic Imbalance: Role in Allergy and Asthma

Rosalind J. Wright

Channing Laboratory, Department of Medicine, Brigham and Women's Hospital, Harvard Medical School, and Department of Environmental Health, Harvard School of Public Health, Boston, Mass., USA

Abstract

Evidence linking psychological stress to allergy has grown with our increased understanding of the natural history and pathophysiology of these disorders and the neurobiology of stress vulnerability. However, the specific pathways that increase vulnerability to developing allergy and associated disorders remain to be elucidated. Autonomic nervous system functioning (autonomic balance) has been implicated in allergy for some time albeit links between autonomic balance and immune function in early development have been under studied. Starting in utero, stress may influence the programming of brain neurotransmitter systems, sympathetic and parasympathetic nervous system functioning, and the hypothalamic-pituitary-adrenal axis, which in turn may alter neural regulation of immune function. Epigenetic dysregulation of gene expression may be a fundamental mechanism for programming of early neural-immune processes.

An important step toward identifying children at risk for chronic allergic and inflammatory conditions is characterizing relevant exposures and mechanisms that lead to and maintain early predisposition. Plasticity is a consequence of environmental exposures during critical life periods (e.g. periods of rapid growth and development) affecting physiological systems that orchestrate underlying developmental processes [1]. Stress experienced during early life, beginning in utero (i.e. maternal stress during fetal ontogeny) can permanently alter the responsiveness of key regulatory systems (i.e. autonomic nervous system (ANS), hypothalamic-pituitary-adrenal (HPA) axis [2–4]) with consequent influences on the developing immune system and enhanced disease risk [5, 6]. Increasingly, evidence suggests that autonomic imbalance or dysfunction, independent of neuroendocrine or hormonal abnormalities [7–9] may be an understudied factor in the expression of a number of disorders, including allergy.

This chapter briefly reviews evidence linking autonomic imbalance and allergy. Given the focus here on the nervous system and allergy, the discussion will then focus more directly on what we know about stress-induced programming of neurological functioning, specifically autonomic balance, that may be related to immune function, allergy and related disorders during early childhood. While mechanisms underlying these relationships are unclear, the involvement of epigenetic dysregulation has gained particular focus and will be discussed [3, 10, 11].

Autonomic Imbalance and Allergy

The etiology of allergic disease (e.g. allergic rhinitis, atopic dermatitis, atopic asthma) is multifactorial with neurological involvement playing an important role [12, 13]. Research linking neural activity and allergy points to bidirectional influences between central and peripheral autonomic nervous system (ANS) activity and both immune responses and allergic symptomatology. Indeed, research implicating autonomic imbalance in the pathogenesis of inflammatory and hypersensitivity reactions in the nose, skin and the lung spans more than four decades [14–16]. While understanding the link between neurological functioning and allergy remains an active area of research, mechanisms operating in early development remain poorly understood.

Our understanding of how the nervous system may be involved in the organization of the immune response continues to evolve [17–20]. Overlapping evidence from various fields demonstrates the bidirectional communication between the brain and immune system with the autonomic nervous system (ANS) playing a central role [21–23]. When immune cells (i.e. T cells, mast cells, dendritic cells) are activated locally (e.g. in the airways) and release proinflammatory molecular mediators, these signals not only influence cells of the innate and adaptive immunological system in the periphery but also activate sensory pathways that relay information to the central nervous system (CNS) [13, 24, 25]. At the same time, CNS-mediated regulation of the peripheral immune response is mediated through vagal output (e.g. suppressing the innate immune defense to pathogens; altering pro-inflammatory cytokine balance). The efferent vagus nerve is proposed as an immune-to-brain pathway that may directly modulate the airway immune response to pathogenic invasion or to injury by irritants and toxins. The cholinergic vagus nerves participate in the regulation of the airway inflammatory response, in part, through efferent vagal endings present in airway smooth muscle. Cholinergic mechanisms represent the predominant constrictor neural pathway in human airways [26]. Differences in expression of muscarinic acetylcholine receptors in asthma suggest that cholinergic system may participate in the molecular framework influencing airway function in this context [27]. Conversely, inflammatory processes may exacerbate allergic cholinergic airway narrowing. A current model of airway narrowing in allergic asthma highlights inflammation-induced damage of m2-autoreceptors which downregulate cholinergic transmission at the level of the postganglionic nerve terminal and thereby limiting the constriction of airway smooth muscles [28, 29]. Notably, animal studies suggest that neural control influencing airway smooth muscle function and these irritant receptor systems are established during the perinatal period [30].

Growing evidence implicates a number of neurotrophins (NTs) as mediators or moderators of allergic disorders [31, 32] and shows that NT expression and signaling may be influenced by stress [33, 34]. One study in subjects with allergic asthma demonstrated that increased psychological stress was correlated with increased levels of brain-derived neurotrophic factor (BDNF) which, in turn, was negatively correlated with percent predicted forced expiratory volume in 1 s (FEV_1) [35]. Notably, stress perception was also positively correlated with the percentage of TNF-α-producing T cells in these subjects. The authors speculated that this may point to a neuro-immunological interaction given the constitutive secretion of BDNF in human peripheral blood monocytes which was enhanced when stimulated with TNF-α [36]. This group has also demonstrated stress-induced increase in tachykinin-like substance P associated with allergic airway inflammation in a mouse model [37]. Thus, it is reasonable to hypothesize that the programmed balance between functional parasympathetic and sympathetic activity in relation to stress, emotional stimuli, and immune function may be important for the expression of allergic sensitization and atopic disorders [38].

Pre- and Postnatal Stress and Physiologic Programming

This section provides an overview of how stress may be involved in the early programming of these systems.

General Stress Paradigm

Stressors are generally thought to influence pathogenesis by causing dysregulated biobehavioral states and lasting effects on physiological processes that influence disease risk [39–41]. In response to stress, physiological systems may operate at higher or lower levels than in normal homeostasis. It is the disturbed balance of these systems is most relevant to disease. Neural and immune defensive biological responses important for the short-term response to stress may produce long-term damage if not checked and terminated [42]. The detrimental cost of such accommodation is conceptualized as 'allostatic load' (i.e. wear-and-tear from chronic under- or overactivity).

One key regulatory system vulnerable to early life programming is the autonomic nervous system (ANS) [4]. As autonomic functioning and the HPA axis act cooperatively to maintain homeostasis, it is important to consider interactions between these systems as well. Disturbed regulation of these stress systems (e.g. ANS, HPA axis) in the mother consequent to her own stress history may modulate offspring immune function beginning in utero [43–45]. Postnatally, nonoptimal early childhood environments and caregiving experiences (e.g. maternal psychopathology, insensitivity) may impact the child's biobehavioral stress response [46–48] with continued effects on immunomodulation.

Perinatal Programming of Autonomic Reactivity

Several animal models as well as human studies support the connection between an adverse intrauterine environment as well as experiences in early postnatal life and alterations of autonomic nervous system balance (e.g. sympathovagal balance) [30, 49–51]. Experimental rat models have shown that prenatal stress is associated with exaggerated cardiovascular reactivity to restraint stress [52]. In humans, infants' autonomic responses show developmental changes with relative stability between 6 and 12 months of age [53]. The balance between functional parasympathetic and sympathetic activity in relation to stress, emotional stimuli, and immune function may be established during this early life period.

The placenta has increasingly been recognized as a key organ involved in fetal programming [54, 55]. Maternal and fetal stress stimulates placental secretion of corticotrophin-releasing hormone (CRH), which in turn is elevated in the neonatal circulation [56–59]. This may stimulate the fetal HPA axis to amplify fetal GC excess as well as activate additional elements of the fetal stress response (i.e. catecholamines and neurotrophins) influencing the developing autonomic nervous system and neural-immune interactions [44].

The caregiving environment is also important to early programming of stress regulatory systems in children. In humans, infants' autonomic responses [53] and the HPA system remain highly reactive and labile in early infancy and start to become organized between 2 and 6 months of age through transactions between the child and caregiver [60]. Studies have consistently demonstrated that the quality of caregiving that the child receives during early development predicts the emergence of later self-regulation abilities, with sensitive caregiving associated with more optimal functioning of the child's stress systems [61]. Not surprisingly then, perinatal maternal stress has been associated with poor stress regulation and other negative outcomes in both animal and human offspring [62–73].

Perinatal Stress and Immunomodulation

Prenatal stress increases allergen-induced airway inflammation [74, 75] and airway hyperresponsiveness (AHR) [76] in mice offspring. Prenatally stressed mice also show dysregulated cellular and humoral immune response upon antigen challenge (e.g. Th2 adaptive response and increased IgE) [76]. In primates, prenatal stress impacts the newborn's antigen response [77]. While these data are suggestive, human studies examining the effects of prenatal stress on airway responses or the developing atopic phenotype in infancy and early childhood are sparse.

While no prospective human study has measured prenatal maternal stress directly in association with child wheeze or other early atopic phenotypes, a few have considered maternal psychological functioning, as a correlate of stress exposure. Lin et al. [78] reported an association between maternal self-reported nervousness during pregnancy and elevated cord blood total IgE and the Avon Longitudinal Study of Parents and Children (ALSPAC) showed associations between maternal anxiety during pregnancy and asthma development in preadolescent children [79]. Reyes et al. [80] reported an association between a composite measure of psychological functioning in pregnancy (maternal demoralization) and increased risk of transient and persistent wheeze in a high-risk New York City sample adjusting for maternal (age, ethnicity, education, history of asthma, and IgE) and child (gender, tobacco smoke exposure) factors.

In a prospective urban pregnancy cohort in Boston [the Asthma Coalition on Community, Environment, and Social Stress (ACCESS) study], my group has documented evidence that prenatal maternal stress is associated with increased cord blood IgE expression in the children [81, 82] and enhanced reactivity to low-dose prenatal allergen exposure as indexed by elevated IgE in cord blood [83] (fig. 1). My group has also prospectively linked early life caregiver stress to dysregulation of immune function in another Boston birth cohort predisposed to allergy [84]. We found the increased maternal caregiving stress was associated with greater antigen-specific TNF-α production in particular. A number of studies have found that stress induces the release of pro-inflammatory cytokines including TNF-α as well as others (e.g., IL-6) [85–87] and that TNF-α is improtant in asthmatic airway inflammation. Continued follow-up of these prospective studies will examine whether stress-induced perinatal immunomodulation impacts the expression of allergic disease in these children.

Factors, including psychological stress, that alter the maturation of local immune networks (e.g. dendritic cells, epithelial cells (ECs), regulatory T cells) may predispose to a Th2 phenotype [88]. Psychological stress has been associated with increased proportions of both natural killer (NK) and NKT cells as well as the altering their functional mechanisms [89, 90].

Chronic psychological stress is known to alter innate- and adaptive-immune responses to a variety of pathogenic challenges with Toll-like receptors (TLRs) playing a key role. Evidence in murine models suggests that psychological stress may operate in a TLR4-dependent manner. Powell et al. [91] have demonstrated that stress modulates Toll-like receptor cytokine secretion in response to unmethylated CpG motif in bacterial deoxyribonucleic acid (DNA) and polyinosinic-polycytidylic acid (Poly I:C) in splenic DCs rendering them resistant to glucocorticoids. Zhang et al. [92] have demonstrated an association between stress and TLR4-mediated P13K/Akt signaling in mice. Notably, recent data from a human pregnancy cohort showed that higher levels of prenatal maternal stress was association with increased IL-8 and TNF-α production following microbial stimulation (e.g. Poly I:C) suggesting that prenatal

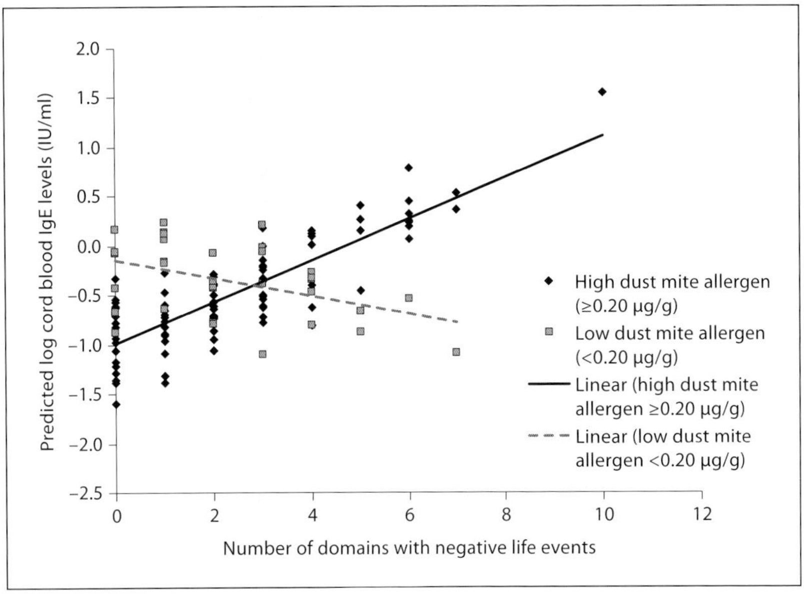

Fig. 1. Association between increasing prenatal maternal stress (negative life events) and cord blood IgE stratified by high vs. low maternal prenatal dust mite exposure.

stress may modify the neonatal immune response through Toll-like receptor (TLR)-dependent pathways [93].

Integration of Systems

Given well documented interactions between the central and peripheral autonomic nervous system, the endocrine system and the immune system starting in early development, future research needs to understand how these systems function in the mothers during pregnancy and in early childhood [94, 95]. For example, no studies to date have examined the influence of prenatal and early life stress on the expression of neuropeptides and their possible role on allergic sensitization and/or airway inflammation and response in early development.

Moreover, as we know that these systems likely act cooperatively to maintain homeostasis, the majority of existing studies examining the impact of stress on physiological systems and subsequent health have examined one system in isolation from others. Recent findings related to HPA axis and ANS functioning highlight the need to consider these systems simultaneously due to their interactive influences on outcomes. Specifically, two recent studies have shown a modifying effect of high vs. low salivary alpha-amylase (as a surrogate marker of sympathetic nervous system functioning) on the influence of high vs. low cortisol on behavioral outcomes in young children [96] and adolescents [97].

Epigenetics – A Fundamental Programming Mechanism

Mechanisms underlying early life programming of neural-immune processes are still not well understood. Growing attention has focused on epigenetic dysregulation of gene expression (i.e. long-lasting changes in gene expression that result from environmental influences) as a programming mechanism [98]. Epigenetics may be at the roots of developmental plasticity in infant stress systems [3, 10, 11]. DNA methylation, the most widely studied epigenetic mechanism, is an adaptable epigenetic mechanism that modifies genome function through the addition of methyl groups to cytosine to form 5-methyl-cytosine (5mC). Increased methylation silences expression. Gene specific DNA methylation changes in response to environmental signals including chemical exposures such as diet and toxins [99, 100]. Recent findings also implicate psychological stress with behavioral studies demonstrating epigenetic changes during fear conditioning [101] and evidence for epigenetic programming related to maternal care [11, 102]. Methylation marks are largely established early in life [98, 103] and may mediate persistent changes in biological and behavioral phenotypes over the lifespan [104]. This is buttressed by human studies demonstrating that prenatal and early life environmental conditions lead to epigenetic changes that may persist throughout life. For example, individuals exposed prenatally to the Dutch famine have reduced DNA methylation of the maternally imprinted insulin-like growth factor II (IGF2) gene compared to their unexposed same-sex siblings when assessed six decades later [105]. In another study, early life experiences of severe psychosocial stress (child abuse) was linked to increased methylation of the hippocampal glucocorticoid receptor (GR) gene (NR3C1 exon 1_F) and reduced GR messenger RNA (i.e. reduced expression) compared to control subjects not exposed to such early stress [106].

As summarized earlier, stress-elicited disruption of interrelated systems – autonomic, neuroendocrine, and immune systems – in mothers prenatally may lead to increased vulnerability in their children. Epigenetics may be at the roots of developmental plasticity in infant stress systems. Given the complexity of these interrelationships, a major challenge will be selecting specific gene pathways through which effects are operating. This brief overview focuses on those pathways that have been identified that may be involved in programming of neural-immune pathways in general and autonomic balance more specifically as summarized in figure 2.

While epigenetics has been proposed as a mediator between prenatal stress and programming of the infant stress response [3], prospective epidemiological studies designed to examine these relationships are sparse. Oberlander et al. [107] reported an association between maternal depression (a correlate of stress) assessed in the 3rd trimester of pregnancy and increased methylation of a region in the GR gene (NR3C1 promoter) – the same region examined in the suicide study [106] and the human homologue of the region Weaver et al. [104] studied in a rodent model of maternal care and programming of the offspring HPA response. Cord blood DNA was used in this sample including 82 subjects. Increased methylation of NR3C1 was

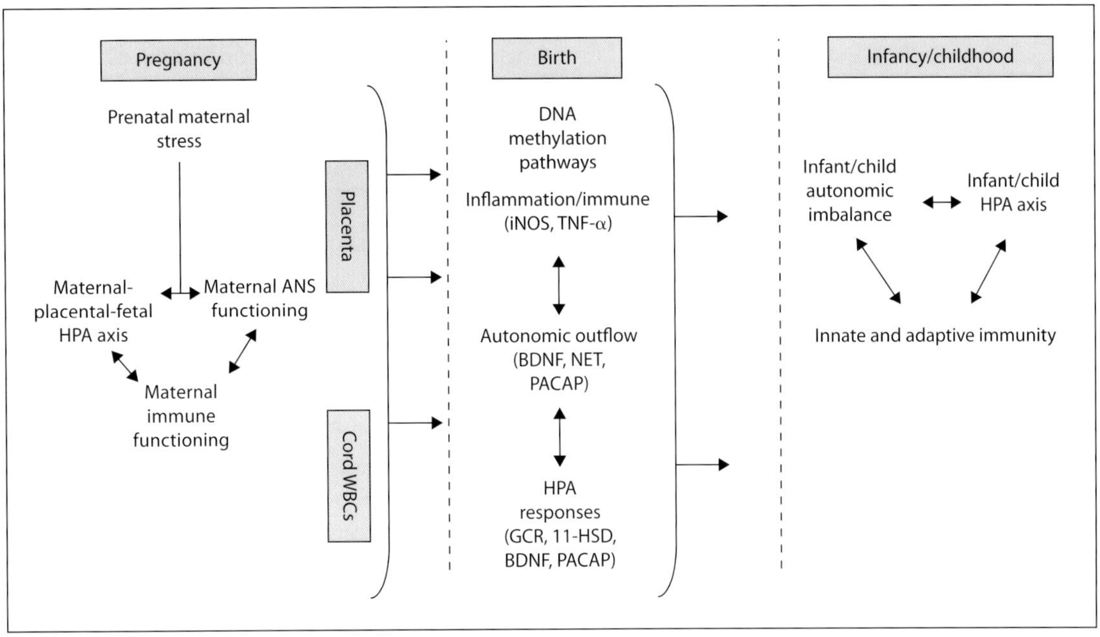

Fig. 2. Potential pathways vulnerable to stress-related methylation changes.

also associated with increased salivary cortisol responses to a standardized stressor (habituation-information processing task) in the 3-month-old infants. The stress response was indexed by a direction of change score between a baseline cortisol and a poststress recovery sample. Infants with an increased cortisol response had significantly higher NR3C1 methylation compared to infants whose cortisol levels declined.

Studies examining the influence of autonomic imbalance in mothers in this context or considering ANS stress reactivity in early life/infancy as well as the infant HPA response as they subsequently relate to early childhood immunophenotypes is needed. Future research should evaluate methylation marks in genes known to control functions modified by stress which are expressed in the target tissues (fig. 2). Some examples from the extant literature are summarized below.

Early life programming of the HPA axis [108–110] may be reflected in the GR gene [111, 112]. In pregnancy, maternal-to-fetal transfer of GCs is regulated by a placental enzyme, 11β-hydroxysteroid deydrogenase type 2 (11β-HSD2) [113, 114]. While 11β-HSD2 provides a protective barrier, approximately 10–20% of maternal GC crosses intact to the fetus [114, 115]. As maternal GC levels are higher than those of the fetus, even subtle changes in placental 11β-HSD2 activity may affect fetal GC exposure [116]. GC receptors are expressed in most fetal tissues from early embryonic stages [117–119] including the placenta where they mediate metabolic and anti-inflammatory effects. 11β-HSD2 is also expressed in the placenta [120], vasculature

[121, 122] and peripheral WBCs [123, 124]. Notably, changes in epigenetic marks in DNA from peripheral WBCs may inform links to adverse outcomes even when the ultimate target tissue is not available. For example, an epigenetic regulatory relationship to hypertension is reported for 11βHSD2 in peripheral WBC DNA [125]. Catecholamines reduce 11β-HSD2 transcription [126] while GCs increase 11β-HSD2 activity [127] in cultured trophoblasts.

Brain-derived neurotrophic factor (BDNF) may be an interesting target gene given animal studies showing that this gene is regulated by methylation and is sensitive to early adverse life experiences, stress [128, 129] and exposure to GCs [130]. Despite its name, BDNF has diverse functions during development and is expressed in a number of tissues including the placenta and peripheral WBCs [131–133]. BDNF is an important component of the HPA pathway and in sympathovagal balance [134, 135]. It is proposed that stress-induced increased cortisol results in the reduced expression and impaired function of BDNF [136]. This gene has been linked to nitric oxide (NO) production [137] and may play a role in the inflammatory stress response as well.

Given increasing evidence that neurotrophins (NTs) may be mediators or moderators of allergic disorders [31, 32] and that NT expression and signaling may be influenced by stress [33, 34] in early development this may be another important pathway. Other research shows that certain NTs involved in the stress axes (e.g. pituitary adenylate cyclase-activating polypeptide; PPACAP) regulates autonomic function by maintaining sympathetic-parasympathetic balance and contributes to peripheral homeostatic maintenance, particularly under stress conditions [138] and are involved in immunity [139].

Inducible nitric oxide synthase (iNOS) is developmentally regulated in the fetus and is likely important in regulating fetal blood flow and sympathetic nerve activity [140–142]. NO is produced in the vasculature, placenta, and peripheral WBCs [143]. NO expression has been linked to arterial reactivity in pregnancy [144]. Emerging evidence suggests oxidative stress and reactive oxygen species (such as NO) play important roles in the modulation of autonomic balance [145], including in pregnancy [146]. NO production is modulated by hormones including cortisol [147]. Stress may influence expression of iNOS through effects on transcription factors such as nuclear factor kappa B which is strongly counterregulated by GR-dependent mechanisms [148].

Norepinephrine transporters (NETs) are membrane proteins that conserve neurotransmitters by transporting them back into the presynaptic neuron. Methylation, and therefore silencing of this gene, may result in increased co-release of epinephrine and decreased norepinephrine reuptake thus creating a mechanism for increasing synaptic and circulating levels of catecholamines. NET expression in peripheral tissues is associated with autonomic outflow [149, 150]. NET is expressed in the placenta [151].

Correlates of stress have also been associated with up-regulation of inflammatory signaling pathways and cytokine expression including TNF-α in the placenta [152].

Elevated proinflammatory cytokines (e.g. TNF-α) assessed systemically or in the placenta have been associated with adverse outcomes including low birth weight, preterm delivery, and effects on the umbilical circulation [153, 154]. Inflammation is considered a central mediator of stress effects on cardiorespiratory and autonomic responses [155]. Based on preliminary studies in our lab, we focus on TNF-α. We have shown an association between maternal stress prenatally and increased expression of TNF-α in stimulated cord blood lymphocytes [93].

Conclusion

Plasticity is a consequence of environmental exposures during critical life periods affecting physiological systems orchestrating underlying developmental processes. The ANS is a putative key regulatory system vulnerable to perinatal stress-related programming toward trajectories of enhanced pediatric and adult disease risk. Given the generalized integration of ANS functioning (e.g. involvement in the modulation of the immune system, disruption of autonomic balance in early development may have long-term health implications for allergic and inflammatory diseases.

Further studies are required to establish the exact contribution of the ANS in the initiation and perpetuation of allergy. Epigenetics may be a fundamental mechanism involved in programming of autonomic balance in early life with implications for the developing immune system and thus should be a focus of research going forward in this area.

Acknowledgements

During preparation of this manuscript Dr. Wright was supported by R01HL080674 and R01HL095606.

References

1 Bateson P, Barker D, Clutton-Brock T, et al: Developmental plasticity and human health. Nature 2004;430:419–421.

2 Thayer JF, Brosschot JF: Psychosomatics and psychopathology: looking up and down from the brain. Psychoneuroendocrinology 2005;30:1050–1058.

3 Harris A, Seckl J: Glucocorticoids, prenatal stress and programming of disease. Horm Behav 2011;59: 279–289.

4 Young JB: Programming of sympathoadrenal function. Trends Endocrinol Metab 2002;13:381–385.

5 Wright RJ: Prenatal maternal stress and early caregiving experiences: implications for childhood asthma risk. Pediatr Perinat Epidemiol 2007;21:8–14.

6 Phillips DIW: Programming of the stress response: a fundamental mechanism underlying the long-term effects of the fetal environment? J Intern Med 2007;261:453–460.

67 DeBellis MD, Baum AS, Birmaher B, et al: Developmental traumatology. 1. Biological stress systems. Biol Psychiatry 1999;9:1259–1270.

68 Heim C, Newport DJ, Heit S, et al: Pituitary-adrenal and autonomic responses to stress in women after sexual and physical abuse in childhood. JAMA 2000;284:592–597.

69 Kaufman J, Birmaher B, Perel J, et al: The corticotropin-releasing hormone challenge in depressed abused, depressed nonabused, and normal control children. Biol Psychiatry 1997;42:669–679.

70 Gunnar MR, Bruce J, Hickman SE: Salivary cortisol response to stress in children. Adv Psychosom Med 2001;22:52–60.

71 Field T: The Effects of Mother's Physical and Emotional Unavailability on Emotions Regulation. Chicago, University of Chicago Press, 1994.

72 Hessl D, Dawson G, Frey K, et al: A longitudinal study of children of depressed mothers: psychobiological findings related to stress; in Hann DM, Huffman LC, Lederhendler KK, et al (eds): Advancing Research on Developmental Plasticity: Integrating the Behavioral Sciences and the Neurosciences of Mental Health. Bethesda, National Institutes of Mental Health, 1998, p 256.

73 Essex MJ, Klein MH, Cho E, et al: Maternal stress beginning in infancy may sensitize children to later stress exposure: effects on cortisol and behavior. Biol Psychiatry 2002;52:776–784.

74 Nogueira PJ, Ferreira HHA, Antunes E, et al: Chronic mild prenatal stress exacerbates the allergen-induced airway inflammation in rats. Mediat Inflamm 1999;8:119–122.

75 Quarcoo D, Pavlovic S, Joachim RA: Stress and airway reactivity in a murine model of allergic airway inflammation Neuroimmunomodulation 2009;16: 318–324.

76 Pincus-Knackstedt MK, Joachim RA, Blois SM, et al: Prenatal stress enhances susceptibility of murine adult offspring toward airway inflammation. J Immunol 2006;177:8484–8492.

77 Coe CL, Lubach GR, Karaszewski JW: Prenatal stress and immune recognition of self and nonself in the primate neonate. Biol Neonate 1999;76:301–310.

78 Lin YC, Wen HJ, Lee YL, et al: Are maternal psychosocial factors associated with cord immunoglobulin E in addition to family atopic history and mother immunoglobulin E? Clin Exp Allergy 2004;34:548–554.

79 Cookson H, Granell R, Joinson C, et al: Mother's anxiety during pregnancy is associated with asthma in their children. J Allergy Clin Immunol 2009;123: 847–853.

80 Reyes M, Perzanowski MS, Whyatt RM, et al: Relationship between maternal demoralization, wheeze, and immunoglobulin E among inner-city children. Ann Allergy Asthma Immunol 2011;107: 42–49.

81 Sternthal MJ, Bosquet Enlow M, Cohen S, et al: Maternal interpersonal trauma and cord blood IgE levels in an inner-city cohort. A life-course perspective. J Allergy Clin Immunol 2009;124:954–960.

82 Sternthal MJ, Coull BA, Chiu Y-HM, et al: Associations among maternal childhood socioeconomic status, cord immunoglobulin E, and repeated wheeze in urban children. J Allergy Clin Immunol 2011;128:337–345.

83 Peters JL, Cohen S, Staudenmayer J, et al: Prenatal negative life events increase cord blood IgE: interactions with dust mite allergen and maternal atopy. Allergy 2012;67:545–551.

84 Wright RJ, Finn PW, Contreras JP, et al: Chronic caregiver stress and IgE expression, allergeninduced proliferation and cytokine profiles in a birth cohort predisposed to atopy. J Allergy Clin Immunol 2004;113:1051–1057.

85 Nakano M, Onozuka K, Yamasu H, et al: Protective effects of cytokines in murine Salmonella. Adv Exp Med Biol 1992;319:89–95.

86 Yamasu K, Shimada Y, Sakaizumi M, et al: Activation of the systemic production of tumor necrosis factor after exposure to acute stress. Eur Cytokine Network 1992;3:391–398.

87 LeMay LG, Vander AJ, Kluger MJ: The effects of pentoxifylline on lipopolysaccharide (LPS) fever, plasma interleukin 6 (IL-6), and tumor necrosis factor (TNF) in the rat. Cytokine 1990;2:300–306.

88 Joachim RA, Handjiski B, Blois SM, et al: Stress-induced neurogenic inflammation in murine skin skews dendritic cells towards maturation and migration. Key role of intercellular adhesion molecule-1/leukocyte function-associated antigen interactions. Am J Pathol 2008;173:1379–1388.

89 Lutgendorf SK, Moore MB, Bradley S, et al: Distress and expression of natural killer receptors on lymphocytes. Brain Behav Immun 2005;19:185–194.

90 Oya H, Kawamura T, Shimizu T, et al: The differential effect of stress on natural killer T (NKT) and NK cell function. Clin Exp Immunol 2000;121: 384–390.

91 Powell ND, Bailey MT, Mays JW, et al: Repeated social defeat activates dendritic cells and enhances Toll-like receptor dependent cytokine secretion. Brain Behav Immun 2009;23:225–231.

92 Zhang Y, Zhang Y, Miao J, et al: Chronic restraint stress promotes immune suppression through toll-like receptor 4-mediated phosphoinositide 3-kinase signaling. J Neuroimmunol 2008;204:13–19.

93 Wright RJ, Visness CM, Calatroni A, et al: Prenatal maternal stress and cord blood innate and adaptive cytokine responses in an inner-city population. Am J Resp Crit Care Med 2010;182:25–33.
94 Wrona D: Neural-immune interactions: an integrative view of the bidirectional relationship between the brain and immune systems. J Neuroimmunol 2006;172:38–58.
95 Butts CL, Sternberg EM: Neuroendocrine factors alter host defense by modulating immune function. Cell Immunol 2008;252:7–15.
96 El-Sheikh M, Erath SA, Buckhalt JA, et al: Cortisol and children's adjustment: the moderating role of sympathetic nervous system activity. J Abnorm Child Psychol 2008;36:601–611.
97 Gordis EB, Granger DA, Susman EJ, et al: Asymmetry between salivary cortisol and alpha-amylase reactivity to stress: relation to aggressive behavior in adolescents. Psychoneuroendocrinology 2006;31:976–987.
98 Gluckman PD, Hanson MA, Cooper C, et al: Effect of in utero and early-life conditions on adult health and disease. N Engl J Med 2008;359:61–73.
99 Jaenisch R, Bird A: Epigenetic regulation of gene expression: how the genome integrates intrinsic and environmental signals. Nat Genet 2003;35:245–254.
100 Baccarelli A, Bollati V: Epigenetics and environmental chemicals. Curr Opin Pediatr 2009;21:243–251.
101 Levenson JM, Sweatt JD: Epigenetic mechanisms: a common theme in vertebrate and invertebrate memory formation. Cell Mol Life Sci 2006;63:1009–1016.
102 Meaney MJ, Szyf M: Maternal care as a model for experience-dependent chromatin plasticity? Trends Neurosci 2005;28:456–463.
103 Feinberg AP: Phenotypic plasticity and the epigenetics of human disease. Nature 2007;447:433–440.
104 Weaver IC, Cervoni N, Champagne FA, et al: Epigenetic programming by maternal behavior. Nat Neurosci 2004;7:847–854.
105 Heijmans BT, Tobi EW, Stein AD, et al: Persistent epigenetic differences associated with prenatal exposure to famine in humans. Proc Natl Acad Sci 2008;105:17046–17049.
106 McGowan PO, Sasaki A, D'Alessio AC, et al: Epigenetic regulation of the glucocorticoid receptor in human brain associated with childhood abuse. Nat Neurosci 2009;12:342–348.
107 Oberlander TF, Weinberg J, Papsdorf M, et al: Prenatal exposure to maternal depression, neonatal methylation of human glucocorticoid receptor gene (NR3C1) and infant cortisol stress responses. Epigenetics 2008;3:97–106.
108 Sanchez MM: The impact of early adverse care on HPA axis development: nonhuman primate models. Horm Behav 2006;50:623–631.
109 Sanchez MM, Noble PM, Lyon CK, et al: Alterations in diurnal cortisol rhythm and acoustic startle response in nonhuman primates with adverse rearing. Biol Psychiatry 2005;15:373–381.
110 Turner JD, Alt SR, Cao L, et al: Transcriptional control of the glucocorticoid receptor: CpG islands, epigenetics and more. Biochem Pharmacol 2010;80:1860–1868.
111 Turner JD, Pelascini LP, Macedo JA, et al: Highly individual methylation patterns of alternative glucocorticoid receptor promoters suggest individualized epigenetic regulatory mechanisms. Nucl Acids Res 2008;36:7207–7218.
112 Radley JJ, Kabbaj M, Jacobson L, Heydendael W, Yehuda R, Herman JP: Stress risk factors and stress-related pathology: europlasticity, epigenetics, and endophenotypes. Stress 2011;14:481–497.
113 Alikhani-Koopaei R, Fouladkou F, Frey FJ, et al: Epigenetic regulation of 11 beta-hydroxysteroid dehydrogenase type 2 expression. J Clin Invest 2004;114:1146–1157.
114 Waddell BJ, Benediktsson R, Brown RW, et al: Tissue-specific messenger ribonucleic acid expression of 11-beta-hydroxysteroid dehydrogenase types 1 and 2 and the glucocorticoid receptor within rat placenta suggests exquisite local control of glucocorticoid action. Endocrinology 1998;139:1517–1523.
115 Benediktsson R, Lindsay R, Noble J, et al: Glucocorticoid exposure in utero: a new model for adult hypertension. Lancet 1993;341:339–341.
116 Edwards C, Benediktsson R, Lindsay R, et al: Dysfunction of placental glucocorticoid barrier – link between fetal environment and adult hypertension. Lancet 1993;341:355–357.
117 Condon J, Gosden C, Gardener D, et al: Expression of type 2 11-beta-hydroxysteroid dehydrogenase and corticosteroid hormone receptors in early human fetal life. J Clin Endocrinol Metab 1998;83:4490–4497.
118 Speirs HJ, Seckl JR, Brown RW: Ontogeny of glucocorticoid receptor and 11 hydroxysteroid dehydrogenase type 1 gene expression identifies potential critical periods of glucocorticoid susceptibilty during development. J Endocrinol 2004;181:105–116.
119 Brown RW, Diaz R, Robson AC, et al: Ontogeny of 11-beta-hydroxysteroid dehydrogenase type 2 and mineralcorticoid receptor gene expression reveal intricate control of glucocorticoid action in development. Endocrinology 1996;137:794–797.

120 McTernan CL, Draper N, Nicholson H, et al: Reduced placental 11-beta-hydroxysteroid dehydrogenase type 2 mRNA levels in human pregnancies complicated by intrauterine growth restriction: an analysis of possible mechanisms. J Clin Endocrinol Metab 2001;86:4979–4983.

121 Takeda Y: Pathophysiological roles of vascular 11-beta-hydroxysteroid dehydrogenase and aldosterone. J Steroid Biochem Mol Biol 2003;85:443–447.

122 Takeda Y, Miyamori I, Yoneda T, et al: Gene expression of 11 beta-hydroxysteroid dehydrogenase in the mesenteric arteries of genetically hypertensive rats. Hypertension 1994;23:577–580.

123 Ferrari P, Sansonnents A, Dick B, et al: In vivo 11 beta-HSD-2 activity: variability, salt sensitivity, and effect of licorice. Hypertension 2001;38:1330–1336.

124 Ferrari P: The role of 11 beta-hydroxysteroid dehydrogenase type 2 in human hypertension. Biochim Biophys Acta 2010;1802:1178–1187.

125 Friso S, Pizzolo F, Choi SW, et al: Epigenetic control of 11-beta-hydroxysteroid dehydrogenase 2 gene promoter is related to human hypertension. Atherosclerosis 2008;199:323–327.

126 Sarkar S, Tsai SW, Nguyen TT, et al: Inhibition of placental 11 beta-hydroxysteroid dehydrogenase type 2 by catecholamines via alpha-adrenergic signaling. Am J Physiol Regul Integr Comp Physiol 2001;281:R1966–R1974.

127 van Beck JP, Guan H, Julan L, et al: Glucocorticoids stimulate the expression of 11 beta-hydroxysteroid dehydrogenase type 2 in cultured human placental trophoblast cells. J Clin Endocrinol Metab 2004;89: 5614–5621.

128 Roth TL, Lubin FD, Funk AJ, et al: Lasting epigenetic influence of early-life adversity on the BDNF gene. Biol Psychiatry 2009;65:760–769.

129 Givalois L, Arancibia S, Alonso G, et al: Expression of brain-derived neurotrophic factor and its receptors in the median eminence cells with sensitivity to stress. Endocrinology 2004;145:4737–4747.

130 Yang JT, Chang CN, Lee TH, et al: Effect of dexamethasone on the expression of brain-derived neurotrophic factor and neurtotrophin-3 messenger ribonucleic acids after forebrain ischemia in the rat. Crit Care Med 2002;30:913–918.

131 Mayeur S, Silog M, Moitrot E, et al: Placental BDNF/TrkB signaling system is modulated by fetal growth disturbances in rat and human. Placenta 2010;31: 785–790.

132 Gilmore JH, Jaskog LF, Vadlamudi S: Maternal poly I:C exposure during pregnancy regulates TNF alpha, BDNF, and NGF expression in neonatal brain and the maternal-fetal unit of the rat. J Neuroimmunol 2005;159:106–112.

133 Devlin AM, Brain U, Austin J, et al: Prenatal exposure to maternal depressed mood and the MTHFR C677T variant affect SLC6A4 methylation in infants at birth. PLoS One 2010;5:e12201.

134 Kohn J, Aloyz RS, Toma JG, et al: Functionally antagonistic interactions between the TrkA and p75 neurotrophin receptors regulate sympathetic neuron growth and target innervation. J Neurosci 1999; 19:5393–5408.

135 Yang AC, Chen TJ, Tsai SJ, et al: BDNF Val66Met polymorphism alters sympathovagal balance in healthy subjects. Am J Med Genet Neuropsychiatr Genet 2010;153B:1024–1030.

136 Kunugi H, Hori H, Adachi N, et al: Interface between hypothalamic-pituitary-adrenal axis and brain-derived neurotrophic factor in depression. Psychiatry Clin Neurosci 2010;64:447–459.

137 Benedick Kahn L, Gustafsson LE, Olgart Hoglund C: Brain-derived neurotrophic factor enhances histamine-induced airway responses and changes levels of exhaled nitric oxide in guinea pigs in vivo. Eur J Pharmacol 2008;595:78–83.

138 Tanida M, Shintani N, Morita Y, et al: Regulation of autonomic nerve activities by central pituitary adenylate cyclase-activating polypeptide. Regul Peptides 2010;161:73–80.

139 Ganea D, Rodriguez R, Delgado M: Vasoactive intestinal peptide and pituitary adenylate cyclase-activating polypeptide: players in innate and adaptive immunity. Cell Mol Biol 2003;49:127–142.

140 Kumagai H, Averill DB, Khosia MC, et al: Role of nitric oxide and angiotensin II in the regulation of sympathetic nerve activity in spontaneously hypertensive rats. Hypertension 1992;21:476–484.

141 Weiner CP, Thompson LP: Nitric oxide and pregnancy. Semin Perinatol 1997;21:367–380.

142 Brooks VL, Dampney AL, Heesch CM: Pregnancy and the endocrine regulation of the baroreceptor reflex. Am J Physiol Regul Integr Comp Physiol 2010;299:R439–R451.

143 McLaughlin MK, Conrad KP: Nitric oxide biosynthesis during pregnancy: implications for circulatory changes. Clin Exp Pharmacol Physiol 1995;22: 164–171.

144 Barron C, Mandala M, Osol G: Effects of pregnancy, hypertension and nitric oxide inhibition on rat uterine artery reactivity. J Vasc Res 2010;47:463–471.

145 Danson EJ, Li D, Wang L, et al: Targeting cardiac sympatho-vagal imbalance using gene transfer of nitric oxide synthase. J Mol Cell Cardiol 2009;46: 482–489.

146 Myatt L: Review: Reactive oxygen and nitrogen species and functional adaptation of the placenta. Placenta 2010;31(suppl):S66–S69.

147 Duckles SP, Miller VM: Hormonal modulation of endothelial NO production. Pflügers Arch 2010; 459:841.
148 Miller GE, Chen E, Sze J, et al: A functional genomic fingerprint of chronic stress in humans: blunted glucocorticoid and increased NF-kappaB signaling. Biol Psychol 2008;64:266–272.
149 Shannon JR, Flattem NL, Jordan J, et al: Orthostatic intolerance and tachycardia associated with norepinephrine-transporter deficiency. N Engl J Med 2000;342:541–549.
150 Esler M, Eikelis N, Schlaich M, et al: Human sympathetic nerve biology: parallel influences of stress and epigenetics in essential hypertension and panic disorder. Ann NY Acad Sci 2008;1148:338–348.
151 Bottalico B, Larsson I, Brodszki J, et al: Norepinephrine transporter (NET), serotonin transporter (SERT), vesicular monoamine transporter (VMAT2) and organic cation transporters (OCT1, 2 and EMT) in human placenta from preeclamptic and normotensive pregnancies. Placenta 2004;25:518–529.
152 Zhu MJ, Du M, Hathanielsz PW, et al: Maternal obesity up-regulates inflammatory signaling pathways and enhances cytokine expression in the midgestation sheep placenta. Placenta 2010;1:387–391.
153 Wang X, Athayde N, Trudinger B: A proinflammatory cytokine response is present in the fetal placental vasculature in placental insufficiency. Am J Obstet Gynecol 2003;189:1445–1451.
154 Challis JR, Lockwood CJ, Myatt L, et al: Inflammation and pregnancy. Reprod Sci 2009;16: 206–215.
155 Donaldson K, Stone V, Seaton A, et al: Ambient particle inhalation and the cardiovascular system: potential mechanisms. Environ Health Persp 2001; 109(suppl 4):523–527.

Dr. Rosalind J. Wright
Channing Laboratory, Harvard Medical School
181 Longwood Ave.
Boston, MA 02115 (USA)
Tel. +1 617 525 0867, E-Mail rosalind.wright@channing.harvard.edu

Bienenstock J (ed): Allergy and the Nervous System.
Chem Immunol Allergy. Basel, Karger, 2012, vol 98, pp 48–69

Role of Parasympathetic Nerves and Muscarinic Receptors in Allergy and Asthma

Gregory D. Scott[a] · Allison D. Fryer[a,b]

[a]Division of Pulmonary and Critical Care Medicine, and [b]Department of Physiology and Pharmacology, Oregon Health and Science University, Portland, Oreg., USA

Abstract

Parasympathetic nerves control the symptoms and inflammation of allergic diseases primarily by signaling through peripheral muscarinic receptors. Parasympathetic signaling targets classic effector tissues such as airway smooth muscle and secretory glands and mediates acute symptoms of allergic disease such as airway narrowing and increased mucus secretion. In addition, parasympathetic signaling modulates inflammatory cells and non-neuronal resident cell types such as fibroblasts and smooth muscle contributing to chronic allergic inflammation and tissue remodeling. Importantly, muscarinic antagonists are experiencing a rebirth for the treatment of asthma and may be useful for treating other allergic diseases.

The past century of research has identified common characteristics of allergic disease including increased smooth muscle contraction, hypersecretion, neuroplasticity and inflammation. The parasympathetic nervous system, a division of the autonomic nervous system, controls all of these events.

Although often unappreciated in the current literature, early studies highlight the importance of the parasympathetic nervous system in allergic disease by showing that surgical and pharmacologic denervation of parasympathetic nerves prevents disease establishment, disease progression, and symptom manifestation. Cutting nerve supply to the nose (vidian nervectomy) prevents allergy-associated overactive secretion [1] and cutting nerves supplying the airway (vagotomy) eliminated asthma symptoms and reduced inflammation [2]. Symptoms and allergic inflammation are also prevented by pharmacologic blockade of parasympathetic nerve signaling. Inhibition of parasympathetic nerves is accomplished by anticholinergic drugs, including ipratropoium and atropine, that block muscarinic receptors. Culminating decades of research, the first antagonist selective for a specific muscarinic receptor subtype, tiotropium, was recently proven to be clinically effective and was approved for treatment of poorly controlled asthma [3]. Here, we will discuss evidence that parasympathetic nerves represent an important common pathway for producing the symptoms of allergy and contributing to allergic disease progression.

Parasympathetic Signaling Controls Organ Functions Relevant to Allergy

Allergy is defined as a hypersensitivity reaction initiated by immunological mechanisms [3]. Allergens, or antigens that cause allergy, are typically foreign proteins that include pollen, pet dander, food, cockroach excrement, and fungal spores. The development of allergic disease in different organs often occurs together in the same person. Numerous studies have found positive associations between allergic rhinitis, asthma, atopic dermatitis, allergic conjunctivitis, and food allergies [4–12]. Irritable bowel syndrome (IBS) is also associated with allergy/atopy [9, 13–15]. Atopy is defined as the tendency, usually in childhood or adolescence, to develop sensitivity to common allergens [3]. The chronic-exposure allergies of the nose (rhinitis), airway (asthma), eye (conjunctivitis), gastrointestinal tract (food allergy, irritable bowel syndrome), and skin (atopic dermatitis, eczema) are characterized by acute and chronic symptoms including itch, pain, limited airflow, hypersecretion, intestinal dysmotility, and tissue remodeling. These manifestations of allergy are each wholly or partially under the control of the parasympathetic nervous system.

General Anatomy and Signaling of the Parasympathetic Nervous System

Parasympathetic nerves travel to end organs via a two-nerve pathway interrupted by the cell body of the second nerve. These cell bodies are ganglia and autonomic nerves are labeled anatomically as either pre- or postganglionic nerves depending on whether they supply the ganglia (preganglionic) or originate at the ganglia (postganglionic). It is the postganglionic nerves that release neurotransmitter onto end organs. Postganglionic nerves signal effector organs including submucosal glands, smooth muscle, and epithelial cells. The principle signaling mechanism between postganglionic parasympathetic nerves and effector target tissues is neuronal release of the neurotransmitter, acetylcholine, onto receptors sensitive to muscarine (muscarinic receptors) [16]. ACh activity is normally terminated by acetylcholinesterase [17].

It is worth noting that parasympathetic nerves also signal through nicotinic acetylcholine receptors and also release nonacetylcholine (noncholinergic) neurotransmitters such as vasoactive intestinal peptide (VIP) and nitric oxide (NO). Although VIP and NO contribute to vasodilation and mucus secretion in some organs, acetylcholine and muscarinic receptors typically provide dominant control of smooth muscle contraction and secretion caused by parasympathetic signaling.

Muscarinic receptors are also present on cells not innervated by the parasympathetic nerves including fibroblasts, and inflammatory cells [18, 19]. These cells may receive ACh that is released from non-neuronal sources such as epithelial cells [20].

Muscarinic receptors are a five-member family that belongs to the larger group of G protein-coupled receptors (GPCRs). For a more in depth review refer to muscarinic receptor classification by the International Union of Pharmacology [21]. The canonical intracellular signaling pathway of odd-numbered muscarinic receptors (M_1, M_3, M_5) is through G_q to activate phospholipase C whereas the canonical signaling pathway of even-numbered receptors (M_2, M_4) is via G_i to inhibit adenylyl cyclase.

Parasympathetic Control of the Lung

Parasympathetic nerves supplying the lung, travel in the vagus nerve, maintain airway tone and play a prominent role in airway narrowing (bronchoconstriction) and in mucus secretion [22]. Action potentials generated in postganglionic nerves travel along short postganglionic fibers to smooth muscle and submucosal glands. Neuronal acetylcholine stimulates M_3 postjunctional muscarinic receptors on smooth muscle and mucus glands. Although M_2 receptors are also present on airway smooth muscle and M_1 receptors are on submucosal glands, cholinergic, M_3 receptor signaling is considered the principle mechanism for neuronally mediated bronchoconstriction and mucus secretion [22, 23]. This is supported in humans since the kinetically selective M_3 muscarinic antagonist, tiotropium, prevents methacholine-induced bronchoconstriction [24]. Non-neuronal epithelial release of acetylcholine stimulates airway epithelial ciliary transport via M_3 receptors to clear the airways but the contribution of parasympathetic nerves to this mechanism remains unknown [25]. M_2 receptors were also shown using knockout mice to inhibit acetylcholine- and M_3-mediated ciliary transport [25].

Inhibition of parasympathetic signaling is provided by M_2 muscarinic receptors on the parasympathetic nerves and by postjunctional VIP/NO signaling. M_2 receptors on nerves at the neuroeffector junction limit further acetylcholine release and thus provide negative feedback, limiting neurotransmission and bronchoconstriction [26, 27]. This was first demonstrated in guinea pigs by administering the selective M_2 receptor antagonist, gallamine, which blocked autoinhibition of acetylcholine release from parasympathetic nerves and in a dose dependent manner potentiated airway smooth muscle contraction induced by stimulating the vagus nerves [27]. The presence of inhibitory M_2 receptors on parasympathetic nerves supplying the lungs has been shown in all species studied so far including mice, guinea pigs, monkeys and humans [28, 29]. Parasympathetic nerves also release VIP and NO that can inhibit airway contraction and mucus secretion as shown in knockout mice, ex vivo airway tissue and release assays [30–34].

Muscarinic Receptor Changes on Airway Smooth Muscle

Whether changes in smooth muscle muscarinic receptor expression or function directly contribute to increased contractility in allergic diseases is controversial.

Multiple studies found that airway smooth muscle isolated from asthmatics does not exhibit increased sensitivity to muscarinic agonists, suggesting that increased muscle contraction seen in vivo is not due to increased responsiveness to muscarinic signaling at the level of the smooth muscle [28, 35, 36]. In contrast, a few authors have shown airway smooth muscle from asthmatics exhibit increased contractile responses to direct stimuli in vitro presumably bypassing parasympathetic nerve signaling [37–39]. The authors speculate that the differences between these studies and those that did not report a difference in asthmatic smooth muscle might be due to differences in the smooth muscle contractile agonist used (carbachol, ACh, histamine, adenosine) and the method of tissue harvest (bronchoscopic biopsy, postmortem harvest); however, a definitive study of muscarinic signaling that includes selective muscarinic antagonists and direct muscle depolarizing agents (e.g. potassium chloride) have not been reported.

Animal studies of allergy have in some cases also reported increased airway smooth muscle contractility and mechanisms involving muscarinic signaling on the muscle. However, despite increased contractility to ACh, a rat model of allergic asthma showed no change in smooth muscle acetylcholinesterase activity, muscarinic receptor density or the ACh dissociation constant, and were unable to provide a physiological explanation of the increased contraction. However, there are low and high agonist affinity sites on muscarinic receptors and when studied in detail, ACh's affinity for the high-affinity muscarinic receptor-binding site was significantly greater in antigen challenged rats [40]. This selective increase in the high affinity ACh site on muscarinic receptors (presumably M_3) with no change in K_d could potentially increase G protein coupling which could increase bronchoconstriction, but this has not yet been linked to physiologic changes. An additional mechanism of increased ACh contraction was discovered in antigen-challenged dogs where isolated tracheal smooth muscle exhibited lower acetylcholinesterase activity than control animals [41]. Decreased acetylcholinesterase activity could increase acetylcholine levels seen by muscle and increase contraction. If inherent smooth muscle responsiveness is increasing it may also occur downstream of muscarinic receptors. This is supported by data that despite no change in muscarinic receptor density or K_d (shown above), airway smooth muscle from rats with airway hyperreactivity exhibit greater intracellular calcium levels (a surrogate measurement for myosin phosphorylation and smooth muscle contraction) in response to histamine [42]. Thus, while there is some evidence in vitro that contraction induced by muscarinic receptor agonists may be greater in muscle from asthmatic humans and antigen challenged animals, no clear mechanisms have been identified as yet, and in vivo, in animals, data supporting increased contraction is less compelling.

Dysfunctional Parasympathetic Nerve Control of Airway Smooth Muscle

Exposure of sensitized individuals to antigens increases contraction of airway smooth muscle mediated by parasympathetic nerves in humans and in animal models of disease [43]. In asthma, cutting the parasympathetic nerve supply to the airway (vagotomy) prevents increased smooth muscle contraction [2]. These findings in humans were replicated in animal models of disease. Multiple studies show that guinea pigs and mice that were sensitized to an antigen (ovalbumin or fungus) and subsequently exposed to that antigen, exhibit increased airway narrowing which is prevented by vagal section or by anticholinergic drugs [43–45]. In virally infected human asthmatics, anticholinergic treatment prevents increased bronchoconstriction and cough suggesting there is increased parasympathetic nerve activity in viral exacerbations of asthma [46, 47].

Studies have shown that autoinhibition of ACh release that is normally provided by inhibitory M_2 receptors on parasympathetic nerves, is disrupted in humans with asthma. Pilocarpine stimulates M_2 receptors and prevents reflex bronchoconstriction initiated by inhaled sulfur dioxide in healthy controls. However, pilocarpine has no protective effect in subjects with asthma, demonstrating that the neuronal M_2 receptors are not responding to an agonist [26]. Similar to humans, animal models of airway hyperreactivity exhibit dysfunctional M_2 receptors in the airway. In control guinea pigs, blocking M_2 receptors with a selective antagonist potentiates vagally induced bronchoconstriction, but in guinea pig models of allergen-, virus-, or ozone-induced airway hyperreactivity, blocking M_2 receptors does not potentiate vagally induced bronchoconstriction demonstrating that neuronal M_2 muscarinic receptors no longer respond to ACh [18, 48–50]. Subsequent studies uncovered several mechanisms that result in loss of M_2 function including a role for inflammatory cells.

Eosinophils, seen commonly in asthma and allergy, produce and release cationic granule proteins including eosinophil major basic protein. Major basic protein is an allosteric antagonist for M_2 muscarinic receptors [51]. In animal models of allergic asthma, it appears that eosinophils are actively recruited to the lung and to airway nerves including parasympathetic ganglia [52] where they are activated. Disrupting eosinophil association with nerves or blocking eosinophil major basic protein prevents neuronal M_2 muscarinic dysfunction in vivo and prevents associated airway hyperreactivity in antigen-challenged, sensitized animals [50, 53, 54]. Thus, release of eosinophil major basic protein onto M_2 muscarinic receptors results in increased ACh and increased bronchoconstriction in allergic guinea pigs. New data show that blocking IL-5 with an antibody inhibits eosinophil recruitment to the lungs and prevents asthma exacerbations supporting that a similar 'eosinophil-major basic protein-M_2 blockade-increased ACh release' mechanism is present in humans with allergic asthma [55, 56].

Alternative mechanisms of M_2 dysfunction have been identified with other models of airway hyperreactivity. For example, viral neuraminidase decreases agonist affinity for M_2 receptors [57], and macrophages release interferon-gamma that decreases neuronal M_2 muscarinic receptor expression [49, 58]. While these have not been demonstrated in allergic asthma, these mechanisms may contribute to the heterogeneity of asthma, a disease difficult to subtype clinically without histologic analysis

[59]. Despite asthma's heterogeneity, in both humans and animal models most if not all disease response can be blocked by adequately inhibiting parasympathetic control with muscarinic antagonists [43].

Another intriguing mechanism of muscarinic antagonists is their ability to inhibit release of the inflammatory mediator, thromboxane A2 [60]. This is important because thromboxane A2 binds thromboxane receptors and potentiates the contraction caused by methacholine stimulation of M_3 receptors [60]. This is an additional mechanism whereby anticholinergic treatment could be beneficial.

Dysfunctional Parasympathetic Signaling and Airway Hypersecretion

Excessive mucus secretion in asthmatics contributes to airway obstruction and is also under parasympathetic control [22]. There is evidence of increased mucus glands (hyperplasia), increased mucus gland size (hypertrophy), and increased mucus secretion in asthma and allergy [59]. A link in humans between muscarinic receptors and mucus glands is shown in isolated airway tissue by administration of the muscarinic agonist, carbachol, which increases expression of mucin-related genes (e.g. MUC5AC) by PCR and protein by ELISA [61]. In two different studies, muscarinic antagonists, ipratropium and oxitropium bromide, inhibited the volume of airway mucus produced by patients with reversible airways obstruction and chronic bronchitis [62]. It is important to note that the effect of muscarinic antagonists on mucus production remains controversial. Some studies report no change in mucus production after tiotropium treatment [63] but cite difficulty in separating mucus production from cough and mucociliary clearance [62]. However, in a mouse model of asthma, increased mucin gene production and decreased airway compliance (presumably due to increased mucus secretion) are prevented by a M_3 muscarinic receptor antagonist, aclidinium bromide [43]. Blocking M_3 with tiotropium in sensitized and antigen challenged guinea pigs also completely prevented the increase in mucus gland hypertrophy [64].

Parasympathetic Nerves and Muscarinic Signaling as Therapeutic Targets for Asthma

Historically, the widespread use of muscarinic antagonists has been tempered by problems including: under dosing, off target bioavailability, receptor subtype nonspecificity, and short dissociation half-lives. In addition, beta-agonists and steroids have been beneficial in asthma [59, 65, 66]. Muscarinic antagonists have been reintroduced into therapeutic use as new and more selective drugs are developed coincident with a greater understanding of the role of muscarinic subtypes in disease.

Older studies demonstrated that nonselective muscarinic antagonists (e.g. atropine) cause significant reversal of airway narrowing in asthma [67]; however, they also produced unacceptable off-target side effects (e.g. dry mouth, tachycardia, confusion). Ipratropium, a newer nonselective anticholinergic drug, was developed to limit systemic bioavailability and decrease side effects but it did not significantly improve lung function in humans with COPD [68]. Importantly, although this lack of efficacy was probably caused by under-dosing ipratropium [18], the lack of effect was used for many years by the research community to discount the parasympathetic nerves contribution to asthma. Ipratropium's clinical dose had been determined using inhibition of bronchoconstriction induced by inhaled ACh rather than vagally released acetylcholine even though the later in humans represents physiologic control of airway smooth muscle. This is important because animal studies show that muscarinic antagonists in doses sufficient to block inhaled ACh-induced bronchoconstriction are not sufficient to block vagally-induced bronchoconstriction, demonstrating that ipratropium dosing is too low to block physiologic bronchoconstriction [69]. In patients with asthma, higher doses of ipratropium, 10-fold above current FDA recommended doses, significantly bronchodilated their airways [18, 70]. As a result, current expert opinion now recommends higher dose ipratropium for acute asthma exacerbations [66].

Under-dosing of cholinergic antagonists continues to be a major problem when evaluating studies of muscarinic antagonists, thus their therapeutic potential is still not fully realized. The newer generation muscarinic antagonists were developed to exhibit selectivity for M_3 over M_2 muscarinic receptors to minimize heart-related side effects [43], but additionally they also spare neuronal M_2 receptors. Tiotropium, a newer muscarinic antagonist with M_3 kinetic selectivity, was the first approved anticholinergic drug specifically shown to treat poorly controlled asthma. Remarkably, tiotropium was more effective at improving peak expiratory flow than steroids alone and was equivalent to combined steroid and long acting beta-agonist treatment [65]. Since dosing was determined similarly to ipratropium [18] this suggests that tiotropium at higher doses than used in this study may further improve therapeutic efficacy [65]. Newer M_3 selective antagonists, bencycloquidium bromide and aclidinium bromide, have been tested in mouse and guinea pig models of allergic asthma and are equally, but not additively, effective as tiotropium. However, these new M_3 antagonists demonstrated faster onset of action, faster off rates (particularly at M_2), and rapid plasma hydrolysis important for limiting side effects [43–45, 71]. Aclidinium bromide is effective and well tolerated in COPD in a phase III trial [72], suggesting that it and other new antagonists could also be developed for treatment of asthma.

Parasympathetic Control of the Nose

The nose is supplied by parasympathetic nerves that control mucus secretion and nasal congestion due to edema, vasodilation, and sinusoidal engorgement [73]. Nasal preganglionic parasympathetic nerves travel in the petrosal and vidian nerves to synapse onto postganglionic nerves in the sphenopalatine ganglia. These postganglionic nerves project to the nasal cavity arteries, venous sinusoids, mucus-producing (seromucous) acinar glands, and goblet cells in nasal respiratory epithelium [73, 74]. Acetylcholine increases mucus secretion and nasal congestion and, as in the lungs,

M_3 muscarinic receptors are the dominant subtype mediating secretion in the nose [26].

As in the lungs, M_2 receptor mRNA has been detected in human nasal mucosa and early pharmacologic data suggest M_2 receptors inhibit secretory reflexes [75]. Non-cholinergic parasympathetic neurotransmitters, VIP, PHM, and nitric oxide are also thought to cause nasal vasodilation and subsequent nasal congestion [73].

Dysfunctional Parasympathetic Signaling Causes Hypersecretion in the Nose

Hypersecretion (rhinorrhea) in allergic rhinitis is under neural control demonstrated most readily by a unilateral antigen challenge, to one side of the nose, causing a bilateral increase in secretion responses [76]. In humans with nasal allergy and in guinea pig models, studies report increased muscarinic receptors that correlate with hypersecretion following administration of muscarinic agonists, and in human's self-reported nose blowing frequency [1, 77, 78]. It is interesting to note that after sensitization to antigen, muscarinic receptor density decreases in nasal mucosa of guinea pigs [1]. However, this decrease in muscarinic receptors may be offset by increased agonist affinity as was shown in one study of nasal mucosa of humans with nasal allergy [77]. Increased agonist affinity was not however, found in an animal study [1]. Allergic rhinitis is also associated with increased activity of the enzyme responsible for acetylcholine synthesis, cholineacetyltransferase [1], so that ACh levels may be increased in nerves.

One potentially important mechanism of muscarinic receptor signaling in the nose is the hypertrophy and hyperplasia of mucus secretory cells. Repeated administration of muscarinic agonists (pilocarpine, methacholine) increased mucus cell hypertrophy and hyperplasia [30]. Muscarinic agonists may stimulate mucus cells via transactivation of epidermal growth factor that causes mucus cell and goblet cell activation and remodeling (hyperplasia and hypertrophy) [79].

Anticholinergic therapy for allergic rhinitis (discussed below) markedly reduced the daily duration and severity of rhinorrhea [80–82]. However, there are data that noncholinergic neurotransmission may also be important. For example, people with nasal allergies have more VIP-positive nerves in the nasal mucosa and also increased VIP release into nasal secretions [83, 84]. Increased VIP may contribute to increased nasal congestion in allergic rhinitis but this has not been directly tested.

Parasympathetic Dysregulation of Vasodilation and Vascular Permeability

In allergic rhinitis nasal congestion is not only produced by secretions but also by increased vasodilation that is under neural control. Administration of antigen or histamine to allergic patients on one side of the nasal mucosa led to closure of the opposite (contralateral) side of the nose demonstrating a neural reflex [76]. The muscarinic receptor antagonist, oxitropium, blocked histamine-induced nasal closure in allergic rhinitis patients demonstrating that muscarinic receptors are critical to this vasodilator response [85].

Parasympathetic Nerves and Muscarinic Receptor Signaling as Therapeutic Targets for Allergic Rhinitis

Allergic rhinitis is typically treated with antihistamines and sympathomimetics. However these have side effects including drowsiness and rebound congestion. Since the antihistamines, diphenhydramine and hydroxyzine, have beneficial off-target anticholinergic effects, specific muscarinic antagonists have been tested for rhinitis. In patients with perennial allergic rhinitis both the severity and duration of rhinorrhea was reduced after treatment with the anticholinergic drug, ipratropium bromide [81, 82], suggesting that anticholinergic drugs, especially the newer muscarinic receptor subtype selective drugs, may be added to the pharmacological options for rhinitis in the future.

Parasympathetic Control of the Eye

Parasympathetic control of the eye includes lens accommodation (focusing), pupil contraction, and production of the protective mucus layer of tear film [86–88]. Preganglionic parasympathetic nerves from the oculomotor nerve synapse with postganglionic nerves in the ciliary ganglion which project to eye muscles and conjunctival goblet cells [89]. Additionally, roughly 20% of cholinergic nerves innervating the conjunctiva project from a different parasympathetic ganglia called the pterygopalatine (sphenopalatine) ganglia. Accommodation, pupil contraction, and tear film production are thought to be mediated primarily by acetylcholine acting at M_3 muscarinic receptors. Tear production is increased by muscarinic agonists (carbachol, oxotremorine) and is blocked by M_3 antagonists both in vivo and in isolated lacrimal glands [90, 91]. Similarly, accommodation and pupil contraction both in vivo and in isolated ciliary muscle were stimulated by muscarinic agonists and inhibited by M_3 antagonists [92, 93].

Most noncholinergic parasympathetic innervation of the eye comes from the pterygopalatine ganglia (via the greater petrosal nerve), with a minority coming from the ciliary ganglion [94]. Noncholinergic nerves primarily release VIP and control intraocular pressure and blood flow [89, 95]. VIP has also been shown to stimulate mucus production and VIP receptors are located on mucus-producing goblet cells [87]. In addition to VIP-containing nerves, the eye contains a dense network of parasympathetic nerves that release nitric oxide. These nerves have been demonstrated next to choroidal and scleral limbal blood vessels and presumably regulate blood supply [96].

Dysfuctional Parasympathetic Control of Lacrimation

Vernal keratoconjunctvitis is a seasonal eye allergy associated with atopy, elevated serum IgE, and increased tear production. Very little research has studied whether parasympathetic signaling or dysfunction may underlie increased tear production.

However, one histologic study of nerves and muscarinic receptors has reported decreased M_1 receptors, decreased nerves, and disorganized expression of M_2/M_3 receptors (assessed by staining morphology) in conjunctival biopsies from vernal keratoconjunctivitis patients [97]. However, this is only one study and additional data are required. This same study reported increased VIP as another potential parasympathetic (but non-cholinergic) contributory mechanism to increased tear production [97]. The potential importance of VIP was also shown in one human trial where neuropeptides were quantified in tear film. Patients with allergic conjunctivitis had increased VIP in tear film as compared to healthy controls, but only after and not before conjunctival antigen provocation [98].

Parasympathetic Control of the Intestine

Intestinal parasympathetic nerves modulate peristalsis through control of the enteric nervous system [99]. Electrical stimulation of the vagal nerves or pelvic efferents innervating the stomach and intestine caused muscle contractions which were inhibited by muscarinic receptor antagonists and blockers of neuronal depolarization [100, 101]. Studies with selective muscarinic antagonists and muscarinic receptor knockout mice concluded M_3 muscarinic receptors are the dominant subtype mediating intestinal motility [102, 103]. In contrast, neuronal M_2 muscarinic receptors and noncholinergic neurotransmission typically inhibit intestinal motility [102, 103].

Parasympathetic Causes of Intestinal Dysmotility

Gastrointestinal allergy and irritable bowel syndrome (IBS), which are associated with allergy/atopy [13–15], manifest in part through dysmotility of the intestine in humans as well as in animal models of the disease [13, 104, 105]. Parasympathetic dysfunction results in increased or decreased sensitivity to muscarinic agonists depending on the smooth muscle layer (inner circular vs. outer longitudinal), segment of the gastrointestinal tract, and disease model studied. The inner, circular, muscle layer of the jejunum and ileum in antigen-challenged mice and guinea pigs with ileitis are less sensitive to muscarinic agonist (carbachol)-induced contraction [106, 107]. In contrast, the outer longitudinal muscle layer exhibits hypersensitivity to carbachol in the same guinea pig ileitis model and also in a parasitic infection model [107, 108]. These data suggest that there may be a mismatch in activity of the inner and outer muscle layers that could lead to dysmotility. Furthermore, this could be mediated by the M_3 muscarinic receptor subtype. In a radiation-induced enteric inflammation model, intestinal dysmotility was prevented by chemical vagotomy of the small intestine using tetrodotoxin, blockade of ganglionic transmission with hexamethonium, blockage of all muscarinic receptors with atropine, and blockade of M_3 muscarinic receptors on the muscle with the M_3 selective antagonist, 4-DAMP [109]. A change in muscarinic binding affinity, discussed above for asthma, represents a potential mechanism for increased muscarinic signaling in gastrointestinal dysmotility. In animal inflammation models, there was a selective increase in the high-affinity muscarinic binding site for carbachol which potentially increases smooth muscle contractility to acetylcholine [110].

Recent data has shown that crosstalk between eosinophils and parasympathetic nerves as discussed in asthma might also occur in gastrointestinal diseases [111, 112]. In intestinal biopsies from humans, mucosal eosinophils and eosinophil granule proteins are co-localized with nerves and myenteric ganglia. The authors speculate that eosinophils may contribute to intestinal dysmotility through a similar mechanism as seen in asthma, but this has not been directly tested [113].

Parasympathetic Nerves and Muscarinic Signaling as Therapeutic Targets for IBS
Several muscarinic receptor antagonists block intestinal dysmotility and provide relief with irritable bowel syndrome [114]. Muscarinic M_3 antagonists (zamifenacin, darifenacin) effectively inhibit intestinal motility and increase gastric emptying in diarrhea-predominant irritable bowel syndrome [114]. However, muscarinic antagonists alleviate pain which could confound mechanistic studies [114]. More selective muscarinic antagonists will help isolate the beneficial gastrointestinal motility effects versus nociceptive effects similar to treatment for chronic pain where M_4 agonists alleviate pain without eliciting cardiovascular side effects of M_2 stimulation [114].

Parasympathetic Control of the Skin

The skin is considered one of the three organs free from parasympathetic nerve control, however there is a small body of evidence showing direct parasympathetic control of facial blood vessels and sweat glands, and the presence of cholinergic, muscarinic, and VIP-ergic regulation of skin vasodilation and sweat secretion [115, 116]. Facial parasympathetic innervation was shown by tracing studies and immunostaining for vesicular choline acetylcholine transferase (marker for ACh synthesis), VIP, and acetylcholinesterase. Parasympathetic and sympathetic nerve fibers projecting to blood vessels in the lower lip are from the otic ganglion, a parasympathetic ganglion [116–119]. Stimulation of the lingual nerve in the presence of a sympathetic nervous system blocker (guanethidine; that depletes neurotransmitters in the sympathetic nerves and thus isolates the effects of stimulation to parasympathetic nerves) caused dose-dependent increases in lower lip blood flow which were prevented by blocking ganglionic transmission with hexamethonium [118]. Although evidence for parasympathetic nervous function in the skin is limited to the lower lip, cholinergic nerves are capable of migrating into shallower layers of injured skin. Following sensory denervation, cholinergic (vesicular choline acetyltransferase positive) nerves were shown to migrate into the upper dermis past their normal depth and persist for at least 8 weeks

[120, 121]. Whether these sprouting nerves are cholinergic sympathetic or parasympathetic nerves remain unknown.

In terms of atopic dermatitis which involves flexural skin locations (elbows, behind the knees) there is controversial data suggesting that cholinergic and noncholinergic signaling plays a role. In non-facial skin there are VIP-containing nerves and acetylcholinesterase-containing nerves and both have been shown to increase in nonlesional skin and decrease in lesional skin from patients with atopic dermatitis [122, 123]. However, other studies found no change in VIP levels in the skin from people with atopic dermatitis [124, 125]. Recent data has demonstrated that itch, the primary symptom of atopic dermatitis, probably involves M_3 muscarinic signaling in the skin. Itch induced by intradermal carbachol injection was prevented both atropine and 4-DAMP, an M_3 muscarinic antagonist [126]. A separate study showed a marked increased in ACh levels in the skin biopsies from atopic dermatitis patients, but choline acetyltransferase immunostaining was limited to non-neuronal cells (keratinocyptes, hair papilla, glands, endothelial cells, and mast cells) suggesting the increased ACh is due to increased non-neuronal ACh production [127].

Role of Parasympathetic Nerves in Inflammation and Disease Progression

Parasympathetic Proinflammatory Signaling, Recruitment, and Cell Adhesion

In allergic asthma increased parasympathetic nerve activity is correlated with airway inflammation and airway hyperreactivity [30, 43]. In addition, specific inflammatory cells are associated with nerves in allergic disease. In general muscarinic signaling is pro-inflammatory and results in production of inflammatory cytokines, chemokines, recruitment of inflammatory cells, and leukocyte adhesion. Therefore, muscarinic receptors and parasympathetic nerves may help establish allergic disease or may further disease progression.

In humans and animal models of asthma, eosinophils reside along nerves, inside nerve bundles, and adjacent to parasympathetic ganglia [128]. In a mouse model of allergic asthma, dendritic cells were also colocalized next to intrinsic (parasympathetic) ganglia and additionally airway sensory nerves [129]. Eosinophil recruitment to parasympathetic nerves in the airway involves cytokines (tumor necrosis factor), chemokines (eotaxin, MCP-3), neuropeptides (VIP, substance P, calcitonin gene-related peptide), and lipid mediators (leukotriene B4, platelet-activating factor) [130]. Eosinophil adherence to parasympathetic nerves is mediated by nerve expression of cell adhesion molecules that results in eosinophil activation and degranulation. Less is known about the recruitment of dendritic cells to parasympathetic nerves, but a recent study suggests nerves might activate dendritic cells. In a mouse model of allergic asthma, dendritic cell-nerve co-localization was associated with sites of T cell proliferation [131].

In studies of gastrointestinal disease and atopic dermatitis, eosinophils and mast cells are found near nerves; likely sensory nerves based upon the location and neurotransmitter content of the nerves. In a mouse model of eosinophilic gastrointestinal disease, electron microscopy demonstrated that eosinophils resided next to damaged small unmyelinated nerve axons [132] while in the skin of patients with atopic dermatitis, eosinophils and mast cells are increased and are in close proximity to nerves containing sensory-enriched neuropeptides [133, 134].

Inflammatory cells all express muscarinic receptors though the function of these receptors is not well studied. Mast cells contain M_1 [18], macrophages contain M_3/M_5 [18, 19], alveolar macrophages contain $M_1/M_2/M_3$ [19, 128], neutrophils contain M_4/M_5 [18] and eosinophils contain $M_3/M_4/M_5$ [18, 19]. In addition to the neuronal sources of ACh, many non-neuronal cells are now known to make and release ACh including epithelial and endothelial cells. For a more complete review, refer to Wessler and Kirkpatrick [20]. It is important to note that in allergic disease or following treatment with muscarinic antagonists, inflammatory cells can change muscarinic receptor subtype expression on their cell surface. For example, peripheral blood lymphocytes isolated from patients with asthma or allergic rhinitis had increased M_2/M_5 receptor expression. In contrast, M_3 receptors are not changed except in patients with severe allergy or with severe asthma in which case M_3 muscarinic receptors on inflammatory cells are decreased [135, 136]. In patients treated with tiotropium for 12 weeks sputum cells had responded to the M_3 antagonist by internalizing their M_3 receptors [137]. These studies suggest the response of inflammatory cells to neuronal or non-neuronal ACh may change in allergy and following treatment.

In some cells muscarinic receptors induce migration of inflammatory cells. For example, ACh causes macrophages to release a substance that is pro-migratory for neutrophils, an effect which is inhibited by M_3 receptor antagonists (4-DAMP, tiotropium) but not M_2 antagonists [18, 128]. Stimulation of macrophage muscarinic receptors with carbachol also increased migration of macrophages [19]. In obstructive airway diseases, muscarinic antagonists decrease eosinophil influx [43] which could indicate that muscarinic signaling mediates eosinophil migration. In one of the original studies of intractable asthma, surgically severing the vagus nerves resulted in a significant reduction of eosinophils in sputum and blood [2]. Mast cell recruitment is also associated with parasympathetic signaling. Cutting the parasympathetic supply to the nose significantly reduced mast cell density in the respiratory mucosa [138].

Depending on the inflammatory cell type and experimental setup, muscarinic receptor signaling either stimulates or inhibits release of pro-inflammatory mediators. Exogenous ACh stimulates peripheral blood monocytes to secrete leukotriene B4, a proinflammatory lipid mediator [139]. In alveolar macrophages, release of TNF-alpha, a potent inflammatory cytokine, and release of reactive oxygen species are stimulated by muscarinic agonists (carbachol) and are inhibited by the M_3 antagonist, tiotropium [128]. In contrast, muscarinic receptor signaling in mast cells may inhibit release of pro-inflammatory mediators although there is disagreement between in vivo and in vitro studies. Histamine release in isolated human airways, presumably by mast cells, is inhibited by exogenous ACh, a muscarinic agonist (oxotremorine), and by an acetylcholinesterase inhibitor (physostigmine). A role for muscarinic receptors was demonstrated since atropine reversed the ACh-induced inhibition of mast cell histamine release [140]. In contrast, an in vivo study of nasal allergy showed parasympathetic signaling might promote mast cell histamine release. When cutting the vidian nerve supplying parasympathetic nerves to the nose in patients with rhinitis, both the density of mast cells and histamine concentration in the nose were significantly reduced [138].

Muscarinic receptor signaling, through a host of different pathways, releases pro-inflammatory mediators from resident non-neuronal (noninflammatory) cells. For example, muscarinic receptor activation increases release of kinins, a family of pro-inflammatory mediators. In both humans with allergic rhinitis and antigen-challenged guinea pigs, methacholine administration leads to production of kinins, increased cytokine levels, and eosinophil infiltration [141, 142]. Ipratropium bromide inhibits this effect suggesting that muscarinic signaling indirectly increases cytokine (e.g. kinin) production and eosinophil influx [142]. For a complete review of the role of muscarinic receptors in airway inflammation, see Gosens et al. [30].

Muscarinic receptor signaling also stimulates proliferation and apoptosis of different inflammatory cells which potentially changes the overall inflammatory response. In isolated T and B cells, exogenous ACh promotes survival and stimulates proliferation [30]. This stimulatory effect of ACh may be through M_3 receptors and act differently on unique T cell subtypes. For example, blocking M_3 receptors on isolated human peripheral blood T cells with tiotropium reduced apoptosis of CD4+ but increased apoptosis of CD8+ T cells [143].

Parasympathetic signaling through nicotinic receptors also produces anti-inflammatory effects in humans with allergy and animal models [144]. In a mouse model of allergic asthma, a nicotinic agonist (1,1-dimethyl-4-phenylpiperazinium, DMPP), reduced inflammation and bronchoconstriction caused by the muscarinic agonist, methacholine [145]. However, exogenous nicotine administered to a rat model of allergic asthma decreases eosinophil influx and cytokine production but nicotine did not affect goblet cell metaplasia [146]. Thus, nicotinic signaling appears to be specific for inflammation and not for tissue remodeling or for mucus production. Nicotinic signaling might directly inhibit the influx of specific inflammatory cells since the nicotinic agonist, DMPP, has been shown to dramatically reduce chemotaxis and inflammatory cytokine release in isolated human eosinophils [147].

Involvement of Parasympathetic Nerves in Tissue Remodeling

Parasympathetic and muscarinic signaling has also been linked to underlying tissue remodeling seen in chronic allergic diseases. In general, muscarinic signaling promotes both the proliferation of smooth muscle and promotes phenotypic differentiation of mesenchymal cells and fibroblasts into a contractile phenotype.

In antigen-challenged guinea pigs, repeated challenge with antigen increased airway smooth muscle mass and smooth muscle myosin heavy chain expression in the main bronchi and this was replicated, ex vivo, in isolated smooth muscle [148]. In this study, the proliferative effect of muscarinic signaling likely acts through M_3 muscarinic receptors since tiotropium prevented antigen-induced airway smooth muscle proliferation [148]. Muscarinic receptor signaling also potentiated smooth muscle remodeling in human and bovine airways, an effect inhibited only by M_3 muscarinic receptor antagonists. As described in the nose, the proliferative effect of M_3 receptor signaling on smooth muscle is thought to involve epidermal growth factor and platelet-derived growth factor [30].

Stimulation of muscarinic receptors also increases fibroblast/mesenchymal proliferation [30] and importantly muscarinic receptors mediate the change of these non-contractile cells to acquire a contractile phenotype [30]. Inhalation of methacholine in humans in vivo causes myofibroblast proliferation and migration into the submucosa that occurs over a period of 2 weeks [149]. The mechanism of phenotypic transitioning by muscarinic signaling was shown to involve M_3 muscarinic receptors and various intracellular signaling molecules. In human fibroblasts the muscarinic agonist, carbachol, activates intracellular ERK1/2 and RhoA-GTP and upregulates collagen type I and α-smooth muscle actin consistent with transitioning to a myofibroblast contractile phenotype. These phenotype transitions caused by carbachol were dose-dependently inhibited by the M_3 antagonist, aclidinium bromide [150].

Indirectly M2-induced muscle contraction can increase muscle proliferation and switch non-muscle cells to a contractile phenotype. For example, muscle strain increases expression of smooth muscle actin and myosin heavy chain [30]. Since muscle strain is mediated by muscarinic receptor activation, this presents a physical rather than biochemical mechanism to increase muscle mass and contraction. Since different GPCR agonists, for example cys-leukotrienes, also increase airway muscle remodeling, an effect that is prevented by a leukotriene antagonist, suggests that remodeling is a function of contraction and not activation of one specific GPCR [30].

Caveolin 3, a component of endocytosis, also represents an untested link between M_2 receptor signaling and muscle proliferation [151]. Cav3 knock-out mice show increased cardiac hypertrophy suggesting that caveolin 3 somehow prevents muscle proliferation [151] although this has not been tested in smooth muscle. Inhibition of caveolin 3 with methyl-beta-cyclodextrin inhibits M_2-mediated muscle contraction which could subsequently prevent contraction-induced muscle proliferation [152].

Muscarinic receptor signaling may also contribute to the barrier dysfunction of skin cells in atopic dermatitis by inducing early-in-life remodeling. Binding experiments and cAMP accumulation assays have shown muscarinic receptors are functional only in fetal skin fibroblasts and not adult fibroblasts [153]. Recent studies demonstrated that pilocarpine stimulates apoptosis in cultured neonatal skin fibroblasts through M_1 and M_3 muscarinic receptors [68].

Concluding Remarks

Parasympathetic nerves supply every major organ system associated with allergy and inflammation including muscle, glands and inflammatory cells. Thus, they are capable of inducing and modulating smooth muscle dysfunction or increased contraction, and increased mucus secretion. Importantly, the influence of the parasympathetic nerves extends to inflammatory cells which all express muscarinic receptors. Thus, parasympathetic nerves may modulate inflammation. Indeed, sectioning parasympathetic nerves decreases inflammation in the lungs and nose of asthmatic and allergic rhinitis patients respectively. Furthermore, parasympathetic nerves may also contribute to smooth muscle remodeling. New therapies that target muscarinic receptors are in development for the treatment of COPD and asthma and they may also show promise in the treatment of allergic disease.

References

1 Kubo N, Minami T, Hori Y, Yamashita T, Kumazawa T: Enhanced parasympathetic nerve activities in experimentally-induced nasal hypersensitivity. Acta Otolaryngol Suppl 1989;463:14–20.

2 Balogh G, Dimitrov-Szokodi D, Husveti A: Lung denervation in the therapy of intractable bronchial asthma. J Thorac Surg 1957;33:166–184.

3 Johansson SG, Bieber T, Dahl R, Friedmann PS, Lanier BQ, Lockey RF, Motala C, Ortega Martell JA, Platts-Mills TA, Ring J, Thien F, Van Cauwenberge P, Williams HC. Revised nomenclature for allergy for global use: report of the Nomenclature Review Committee of the World Allergy Organization, October 2003. J Allergy Clin Immunol 2004;113: 832–836.

4 Bieber T, Leung D, Ivancevich JC, Gamal YE: Atopic eczema and contact dermatitis; in Pawankar R, et al (eds): World Allergy Organization (WAO) White Book on Allergy. London, World Allergy Organization, 2011.

5 Woods RK, Thien F, Raven J, Walters EH, Abramson M: Prevalence of food allergies in young adults and their relationship to asthma, nasal allergies, and eczema. Ann Allergy Asthma Immunol 2002;88: 183–189.

6 Sahin-Yilmaz A, Nocon CC, Corey JP: Immunoglobulin E-mediated food allergies among adults with allergic rhinitis. Otolaryngol Head Neck Surg 2010;143:379–385.

7 Worth A, Sheikh A: Food allergy and atopic eczema. Curr Opin Allergy Clin Immunol 2010;10:226–230.

8 Spergel JM: From atopic dermatitis to asthma: the atopic march. Ann Allergy Asthma Immunol 2010; 105:99–106, quiz 107–109, 117.

9 Ellman LK, Chatchatee P, Sicherer SH, Sampson HA: Food hypersensitivity in two groups of children and young adults with atopic dermatitis evaluated a decade apart. Pediatr Allergy Immunol 2002;13: 295–298.

10 Pawankar R, Sanchez-Borges M, Bonini S, Kaliner MA: Rhinitis, conjunctivitis, and rhinosinusitis; in Pawankar R, et al (eds): World Allergy Organization (WAO) White Book on Allergy. London, World Allergy Organization, 2011.

11 Holgate ST, Canonica GW, Baena Cagnani CE, Casale T, Zitt M, Nelson H, Vichyanond P: Asthma; in Pawankar R, et al (eds): World Allergy Organization (WAO) White Book on Allergy. London, World Allergy Organization, 2011.

12 Fiocchi A, Sampson HA, Bahna SL, Lack G: Food allergy; in Pawankar R, et al (eds): World Allergy Organization (WAO) White Book on Allergy. London, World Allergy Organization, 2011.

13 Tobin MC, Moparty B, Farhadi A, DeMeo MT, Bansal PJ, Keshavarzian A: Atopic irritable bowel syndrome: a novel subgroup of irritable bowel syndrome with allergic manifestations. Ann Allergy Asthma Immunol 2008;100:49–53.

14 Soares R, Figueiredo HN, Filho PFM, Oliveira RF, Goncalves CD, Micuci AJQ, Parada BA, Bromonschenkel I, Rodrigues CC: The prevalence and clinical characteristics of atopic manifestations in patients with irritable bowel syndrome in a Brazilian urban community. Gastroenterology Insights 2010;2:41–43.

15 Kubo M, Fujiwara Y, Shiba M, Kohata Y, Yamagami H, Tanigawa T, Watanabe K, Watanabe T, Tominaga K, Arakawa T: Differences between risk factors among irritable bowel syndrome subtypes in Japanese adults. Neurogastroenterol Motil 2011;23: 249–254.
16 Dale HH: The action of certain esters and ethers of choline, and their relation to muscarine. J Pharmacol Exp Ther 1914;6:147–190.
17 Rosenberry TL: Acetylcholinesterase. Adv Enzymol Relat Areas Mol Biol 1975;43:103–218.
18 Moulton BC, Fryer AD: Muscarinic receptor antagonists, from folklore to pharmacology: finding drugs that actually work in asthma and COPD. Br J Pharmacol 2011;163:44–52.
19 Kolahian S, Gosens R: Cholinergic regulation of airway inflammation and remodelling: the role of the airway smooth msucle. J Allergy 2012;2012:1–9.
20 Wessler I, Kirkpatrick CJ: Acetylcholine beyond neurons: the non-neuronal cholinergic system in humans. Br J Pharmacol 2008;154:1558–1571.
21 Caulfield MP, Birdsall NJ: International Union of Pharmacology. XVII. Classification of muscarinic acetylcholine receptors. Pharmacol Rev 1998;50: 279–290.
22 Nadel JA, Barnes PJ: Autonomic regulation of the airways. Annu Rev Med 1984;35:451–467.
23 Mak JC, Barnes PJ: Autoradiographic visualization of muscarinic receptor subtypes in human and guinea pig lung. Am Rev Respir Dis 1990;141: 1559–1568.
24 O'Connor BJ, Towse LJ, Barnes PJ: Prolonged effect of tiotropium bromide on methacholine-induced bronchoconstriction in asthma. Am J Respir Crit Care Med 1996;154(4 Pt 1):876–880.
25 Klein MK, Haberberger RV, Hartmann P, Faulhammer P, Lips KS, Krain B, Wess J, Kummer W, Konig P: Muscarinic receptor subtypes in cilia-driven transport and airway epithelial development. Eur Respir J 2009;33:1113–1121.
26 White MV: Muscarinic receptors in human airways. J Allergy Clin Immunol 1995;95:1065–1068.
27 Fryer AD, Maclagan J: Muscarinic inhibitory receptors in pulmonary parasympathetic nerves in the guinea-pig. Br J Pharmacol 1984;83:973–978.
28 Fryer AD, Jacoby DB: Muscarinic receptors and control of airway smooth muscle. Am J Respir Crit Care Med 1998;158:S154–S160.
29 Minette PA, Barnes PJ: Prejunctional inhibitory muscarinic receptors on cholinergic nerves in human and guinea pig airways. J Appl Physiol 1988; 64:2532–2537.
30 Gosens R, Zaagsma J, Meurs H, Halayko AJ: Muscarinic receptor signaling in the pathophysiology of asthma and COPD. Respir Res 2006;7:73.
31 Liu YC, Patel HJ, Khawaja AM, Belvisi MG, Rogers DF: Neuroregulation by vasoactive intestinal peptide (VIP) of mucus secretion in ferret trachea: activation of BK(Ca) channels and inhibition of neurotransmitter release. Br J Pharmacol 1999;126: 147–158.
32 Belvisi MG, Stretton CD, Yacoub M, Barnes PJ: Nitric oxide is the endogenous neurotransmitter of bronchodilator nerves in humans. Eur J Pharmacol 1992;210:221–222.
33 Szema AM, Hamidi SA, Lyubsky S, Dickman KG, Mathew S, Abdel-Razek T, Chen JJ, Waschek JA, Said SI: Mice lacking the VIP gene show airway hyperresponsiveness and airway inflammation, partially reversible by VIP. Am J Physiol Lung Cell Mol Physiol 2006;291:L880–L886.
34 Widdicombe JH: Neuroanatomy of the airways; in Pawankar R, Holgate ST, Rosenwasser LJ (eds): Allergy Frontiers: Classification and Pathomechanisms, 2009, Springer, Tokyo, pp 459–468.
35 Whicker SD, Armour CL, Black JL: Responsiveness of bronchial smooth muscle from asthmatic patients to relaxant and contractile agonists. Pulm Pharmacol 1988;1:25–31.
36 Goldie RG, Spina D, Henry PJ, Lulich KM, Paterson JW: In vitro responsiveness of human asthmatic bronchus to carbachol, histamine, beta-adrenoceptor agonists and theophylline. Br J Clin Pharmacol 1986;22:669–676.
37 de Jongste JC, Mons H, Bonta IL, Kerrebijn KF: In vitro responses of airways from an asthmatic patient. Eur J Respir Dis 1987;71:23–29.
38 Bai TR: Abnormalities in airway smooth muscle in fatal asthma. A comparison between trachea and bronchus. Am Rev Respir Dis 1991;143:441–443.
39 Bjorck T, Gustafsson LE, Dahlen SE: Isolated bronchi from asthmatics are hyperresponsive to adenosine, which apparently acts indirectly by liberation of leukotrienes and histamine. Am Rev Respir Dis 1992;145:1087–1091.
40 Chiba Y, Misawa M: Characteristics of muscarinic cholinoceptors in airways of antigen-induced airway hyperresponsive rats. Comp Biochem Physiol C Pharmacol Toxicol Endocrinol 1995;111:351–357.
41 Mitchell RW, Kelly E, Leff AR: Reduced activity of acetylcholinesterase in canine tracheal smooth muscle homogenates after active immune-sensitization. Am J Respir Cell Mol Biol 1991;5:56–62.
42 Tao FC, Tolloczko B, Eidelman DH, Martin JG: Enhanced Ca(2+) mobilization in airway smooth muscle contributes to airway hyperresponsiveness in an inbred strain of rat. Am J Respir Crit Care Med 1999;160:446–453.

43 Damera G, Jiang M, Zhao H, Fogle HW, Jester WF, Freire J, Panettieri RA Jr: Aclidinium bromide abrogates allergen-induced hyperresponsiveness and reduces eosinophilia in murine model of airway inflammation. Eur J Pharmacol 2010;649:349–353.

44 Jiang JX, Cao R, Deng WD, Jin F, Dong XW, Zhu Y, Chen XP, Xie YC, Bao MJ, Li FF, Xie QM: Characterization of bencycloquidium bromide, a novel muscarinic M(3) receptor antagonist in guinea pig airways. Eur J Pharmacol 2011;655: 74–82.

45 Cao R, Dong XW, Jiang JX, Yan XF, He JS, Deng YM, Li FF, Bao MJ, Xie YC, Chen XP, Xie QM: M(3) muscarinic receptor antagonist bencycloquidium bromide attenuates allergic airway inflammation, hyperresponsiveness and remodeling in mice. Eur J Pharmacol 2011;655:83–90.

46 Kanazawa H, Hirata K, Yoshikawa J: Increased responses to inhaled oxitropium bromide in asthmatic patients with active hepatitis C virus infection. Chest 2004;125:1368–1371.

47 Empey DW, Laitinen LA, Jacobs L, Gold WM, Nadel JA: Mechanisms of bronchial hyperreactivity in normal subjects after upper respiratory tract infection. Am Rev Respir Dis 1976;113:131–139.

48 Nie Z, Scott GD, Weis PD, Itakura A, Fryer AD, Jacoby DB: Role of TNF-alpha in virus-induced airway hyperresponsiveness and neuronal M muscarinic receptor dysfunction. Br J Pharmacol 2011;164: 444–452.

49 Lee AM, Fryer AD, van Rooijen N, Jacoby DB: Role of macrophages in virus-induced airway hyperresponsiveness and neuronal M2 muscarinic receptor dysfunction. Am J Physiol Lung Cell Mol Physiol 2004;286:L1255–L1259.

50 Yost BL, Gleich GJ, Fryer AD: Ozone-induced hyperresponsiveness and blockade of M2 muscarinic receptors by eosinophil major basic protein. J Appl Physiol 1999;87:1272–1278.

51 Jacoby DB, Gleich GJ, Fryer AD: Human eosinophil major basic protein is an endogenous allosteric antagonist at the inhibitory muscarinic M2 receptor. J Clin Invest 1993;91:1314–1318.

52 Costello RW, Schofield BH, Kephart GM, Gleich GJ, Jacoby DB, Fryer AD: Localization of eosinophils to airway nerves and effect on neuronal M2 muscarinic receptor function. Am J Physiol 1997;273: L93–L103.

53 Evans CM, Fryer AD, Jacoby DB, Gleich GJ, Costello RW: Pretreatment with antibody to eosinophil major basic protein prevents hyperresponsiveness by protecting neuronal M2 muscarinic receptors in antigen-challenged guinea pigs. J Clin Invest 1997; 100:2254–2262.

54 Fryer AD, Stein LH, Nie Z, Curtis DE, Evans CM, Hodgson ST, Jose PJ, Belmonte KE, Fitch E, Jacoby DB: Neuronal eotaxin and the effects of CCR3 antagonist on airway hyperreactivity and M2 receptor dysfunction. J Clin Invest 2006;116:228–236.

55 Nair P, Pizzichini MM, Kjarsgaard M, Inman MD, Efthimiadis A, Pizzichini E, Hargreave FE, O'Byrne PM: Mepolizumab for prednisone-dependent asthma with sputum eosinophilia. N Engl J Med 2009;360:985–993.

56 Haldar P, Brightling CE, Hargadon B, Gupta S, Monteiro W, Sousa A, Marshall RP, Bradding P, Green RH, Wardlaw AJ, Pavord ID: Mepolizumab and exacerbations of refractory eosinophilic asthma. N Engl J Med 2009;360:973–984.

57 Fryer AD, el-Fakahany EE, Jacoby DB: Parainfluenza virus type 1 reduces the affinity of agonists for muscarinic receptors in guinea-pig lung and heart. Eur J Pharmacol 1990;181:51–58.

58 Jacoby DB, Xiao HQ, Lee NH, Chan-Li Y, Fryer AD: Virus- and interferon-induced loss of inhibitory M2 muscarinic receptor function and gene expression in cultured airway parasympathetic neurons. J Clin Invest 1998;102:242–248.

59 Peters SP: Heterogeneity in the pathology and treatment of asthma. Am J Med 2003;115(suppl 3A): 49S–54S.

60 Allen IC, Hartney JM, Coffman TM, Penn RB, Wess J, Koller BH: Thromboxane A2 induces airway constriction through an M3 muscarinic acetylcholine receptor-dependent mechanism. Am J Physiol Lung Cell Mol Physiol 2006;290:L526–L533.

61 Cortijo J, Mata M, Milara J, Donet E, Gavalda A, Miralpeix M, Morcillo EJ: Aclidinium inhibits cholinergic and tobacco smoke-induced MUC5AC in human airways. Eur Respir J 2011;37:244–254.

62 Bateman ED, Rennard S, Barnes PJ, Dicpinigaitis PV, Gosens R, Gross NJ, Nadel JA, Pfeifer M, Racke K, Rabe KF, Rubin BK, Welte T, Wessler I: Alternative mechanisms for tiotropium. Pulm Pharmacol Ther 2009;22:533–542.

63 Hasani A, Toms N, Agnew JE, Sarno M, Harrison AJ, Dilworth P: The effect of inhaled tiotropium bromide on lung mucociliary clearance in patients with COPD. Chest 2004;125:1726–1734.

64 Bos IS, Gosens R, Zuidhof AB, Schaafsma D, Halayko AJ, Meurs H, Zaagsma J: Inhibition of allergen-induced airway remodelling by tiotropium and budesonide: a comparison. Eur Respir J 2007; 30:653–661.

65 Peters SP, Kunselman SJ, Icitovic N, et al: Tiotropium bromide step-up therapy for adults with uncontrolled asthma. N Engl J Med 2010;363:1715–1726.

66 Expert Panel Report 3 (EPR-3): Guidelines for the Diagnosis and Management of Asthma – Summary Report 2007. J Allergy Clin Immunol 2007; 120(5 suppl):S94–S138.
67 Sheppard D, Epstein J, Holtzman MJ, Nadel JA, Boushey HA: Dose-dependent inhibition of cold air-induced bronchoconstriction by atropine. J Appl Physiol 1982;53:169–174.
68 Anthonisen NR, Connett JE, Kiley JP, et al: Effects of smoking intervention and the use of an inhaled anticholinergic bronchodilator on the rate of decline of FEV1. The Lung Health Study. JAMA 1994;272: 1497–1505.
69 Holtzman MJ, McNamara MP, Sheppard D, Fabbri LM, Hahn HL, Graf PD, Nadel JA: Intravenous versus inhaled atropine for inhibiting bronchoconstrictor responses in dogs. J Appl Physiol 1983;54: 134–139.
70 Rodrigo GJ, Rodrigo C: First-line therapy for adult patients with acute asthma receiving a multiple-dose protocol of ipratropium bromide plus albuterol in the emergency department. Am J Respir Crit Care Med 2000;161:1862–1868.
71 Gavalda A, Miralpeix M, Ramos I, Otal R, Carreno C, Vinals M, Domenech T, Carcasona C, Reyes B, Vilella D, Gras J, Cortijo J, Morcillo E, Llenas J, Ryder H, Beleta J: Characterization of aclidinium bromide, a novel inhaled muscarinic antagonist, with long duration of action and a favorable pharmacological profile. J Pharmacol Exp Ther 2009;331: 740–751.
72 Jones PW, Agusti A, Bateman ED, Singh D, Lamarca R, de Miquel G, Garcia Gil E: Aclinidium bromide in patients with chronic obstructive pulmonary disease: efficacy and safety results from Attain; in: America Thoracic Society Thematic Poster Session: A45 Bronchodilators for COPD: Old Faithfuls and Novel Compounds. Colorado Convention Center, Denver, 2011.
73 Kaliner MA: The physiology and pathophysiology of the parasympathetic nervous system in nasal disease: an overview. J Allergy Clin Immunol 1992; 90(6 Pt 2):1044–1045.
74 Baraniuk JN: Sensory, parasympathetic, and sympathetic neural influences in the nasal mucosa. J Allergy Clin Immunol 1992;90:1045–1050.
75 Sheahan P, Thornton M, Walsh RM, Walsh MA, Costello RW: Role of the muscarinic M2 receptor in human nasal mucosa. Rhinology 2007;45:229–234.
76 Sheahan P, Walsh RM, Walsh MA, Costello RW: Induction of nasal hyper-responsiveness by allergen challenge in allergic rhinitis: the role of afferent and efferent nerves. Clin Exp Allergy 2005;35:45–51.
77 van Megen YJ, Rodrigues de Miranda JF, Klaassen AB: Alterations of neuroreceptors in nasal hyperreactivity. Br J Clin Pharmacol 1990; 30(suppl 1): 162S–164S.
78 Ishibe T, Yamashita T, Kumazawa T, Tanaka C: Adrenergic and cholinergic receptors in human nasal mucosa in cases of nasal allergy. Arch Otorhinolaryngol 1983;238:167–173.
79 Burgel PR, Nadel JA: Roles of epidermal growth factor receptor activation in epithelial cell repair and mucin production in airway epithelium. Thorax 2004;59:992–996.
80 Becker B, Borum S, Nielsen K, Mygind N, Borum P: A time-dose study of the effect of topical ipratropium bromide on methacholine-induced rhinorrhoea in patients with perennial non-allergic rhinitis. Clin Otolaryngol Allied Sci 1997;22:132–134.
81 Finn AF Jr, Aaronson D, Korenblat P, Lumry W, Settipane G, Spector S, Woehler T, Drda K, Wood CC: Ipratropium bromide nasal spray 0.03% provides additional relief from rhinorrhea when combined with terfenadine in perennial rhinitis patients; a randomized, double-blind, active-controlled trial. Am J Rhinol 1998;12:441–449.
82 Georgitis JW: The anticholinergic treatment of allergic perennial rhinitis. J Allergy Clin Immunol 1992;90(6 Pt 2):1071–1076.
83 Chaen T, Watanabe N, Mogi G, Mori K, Takeyama M: Substance P and vasoactive intestinal peptide in nasal secretions and plasma from patients with nasal allergy. Ann Otol Rhinol Laryngol 1993; 102:16–21.
84 Fischer A, Wussow A, Cryer A, Schmeck B, Noga O, Zweng M, Peiser C, Dinh QT, Heppt W, Groneberg DA: Neuronal plasticity in persistent perennial allergic rhinitis. J Occup Environ Med 2005;47:20–25.
85 Birchall MA, Henderson JC, Pride NB, Fuller RW: A comparison of the effects of an alpha-agonist, an anti-muscarinic agent and placebo on intranasal histamine challenge in allergic rhinitis. Clin Otolaryngol Allied Sci 1996;21:212–217.
86 Rios JD, Forde K, Diebold Y, Lightman J, Zieske JD, Dartt DA: Development of conjunctival goblet cells and their neuroreceptor subtype expression. Invest Ophthalmol Vis Sci 2000;41:2127–2137.
87 Rios JD, Zoukhri D, Rawe IM, Hodges RR, Zieske JD, Dartt DA: Immunolocalization of muscarinic and VIP receptor subtypes and their role in stimulating goblet cell secretion. Invest Ophthalmol Vis Sci 1999;40:1102–1111.
88 Dartt DA, McCarthy DM, Mercer HJ, Kessler TL, Chung EH, Zieske JD: Localization of nerves adjacent to goblet cells in rat conjunctiva. Curr Eye Res 1995;14:993–1000.

89 Cavallotti C, Frati A, Sagnelli P, Pescosolido N: Re-evaluation and quantification of the different sources of nerve fibres supplying the rat eye. J Anat 2005;206:217–224.

90 Nakamura M, Tada Y, Akaishi T, Nakata K: M3 muscarinic receptor mediates regulation of protein secretion in rabbit lacrimal gland. Curr Eye Res 1997;16:614–619.

91 Howell G 3rd, West L, Jenkins C, Lineberry B, Yokum D, Rockhold R: In vivo antimuscarinic actions of the third generation antihistaminergic agent, desloratadine. BMC Pharmacol 2005;5:13.

92 Poyer JF, Gabelt BT, Kaufman PL: The effect of muscarinic agonists and selective receptor subtype antagonists on the contractile response of the isolated rhesus monkey ciliary muscle. Exp Eye Res 1994;59:729–736.

93 Gabelt BT, Kaufman PL: Inhibition of aceclidine-stimulated outflow facility, accommodation and miosis in rhesus monkeys by muscarinic receptor subtype antagonists. Exp Eye Res 1994;58:623–630.

94 Elsas T, Edvinsson L, Sundler F, Uddman R: Neuronal pathways to the rat conjunctiva revealed by retrograde tracing and immunocytochemistry. Exp Eye Res 1994;58:117–126.

95 Kuchiiwa S: Intraocular projections from the pterygopalatine ganglion in the cat. J Comp Neurol 1990;300:301–308.

96 Yamamoto R, Bredt DS, Snyder SH, Stone RA: The localization of nitric oxide synthase in the rat eye and related cranial ganglia. Neuroscience 1993;54:189–200.

97 Motterle L, Diebold Y, Enríquez de Salamanca A, Saez V, Garcia-Vazquez C, Stern ME, Calonge M, Leonardi A: Altered expression of neurotransmitter receptors and neuromediators in vernal keratoconjunctivitis. Arch Ophthalmol 2006;124:462–468.

98 Sacchetti M, Micera A, Lambiase A, Speranza S, Mantelli F, Petrachi G, Bonini S: Tear levels of neuropeptides increase after specific allergen challenge in allergic conjunctivitis. Mol Vis 2011;17:47–52.

99 Richard S: Epidural Anesthesia and Gastrointestinal Motility. Anesth Analg 1998;86:837–844.

100 Blanquet F, Gonella J: Role of M1 muscarinic receptors in the parasympathetic control of colonic motility in cats and rabbits. J Physiol 1992;458:655–666.

101 Sevcencu C: Gastrointestinal mechanisms activated by electrical stimulation to treat motility dysfunctions in the digestive tract: a review. Neuromodulation 2007;10:100–112.

102 Blanquet F, Abysique A, Gonella J: In vivo study of the role of muscarinic receptors in the parasympathetic control of rabbit colonic motility. J Auton Nerv Syst 1994;46:217–227.

103 Takeuchi T, Tanaka K, Nakajima H, Matsui M, Azuma YT: M2 and M3 muscarinic receptors are involved in enteric nerve-mediated contraction of the mouse ileum: findings obtained with muscarinic-receptor knockout mouse. Am J Physiol Gastrointest Liver Physiol 2007;292:G154–G164.

104 Saavedra Y, Vergara P: Hypersensitivity to ovalbumin induces chronic intestinal dysmotility and increases the number of intestinal mast cells. Neurogastroenterol Motil 2005;17:112–122.

105 Arslan G, Gilja OH, Lind R, Florvaag E, Berstad A: Response to intestinal provocation monitored by transabdominal ultrasound in patients with food hypersensitivity. Scand J Gastroenterol 2005;40:386–394.

106 Valeur J, Lappalainen J, Rita H, Lin AH, Kovanen PT, Berstad A, Eklund KK, Vaali K: Food allergy alters jejunal circular muscle contractility and induces local inflammatory cytokine expression in a mouse model. BMC Gastroenterol 2009;9:33.

107 Martinolle JP, Garcia-Villar R, Fioramonti J, Bueno L: Altered contractility of circular and longitudinal muscle in TNBS-inflamed guinea pig ileum. Am J Physiol 1997;272(5 Pt 1):G1258–G1267.

108 Vermillion DL, Collins SM: Increased responsiveness of jejunal longitudinal muscle in *Trichinella*-infected rats. Am J Physiol 1988;254:G124–G129.

109 Frisby CL, Fraser RJ, Schirmer MB, Yeoh EK, Blackshaw LA: Roles of muscarinic receptor subtypes in small intestinal motor dysfunction in acute radiation enteritis. Am J Physiol Gastrointest Liver Physiol 2007;293:G121–G127.

110 Akiho H, Khan WI, Al-Kaabi A, Blennerhassett P, Deng Y, Collins SM: Cytokine modulation of muscarinic receptors in the murine intestine. Am J Physiol Gastrointest Liver Physiol 2007;293:G250–G255.

111 Murch S: Allergy and intestinal dysmotility – evidence of genuine causal linkage? Curr Opin Gastroenterol 2006;22:664–668.

112 Attwood SE: Eosinophils and gut dysmotility. Eur J Gastroenterol Hepatol 2005;17:891–892.

113 Zuo L, Rothenberg ME: Gastrointestinal eosinophilia. Immunol Allergy Clin North Am 2007;27:443–455.

114 Eglen RM: Muscarinic receptor subtypes in neuronal and non-neuronal cholinergic function. Auton Autacoid Pharmacol 2006;26:219–233.

115 Reina S, Sterin-Borda L, Passafaro D, Borda E: Muscarinic cholinoceptor activation by pilocarpine triggers apoptosis in human skin fibroblast cells. J Cell Physiol 2011;222:640–647.

116 Izumi H, Ishii H, Niioka T: Parasympathetic vasodilator fibers in the orofacial region. J Oral Biosci 2006;48:30–41.

117 Izumi H: Reflex parasympathetic vasodilatation in facial skin. Gen Pharmacol 1995;26:237–244.
118 Watanabe H, Ishii H, Niioka T, Yamamuro M, Izumi H: Occurrence of parasympathetic vasodilator fibers in the lower lip of the guinea-pig. J Comp Physiol B 2008;178:297–305.
119 Kaji A, Shigematsu H, Fujita K, Maeda T, Watanabe S: Parasympathetic innervation of cutaneous blood vessels by vasoactive intestinal polypeptide-immunoreactive and acetylcholinesterase-positive nerves: histochemical and experimental study on rat lower lip. Neuroscience 1988;25:353–362.
120 Ramien M, Ruocco I, Cuello AC, St-Louis M, Ribeiro-Da-Silva A: Parasympathetic nerve fibers invade the upper dermis following sensory denervation of the rat lower lip skin. J Comp Neurol 2004;469:83–95.
121 Taylor AM, Ribeiro-da-Silva A: GDNF levels in the lower lip skin in a rat model of trigeminal neuropathic pain: implications for nonpeptidergic fiber reinnervation and parasympathetic sprouting. Pain 2010;152:1502–1510.
122 Fantini F, Pincelli C, Romualdi P, Donatini A, Giannetti A: Substance P levels are decreased in lesional skin of atopic dermatitis. Exp Dermatol 1992;1:127–128.
123 Pincelli C, Fantini F, Romualdi P, Lesa G, Giannetti A: Skin levels of vasoactive intestinal polypeptide in atopic dermatitis. Arch Dermatol Res 1991;283: 230–232.
124 Ostlere LS, Cowen T, Rustin MH: Neuropeptides in the skin of patients with atopic dermatitis. Clin Exp Dermatol 1995;20:462–467.
125 Pincelli C, Fantini F, Massimi P, Girolomoni G, Seidenari S, Giannetti A: Neuropeptides in skin from patients with atopic dermatitis: an immunohistochemical study. Br J Dermatol 1990;122:745–750.
126 Miyamoto T, Nojima H, Kuraishi Y: Intradermal cholinergic agonists induce itch-associated response via M3 muscarinic acetylcholine receptors in mice. Jpn J Pharmacol 2002;88:351–354.
127 Wessler I, Reinheimer T, Kilbinger H, Bittinger F, Kirkpatrick CJ, Saloga J, Knop J: Increased acetylcholine levels in skin biopsies of patients with atopic dermatitis. Life Sci 2003;72:2169–2172.
128 Vacca G, Randerath WJ, Gillissen A: Inhibition of granulocyte migration by tiotropium bromide. Respir Res 2010;12:24.
129 Veres TZ, Rochlitzer S, Shevchenko M, Fuchs B, Prenzler F, Nassenstein C, Fischer A, Welker L, Holz O, Muller M, Krug N, Braun A: Spatial interactions between dendritic cells and sensory nerves in allergic airway inflammation. Am J Respir Cell Mol Biol 2007;37:553–561.
130 Scott GD, Fryer AD: Eosinophil and nerve interactions; in Lee JJ, Rosenberg HF (eds): Eosinophils in Health and Disease. New York, International Eosinophil Society: Elsevier, 2011.
131 Veres TZ, Shevchenko M, Krasteva G, Spies E, Prenzler F, Rochlitzer S, Tschernig T, Krug N, Kummer W, Braun A: Dendritic cell-nerve clusters are sites of T cell proliferation in allergic airway inflammation. Am J Pathol 2009;174:808–817.
132 Hogan SP, Mishra A, Brandt EB, Royalty MP, Pope SM, Zimmermann N, Foster PS, Rothenberg ME: A pathological function for eotaxin and eosinophils in eosinophilic gastrointestinal inflammation. Nat Immunol 2001;2:353–360.
133 Theoharides TC, Donelan JM, Papadopoulou N, Cao J, Kempuraj D, Conti P: Mast cells as targets of corticotropin-releasing factor and related peptides. Trends Pharmacol Sci 2004;25:563–568.
134 Foster EL, Simpson EL, Fredrikson LJ, Lee JJ, Lee NA, Fryer AD, Jacoby DB: Eosinophils increase neuron branching in human and murine skin and in vitro. PLoS One 2011;6:e22029.
135 Ricci A, Amenta F, Bronzetti E, Mannino F, Mariotta S, Tayebati SK: Expression of peripheral blood lymphocyte muscarinic cholinergic receptor subtypes in airway hyperresponsiveness. J Neuroimmunol 2002;129:178–185.
136 Ricci A, Mariotta S, Amenta F, Tayebati SK, Terzano C: Changes in muscarinic cholinergic receptor expression in human peripheral blood lymphocytes in allergic rhinitis patients. Pulm Pharmacol Ther 2008;21:79–87.
137 Holownia A, Mroz RM, Skopinski T, Kielek A, Kolodziejczyk A, Chyczewska E, Braszko JJ: Tiotropium increases cytosolic muscarinic M3 receptors and acetylated H3 histone proteins in induced sputum cells of COPD patients. Eur J Med Res 2010;15(suppl 2):64–67.
138 Rucci L, Masini E, Arbi Riccardi R, Giannella E, Fioretti C, Mannaioni PF, Borghi Cirri MB, Fini Storchi O: Vidian nerve resection, histamine turnover and mucosal mast cell function in patients with chronic hypertrophic non-allergic rhinitis. Agents Actions 1989;28:224–230.
139 Profita M, Giorgi RD, Sala A, Bonanno A, Riccobono L, Mirabella F, Gjomarkaj M, Bonsignore G, Bousquet J, Vignola AM: Muscarinic receptors, leukotriene B4 production and neutrophilic inflammation in COPD patients. Allergy 2005;60:1361–1369.
140 Reinheimer T, Baumgartner D, Hohle KD, Racke K, Wessler I: Acetylcholine via muscarinic receptors inhibits histamine release from human isolated bronchi. Am J Respir Crit Care Med 1997;156: 389–395.

141 Turner PJ, Dear JW, Foreman JC: Involvement of kinins in hyperresponsiveness induced by platelet activating factor in the human nasal airway. Br J Pharmacol 2000;129:525–532.

142 Sugahara S, Nabe T, Mizutani N, Takenaka H, Kohno S: Kinins are involved in the development of allergic nasal hyperresponsiveness in guinea pigs. Eur J Pharmacol 2003;476:229–237.

143 Profita M, Riccobono L, Montalbano AM, Bonanno A, Ferraro M, Albano GD, Gerbino S, Casarosa P, Pieper MP, Gjomarkaj M: In vitro anticholinergic drugs affect CD8+ peripheral blood T-cells apoptosis in COPD. Immunobiology 2011 Aug 3 [Epub ahead of print].

144 Pavlov VA, Parrish WR, Rosas-Ballina M, Ochani M, Puerta M, Ochani K, Chavan S, Al-Abed Y, Tracey KJ: Brain acetylcholinesterase activity controls systemic cytokine levels through the cholinergic anti-inflammatory pathway. Brain Behav Immun 2009;23:41–45.

145 Blanchet MR, Israel-Assayag E, Cormier Y: Modulation of airway inflammation and resistance in mice by a nicotinic receptor agonist. Eur Respir J 2005;26:21–27.

146 Mishra NC, Rir-Sima-Ah J, Langley RJ, Singh SP, Pena-Philippides JC, Koga T, Razani-Boroujerdi S, Hutt J, Campen M, Kim KC, Tesfaigzi Y, Sopori ML: Nicotine primarily suppresses lung Th2 but not goblet cell and muscle cell responses to allergens. J Immunol 2008;180:7655–7663.

147 Blanchet MR, Langlois A, Israel-Assayag E, Beaulieu MJ, Ferland C, Laviolette M, Cormier Y: Modulation of eosinophil activation in vitro by a nicotinic receptor agonist. J Leukoc Biol 2007;81:1245–1251.

148 Gosens R, Bos IS, Zaagsma J, Meurs H: Protective effects of tiotropium bromide in the progression of airway smooth muscle remodeling. Am J Respir Crit Care Med 2005;171:1096–1102.

149 Kelly MM, O'Connor TM, Leigh R, Otis J, Gwozd C, Gauvreau GM, Gauldie J, O'Byrne PM: Effects of budes onide and formoterol on allergen-induced airway responses, inflammation, and airway remodeling in asthma. J Allergy Clin Immunol 2011;125: 349–356 e13.

150 Milara J, Serrano A, Peiro T, Gavalda A, Miralpeix M, Morcillo EJ, Cortijo J: Aclidinium inhibits human lung fibroblast to myofibroblast transition. Thorax 2011 Sep 28 [Epub ahead of print].

151 Gazzerro E, Sotgia F, Bruno C, Lisanti MP, Minetti C: Caveolinopathies: from the biology of caveolin-3 to human diseases. Eur J Hum Genet 2010;18: 137–145.

152 Schlenz H, Kummer W, Jositsch G, Wess J, Krasteva G: Muscarinic receptor-mediated bronchoconstriction is coupled to caveolae in murine airways. Am J Physiol Lung Cell Mol Physiol 2011;298: L626–L636.

153 Van Riper DA, Absher MP, Lenox RH: Muscarinic receptors on intact human fibroblasts. Absence of receptor activity in adult skin cells. J Clin Invest 1985;76:882–886.

Dr. Allison D. Fryer
Department of Pulmonary and Critical Care Medicine, Oregon Health and Science University
3181 SW Sam Jackson Park Rd., L334
Portland, OR 97239 (USA)
Tel. +1 503 494 2345, E-Mail fryera@ohsu.edu

Bienenstock J (ed): Allergy and the Nervous System.
Chem Immunol Allergy. Basel, Karger, 2012, vol 98, pp 70–84

Developmental Programming of Allergic Diseases

Maike Pincus[a] · Petra Arck[b]

[a]Department of Pediatrics, Pneumology and Immunology Division, Charité Universitaetsmedizin Berlin, Berlin, and [b]Department for Obstetrics and Prenatal Medicine, Laboratory for Experimental Feto-Maternal Medicine, University Medical Center Hamburg-Eppendorf, Hamburg, Germany

Abstract

Emerging evidence reveals that the incidence of allergic disorders commencing during childhood is influenced by pre-, peri- and early postnatal environmental challenges. We here highlight biomarkers involved in the purported interaction of a challenged intrauterine environment during pregnancy and the risk for allergies in the children later in life. We propose that the identification of biomarkers during pregnancy may allow early detection of children prone to develop allergies and possibly other chronic immune diseases. Subsequently, therapeutic interventions designed to prevent negative consequences of prenatal environmental challenges on children's immune system would be within reach.

The unprecedented rise of atopic disorders observed over the past five decades in the industrialized world has resulted in a wealth of research endeavors to identify its cause. Generally, a genetic predisposition combined with environmental challenges, generally referred to as 'gene × environment interaction' are held responsible for having the risk of developing atopic diseases [1–4]. However, a modification of the human genome seems rather unlikely as it would not cause such a rapid increase of disease. More generations are needed before such a profound increase in disease prevalence will be seen. Hence, a strong alteration in life circumstances and life style has been proposed to be responsible for the increase in allergic diseases. Many environmental factors have been discussed as having an influence on the risk of asthma and atopy especially during childhood [3]. Here, parental smoking, especially maternal smoking, is a very important factor for triggering asthma or lower airway diseases [3, 5, 6]. Air pollution and ozone exposure have also been shown to influence the risk and course of asthma [3, 7–10]. Living close to a highway or major intersection in an urban environment could be linked to airway symptoms, but not to airway hyperresponsiveness itself [3, 11–14]. Allergen exposure has been proposed to induce allergic sensitization, especially dust mite and cat dander [3, 15]. The emotional well-being and the atmosphere at home also seem to be important environmental factors during childhood for the development of asthma and atopy. Chronic stress of a caregiver parent was associated with an atopic immune profile in the children, which predisposed them to atopy-related asthma [16]. Accordingly, domestic violence could be linked to increased early childhood asthma [17]. Last but not least, microbial substances are an important factor in modulating the risk for allergic diseases. Exposure to bacterial micro-organisms as well as mold fungus during childhood has a protective effect on the development of allergic diseases [18].

Most of these studies have focused on risk factors to which an individual is exposed to after birth. Emerging evidence now supports that environmental challenges during the prenatal/fetal period may cause long-lasting negative repercussions on health and disease risks later in life [19]. The time in the womb is characterized on the one hand by a unique protection against external influences but on the other hand it is a time of extreme vulnerability and external influences may exert detrimental and long-lasting changes due to the plasticity of the organism during that period. These observations draw attention to the prenatal period in the context of programming the risk to develop atopic diseases.

Life before 'Life'

The concept of developmental programming of health and diseases was introduced a few decades ago, postulating that fetal development is mainly determined by the maternal state of health. Back then, the key focus was predominantly the nutritional status of the mother. For example, David Barker, a physician and researcher in the UK, described a relation between low weight at birth or infancy and a subsequently increased risk to develop coronary heart disease. Low birth weight is linked to malnutrition in utero [19]. A prolonged phase of malnutrition in utero will lead to fetal growth restriction. Such growth retardation is associated with an altered insulin response to glucose [20]. These profound alterations demonstrate a 'programming' of the fetus on suboptimal nutrient exploitation, leading to a 'thrifty' state of metabolism [21]. This altered metabolism may program the child to expect food shortage and to hoard calories. Hence, these children are more likely to be overweight or obese and are predisposed to an increased risk of type II diabetes as well as coronary heart disease.

Malnutrition in this context is not simply defined as deprivation in calories but also as unbalanced composition of the food. A surplus of protein can be detrimental during pregnancy as it is known to induce obesity and high blood pressure in postnatal life, predominantly in boys [22]. Most of the following studies in this area have concentrated on significantly altered nutrition in utero, but more recently, the list of programming agents during pregnancy has been amended and comprises air/water pollution, endocrine agonists and antagonist, corticosteroid exposure, maternal smoking, bacterial stimuli (endotoxin) and stress perception [6, 7, 23–31]. The in-depth investigation of these programming agents may be pertinent, e.g. in Western Society cohorts. Therefore, we will clarify to which extent timely environmental insults during pregnancy may influence the risk of allergic disease in postnatal life in Western Societies.

Developmental Programming of the Endocrine System

Developmental programming of the endocrine system is best studied for the glucocorticoid system. One reason lies in the fact that glucocorticoids are routinely administered during gestation as a therapeutic intervention. In third-trimester gestation dexamethasone is injected to accelerate lung maturation [32]. Dexamethasone administration throughout pregnancy starting in the first trimester is carried out to attenuate fetal adrenal steroid overproduction in fetuses with congenital adrenal hyperplasia (CAH) [33]. Antenatal exposure to a single course of betamethasone does not alter lung function or the prevalence of wheezing and asthma at age 30 [34]. Fairly sparse information is available on the effect of this treatment on the endocrine response of the developing fetus. Treatment with dexamethasone significantly reduces birth weight in rodents [35] and humans as newborns of mothers with higher cortisol levels in pregnancy had lower birth weights and were shorter at birth. This underlines that maternal cortisol levels in pregnancy influence intrauterine growth [36]. Additionally, treatment with dexamethasone during the last week of gestation in rats increases CRH gene expression in the PVN in rats and is thus thought to alter the 'set point' of the HPA axis in these animals. Alteration of the HPA axis responsiveness as well as the brain monoamine levels is associated with affective disorders in humans [38, 39]. Clinical administration is one way to alter gestational glucocorticoid levels, prenatal stress, maternal deprivation and neonatal handling have also been shown to alter CNS development and have long-term effects on adult brain function [37–46]. Our group could demonstrate – in an experimental model – that prenatal stress lead to a more anxiety prone behavior in female offspring and this was linked to an alteration of the HPA axis. Here prenatal stress was linked to a decrease in CRH mRNA expression in the PVN [47]. Additionally, we could link prenatal stress and the subsequent altered endocrine response to an increased susceptibility for allergic airway inflammation in prenatally stressed female offspring. Buske-Kirschbaum et al. [48] have demonstrated that former pre-terms show significantly higher cortisol levels after awakening accompanied by a significantly suppressed delayed type hypersensitivity response, which suggests that preterm birth may be associated with altered endocrine and immune functions into late childhood. Further, neonates with a positive parental atopic heritage and elevated cord IgE show significantly elevated cortisol responses to the heel prick stress when compared to newborns without a parental atopic history and normal cord IgE values. Hence, not only does exposure to altered levels of glucocorticoids influence the postnatal 'set point' of the HPA axis and the susceptibility to atopic diseases, but obviously this relation may also work in reverse. Atopic disposition itself causes altered responsiveness of the HPA axis to stress leading to an increased vulnerability to develop atopy later in life [49].

Modulation of the HPA axis is only one pathway of developmental influence of the endocrine system of the embryo/fetus, which subsequently changes the risk for atopic diseases later on in life. Epidemiological studies have also shown that maternal hormonal levels have an influence on the child's risk to develop an atopic disease.

Pregnancy is a time of immense immunological adaptation – especially during the first trimester –, which is under the regulation of progesterone [50, 51]. Hence, along with its endocrine effects, progesterone acts as a potent 'immunosteroid' and contributes significantly to the establishment of a pregnancy protective immune milieu, placental formation and fetal development [51, 52] by maintaining the uterine expression of galectin-1 [53], supporting an immature phenotype of dendritic cells (iDC) [54] and homing of natural killer (NK) cells to the fetomaternal interface [52, 55, 56]. Strikingly, emerging evidence arising from studies in humans, mice and other species suggests that maternal levels of progesterone during pregnancy may be suppressed by high perception of stress [50, 57–60], smoking [61, 62] or persistent organic pollutants such as p,p'-dichlorodiphenyltrichloroethane (DDT) [63–65]. Such decrease in progesterone may affect pregnancy outcome by increasing the risk for fetal loss or impaired fetal development. In a cohort study, it could be demonstrated that low levels of maternal progesterone in early pregnancy are associated with an augmented risk to develop atopic dermatitis as well as allergic airway diseases – only in girls. This observation indicates a programming effect of the maternal endocrine system on the fetal immune system, which is gender dependent. Accordingly, prenatal stress increased the susceptibility for an allergic airway inflammation only in female not in male progeny in a mouse model for allergic airway disease. This effect could be abrogated by administration of progesterone prior to the stress exposure. To the reason why the female organism is more susceptible to fetal programming of allergic diseases via prenatal stress and endocrine imbalance is not yet understood. The different connection of the endocrine and the immune system in a female and a male organism might be one explanation.

Developmental Programming of the Immune System

Immunologically, allergy resembles a status of overstimulation of the immune system by reacting on the exposure of generally harmless environmental antigens [66].

Since the human genome has not changed substantially over the past decades, it has become evident that exposure to environmental challenges contributes to the unprecedented increase in allergy prevalence [3, 67]. Recently, it has become more and more recognized that exposure to environmental challenges during pregnancy can already modulate the susceptibility to develop allergies in later life of the children. However, the mechanisms along how these prenatal environmental challenges increase the risk for allergies remain largely elusive and require identification.

As one explanation, the hygiene hypothesis connected the microbial environment and the clinical manifestation of infections during early childhood with the prevalence of allergic diseases later on in life. As the underlying mechanism, a different stimulation of either a Th1 or the Th2 immune response due to the microbial environment and the number of infections were discussed. Within the last years, it became obvious that more immune regulatory mechanisms such as regulatory T cells, Th17 cells, dendritic cells, NKT cells and B cells [68–74] are involved in the development of allergies. The mechanism through which environmental factors exert their influence on the neonatal immune system is not yet understood, but three pathways are discussed [66]. As outlined above, environmental challenges can decrease the levels of progesterone [50, 57–62], which subsequently impairs fetal development. This suggests that progesterone may be a common denominator through which the risk for allergies is programmed prenatally by environmental challenges.

Secondly, a direct allergen exposure via the amniotic fluid or the placenta during pregnancy, which can occur at the 20th week of pregnancy [66, 75, 76], may modulate the atopy risk of the child. A direct dose-response relation between intrauterine allergen exposure and immune response to allergens in cord blood cells has not been described [66, 77]. One reason for this could be an accumulation of allergen in placental tissue [66, 78].

A third explanation how environmental factors influence the child's risk to develop atopy could be a disruption of immune regulatory processes on the maternal side during pregnancy. The growing fetus is semiallogenic and the maternal organism must undergo immunological adaptation in order to not reject the embryonic 'graft'. An orchestra of immune cells is involved in this process such as dendritic cells, uterine NK cells, T cells (CD8 and gd-T cells), regulatory T cells as well as cytokines (TNF-α, IFN-γ, TGF-β, IL-10), integrin pathways (LFA-1/ICAM-1) as well as indolamine-2,3-dioxygenase expression. To which extent this immune adaption process may be different in allergic mothers is not yet explored. The adaptive immune response of the human fetus is developed at a gestational age of 15–20 weeks and here the fetus can react in an antigen-specific manner [66]. Recently, it was described that substantial numbers of maternal cells cross the placental barrier and invade fetal lymph nodes. They induce the development of regulatory T cells, which suppress fetal antimaternal immunity and which persist surprisingly until early adulthood. For the first time, this work reports a crossing of maternal immune cells in the fetal organism and a specific response of the fetal immune system to the maternal cells. In the here described setting, antigen-specific tolerance is induced in utero which actively regulates immune responses after birth [79]. Such a pathway might exist in the presence of maternal allergy inducing not tolerance but eventually an allergic immune response as early as during fetal life. If such a relation exists it must be a matter of future studies. In experimental studies, a close linkage between fetal and maternal immune system has already been demonstrated. Maternal immunization inhibited a specific IgE response of the progeny, when they had been exposed to the same allergen at an early time point [66, 81, 82]. In the mouse, it is possible to transfer an allergic phenotype of the mother on to the progeny allergen by breast milk; however, this pathway is not required for allergen-independent maternal transmission of asthma risk to the progeny [82]. Prenatally different risk factors of mother and child on the immune response of the child at the earliest time point (cord blood) have been described and include ethnicity, smoking, maternal stress perception, nutrition and the APGAR of the neonate.

Analyses of regulatory T cells in the children appear to be a promising candidate to understand mechanisms involved in fetal origin of allergic diseases. Based on the ability of regulatory T cells to, for example, suppress T cell activation and a pathogenic Th2 bias [66, 83–87], prenatally programmed altered frequencies or default function of regulatory T cells may fail to fulfil this task and thereby contribute to the development or progression of allergies. Maternal atopy has been shown to be associated with a reduced number and function of regulatory T cells in the cord blood [66, 88, 89]. These results are predominantly gained after microbial stimulation of the cord blood cells. Hence, it might be possible that a missing microbial stimulation during pregnancy induces a certain 'weakness' of the neonatal and the child's immune system [90] perhaps due to a lack of regulatory function. Going in the same direction is the finding that children with an early egg allergy show an impaired regulatory immune function at birth [91].

Environmental influences on the risk for a child's atopy include maternal smoking, but also maternal stress perception and her living environment. Maternal stress was recently studied in an inner-city cohort in the US and included financial hardship, difficult life circumstances, community violence, and neighborhood/block and housing conditions. This study revealed that prenatal stress was associated with altered innate and adaptive immune responses in cord blood cells, e.g. increased IL-13 after dust mite stimulation [92]. In a mouse model, it could be demonstrated that prenatal stress induced an increased susceptibility towards allergic airway inflammation in the female progeny [47]. Here, prenatal stress resulted in a stronger TH2 response at female adolescent progeny in the setting of an allergic phenotype [47]. In a large British cohort study with over 5,000 participating pregnant women, a linkage between maternal anxiety symptoms and the development of asthma during childhood has been found [93]. By which mechanism maternal stress is transferred to the fetus remain elusive. Next to maternal stress exposure her living condition are of special interest also known as the 'farm effect' [25, 94]. The 'farm effect' is especially strong, if the exposure to a farming environment takes place in utero [25, 66]. As underlying mechanism the specific microbial environment on a farm is thought to be responsible. In the mouse model, the exposure to LPS, a compound of the bacterial wall, can prevent allergic sensitization but interestingly does not affect airway reactivity in a model of induced allergic airway inflammation [26, 27, 66]. It is noteworthy that prenatal stress in the same mouse model predominantly influences airway reactivity and to a much lesser extent airway inflammation, suggesting different pathways of transmission for prenatal stress and prenatal LPS exposure. In a different mouse study maternal intranasal exposure to coshed-derived bacterium *Acinetobacter lwoffii* prevented allergic airway inflammation in the progeny [95].This preventive effect was abolished when the mother did not express TLR2/3/4/7/9 but the child being heterozygous for the knockout mutation did express the TLR receptors [95]. This work indicates that it is the response of the maternal immune system which matters in the context of fetal programming of allergic diseases. The responding counterpart on the fetal side is still needed to be describes. Regulatory T cells could be a candidate responding to maternal immune alterations. In epidemiological studies a farming environment induced function and number of regulatory T cells as early as in the cord blood being accompanied by a reduction of TH2 cytokines [90]. The suppressive phenotype of CD4+CD25+ T cells is associated with expression of the forkhead/winged-helix family transcriptional repressor p3 (FoxP3), which has become a widely used marker for the identification of regulatory T cells. Strikingly, Foxp3, the pivotal marker for regulatory T cell function, has been reported to be under epigenetic regulation [66, 96–98]. Epigenetics is defined as the regulation of gene expression without altering the nucleotide sequence in the genome. Epigenetic mechanisms imprint the activity state of specific gene loci and alterations may remain through cell divisions for the remainder of the cell's life and may also become heritable [99]. An epigenetic demethylation of FOXP3 has been found in children whose mothers had been exposed to a farm environment during pregnancy [90].

A therapeutic approach in order to mimic the 'farm effect' is the administration of probiotics, which are even able to inhibit an allergic airway response in adult mice [100]. Perinatal administration of, for example, LGG prevented LPS airway inflammation but not airway responsiveness [101], and postnatal application of probiotic bacteria inhibited allergic airway diseases interestingly by inducing regulatory T cells and TGF-β production [102] in experimental models. In epidemiological studies, Kalliomäki et al. [103] were the first to demonstrate that the administration of probiotic strains (e.g. *Lactobacilli* GG) significantly reduced the risk for atopic dermatitis in children. Interestingly, Kalliomäki et al. [103] started the immunomodulatory treatment with the probiotics as early as during the third trimester of pregnancy. In a study investigating the use of probiotics only during the last 4 weeks of pregnancy in a high-risk population, the treatment was not associated with any change in cord blood immune markers and was not sufficient to prevent eczema [104]. Many other studies with various study designs have come to very different findings, some report a beneficial effect, others don't. As long as the underlying mechanisms of the immune modulation induced in the fetal organism are not fully understood, it will be difficult to know the best time to start a preventive treatment with probiotics during pregnancy.

Developmental Programming of the Nervous System

Reflecting the developmental origin of allergic diseases one must also draw attention to the peripheral nervous system and potential 'point of attacks' during its development. Neuronal function in young monkeys has been shown to be irreversibly disturbed upon ozone or allergen exposure [105–108]. Neuronal function as well as the development of the peripheral sensory nervous system is dependent on neurotrophin support [107]. Inflammatory diseases such as asthma have been linked to neuronal dysfunction, where at the site of inflammation immune cells can be found in direct contact of neuropeptides and neurotrophins containing nerves [109]. Such neuropeptides and neurotrophins include nerve growth factor (NGF) or substance P. Such neuropeptides are capable of influencing sensory nerve function and hence boosting allergic inflammation and airway reactivity in asthma [110].

Programming of allergic airway disease could be associated with irreversible alterations in neuronal development caused by altered local production of neurotrophins in utero [107]. This idea is supported by the finding that NGF expression in the lung is declining with age and is highest in early life [107, 111, 112]. An overexpression of NGF – as seen after stress exposure – induces hyperinnervation in the lung [107, 113], which may increase susceptibility to airway reactivity. In early childhood, infections with certain viruses such as respiratory syncytical virus are clinically linked to an increased risk for childhood asthma. The infection itself is also often accompanied by severe bronchial obstruction and airway reactivity. By which mechanism the RSV infection panders the child to asthma is not yet fully understood. It has been demonstrated that RSV infection is accompanied by a demonstrative neurogenic inflammation [114] mediated by neurotrophins leading to long-term changes in the distribution and reactivity of sensory nerves within the respiratory tract triggering airway reactivity [107, 112, 115].

Thus, stimuli which are able to trigger neurotrophin production and release during pregnancy may influence – organ dependently – the release of neurotrophins and the maturation and development of the peripheral sensory nervous system. An 'overstimulation' may lead to irreversible sensory hyperreactivity and hyperinnervation and may promote the onset of allergic diseases by neurogenic inflammation [107].

Severe conditions in newborns such as intraventricular hemorrhage have been associated with lower cord blood levels of the neurotrophin called brain-derived nerve factor (BDNF). Interestingly, BDNF as well as neurotrophin 4 were increased in cord blood, when steroids had been administered antenatally [116]. NGF itself can be

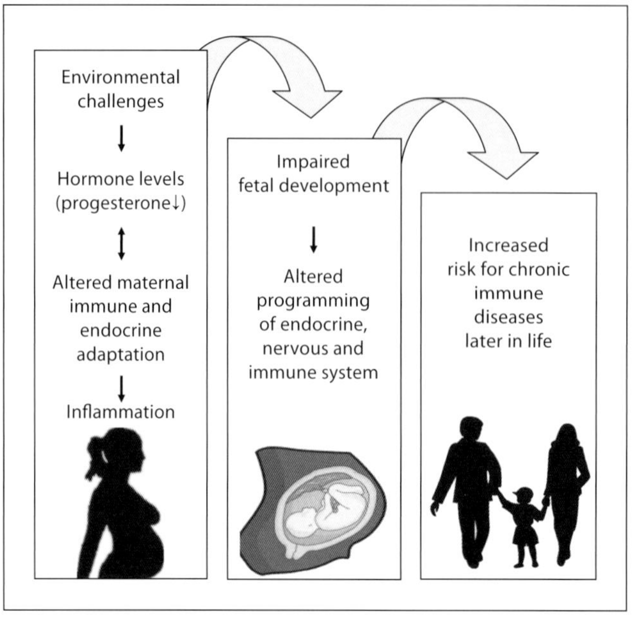

Fig. 1. Hypothetical scenario of developmenal programming of allergic diseases: Fetal development is largely dependent on the mother. However, pregnancy maintenance and consequently fetal development are highly vulnerable and sensitive to disruption, triggered by, for example, environmental challenges. Such challenges can modulate the maternal endocrine and immune responses during pregnancy, for example by decreasing levels of progesterone. Further, fetal development, including the maturation of the immune, endorcine and nervous systems, may be impaired upon prenatal environmental challenges. Such impaired fetal development carries over into postnatal life, rendering the child more prone to developing chronic immune diseases including allergies.

linked to in utero growth as it has been shown that intrauterine growth restriction is accompanied by suppressed levels of NGF [117] indicating that a well-balanced regulation of neurotrophins is important to avoid pathological condition. At the decidua, the fetomaternal interface in pregnancy, stress exposure of the dam as well as injection of substance P increased the expression of NGF and its receptor (TrkA) resulting in early pregnancy in abortion [118]. Unfortunately, data on fetal brain and lung development in regard to neurotrophins in response to maternal stress exposure are lacking.

Conclusions

We have discussed the complex interrelationships which together form the basis of our current knowledge in the factors which influence the developmental programming of allergic disease (fig. 1). Understanding how programming agents are operational in the context of the developmental origin of atopic diseases may lead to the identification of biomarkers, which will then allow the early detection of pregnancies/ neonate with a predisposed risk for atopic diseases. As this provides a platform for the primary prevention or modulation of the risk for atopic diseases, interdisciplinary 'mother-child' research should be progressively more implemented in the context of atopic diseases.

References

1 Bach JF: The effect of infections on susceptibility to autoimmune and allergic diseases. N Engl J Med 2002;347:911–920

2 Center of Disease Control and Prevention Health US 2010: National Center for Disease Control and Prevention, http://www.cdc.gov/nchs/data/hus/hus10.pdf, table 246, p 216.

3 Von Mutius E: Prävalenz und Determinanten des kindlichen Asthma bronchiale. Monatsschr Kinderheilkd 2010;158:121–128.

4 Schlaud M, Atzpodien K, Thierfelder W: Allergic diseases. Results from the German Health Interview and Examination Survey for Children and Adolescents (KiGGS). Bundesgesundheitsbl Gesundheitsforsch Gesundheitsschutz 2007;50:701–710.

5 Strachan DP, Cook DG: Health effects of passive smoking. 6. Parental smoking and childhood asthma: longitudinal and case control studies. Thorax 1998;53:204–212.

6 Keil T, Lau S, Roll S, Grüber C, Nickel R, Niggemann B, Wahn U, Willich SN, Kulig M: Maternal smoking increases risk of allergic sensitization and wheezing only in children with allergic predisposition: longitudinal analysis from birth to 10 years. Allergy 2009;64:445–451.

7 Fedulov AV, Leme A, Yang Z, Dahl M, Lim R, Mariani TJ, Kobzik L: Pulmonary exposure to particles during pregnancy causes increased neonatal asthma susceptibility. Am J Respir Cell Mol Biol 2008;38:57–67.

8 Gilliland FD: Outdoor air pollution, genetic susceptibility, and asthma management: opportunities for intervention to reduce the burden of asthma. Pediatrics 2009;123(suppl 3):S168–S173.

9 Holguin F: Traffic, outdoor air pollution, and asthma. Immunol Allergy Clin North Am 2008;28: 577–588, viii–ix.

10 McCreanor J, Cullinan P, Nieuwenhuijsen MJ, Stewart-Evans J, Malliarou E, Jarup L, Harrington R, Svartengren M, Han IK, Ohman-Strickland P, Chung KF, Zhang J: Respiratory effects of exposure to diesel traffic in persons with asthma. N Engl J Med 2007;357:2348–2358.

11 Oosterlee A, Drijver M, Lebret E, Brunekreef B: Chronic respiratory symptoms in children and adults living along streets with high traffic density. Occup Environ Med 1996;53:241–247.

12 van Vliet P, Knape M, de Hartog J, Janssen N, Harssema H, Brunekreef B: Motor vehicle exhaust and chronic respiratory symptoms in children living near freeways. Environ Res 1997;74:122–132.

13 Venn AJ, Lewis SA, Cooper M, Hubbard R, Britton J: Living near a main road and the risk of wheezing illness in children. Am J Respir Crit Care Med 2001;164:2177–2180.

14 Nicolai T, Carr D, Weiland SK, Duhme H, von Ehrenstein O, Wagner C, von Mutius E: Urban traffic and pollutant exposure related to respiratory outcomes and atopy in a large sample of children. Eur Respir J 2003;21:956–963.

15 Lau S, Illi S, Sommerfeld C, Niggemann B, Bergmann R, von Mutius E, Wahn U: Early exposure to house-dust mite and cat allergens and development of childhood asthma: a cohort study: Multicentre Allergy Study Group. Lancet 2000;356: 1392–1397.

16 Wright RJ, Finn P, Contreras JP, Cohen S, Wright RO, Staudenmayer J, Wand M, Perkins D, Weiss ST, Gold DR: Chronic caregiver stress and IgE expression, allergen-induced proliferation, and cytokine profiles in a birth cohort predisposed to atopy. J Allergy Clin Immunol 2004;113:1051–1057.

17 Suglia SF, Enlow MB, Kullowatz A, Wright RJ: Maternal intimate partner violence and increased asthma incidence in children: buffering effects of supportive caregiving. Arch Pediatr Adolesc Med 2009;163:244–250.

18 Braun-Fahrlander C, Lauener R: Farming and protective agents against allergy and asthma. Clin Exp Allergy 2003;33:409–411.

19 Barker DJ: The developmental origins of adult disease. Eur J Epidemiol 2003;18:733–736.

20 Hales CN, Barker DJ, Clark PM, Cox LJ, Fall C, Osmond C, Winter PD. Fetal and infant growth and impaired glucose tolerance at age 64. BMJ 1991; 303:1019–1022.

21 Hales CN, Barker DJ: The thrifty phenotype hypothesis. Br Med Bull 2001;60:5–20.

22 Thone-Reineke C, Kalk P, Dorn M, Klaus S, Simon K, Pfab T, Godes M, Persson P, Unger T, Hocher B: High-protein nutrition during pregnancy and lactation programs blood pressure, food efficiency, and body weight of the offspring in a sex-dependent manner. Am J Physiol Regul Integr Comp Physiol 2006;291:R1025–R1030.

23 Wittig HJ, McLaughlin ET, Leifer KL, Belloit JD: Risk factors for the development of allergic disease: analysis of 2,190 patient records. Ann Allergy 1978;41:84–88.

24 von Mutius E: The environmental predictors of allergic disease. J Allergy Clin Immunol 2000;105: 9–19.

25 Riedler J, Braun-Fahrländer C, Eder W, Schreuer M, Waser M, Maisch S, Carr D, Schierl R, Nowak D, von Mutius E, ALEX Study Team: Exposure to farming in early life and development of asthma and allergy: a cross-sectional survey. Lancet 2001; 358:1129–1133.

26 Blümer N, Herz U, Wegmann M, Renz H: Prenatal lipopolysaccharide-exposure prevents allergic sensitization and airway inflammation, but not airway responsiveness in a murine model of experimental asthma. Clin Exp Allergy 2005;35:397–402.

27 Gerhold K, Avagyan A, Seib C, Frei R, Steinle J, Ahrens B, Dittrich AM, Blumchen K, Lauener R, Hamelmann E: Prenatal initiation of endotoxin airway exposure prevents subsequent allergen-induced sensitization and airway inflammation in mice. J Allergy Clin Immunol 2006;118:666–673.

28 Gerhold K, Avagyan A, Reichert E, Blumchen K, Wahn U, Hamelmann E: Lipopolysaccharides modulate allergen-specific immune regulation in a murine model of mucosal tolerance induction. Int Arch Allergy Immunol 2008;147:25–34.

29 Lannerö E, Wickman M, Pershagen G, Nordvall L: Maternal smoking during pregnancy increases the risk of recurrent wheezing during the first years of life (BAMSE). Respir Res 2006;7:3.

30 Sternthal MJ, Coull BA, Chiu YH, Cohen S, Wright RJ: Associations among maternal childhood socioeconomic status, cord blood IgE levels, and repeated wheeze in urban children J Allergy Clin Immunol 2011;128:337–345.

31 Pincus M, Keil T, Rücke M, Bruenahl C, Magdorf K, Klapp BF, Douglas AJ, Paus R, Wahn U, Arck P: Fetal origin of atopic dermatitis. J Allergy Clin Immunol 2010;125:273–275.

32 Kattner E, Metze B, Waiss E, Obladen M: Accelerated lung maturation following maternal steroid treatment in infants born before 30 weeks gestation. J Perinat Med 1992;20:449–457.

33 Mercado AB, Wilson RC, Cheng KC, Wei JQ, New MI: Prenatal treatment and diagnosis of congenital adrenal hyperplasia owing to steroid 21-hydroxylase deficiency. J Clin Endocrinol Metab 1995;80: 2014–2020.

34 Dalziel SR, Rea HH, Walker NK, Parag V, Mantell C, Rodgers A, Harding JE: Long term effects of antenatal betamethasone on lung function: 30 year follow up of a randomised controlled trial. Thorax 2006;61:678–683.

35 Welberg LA, Seckl JR, Holmes MC: Prenatal glucocorticoid programming of brain corticosteroid receptors and corticotrophin-releasing hormone: possible implications for behavior Neuroscience 2001;104:71–79.

36 Bolten MI, Wurmser H, Buske-Kirschbaum A, Papoušek M, Pirke KM, Hellhammer D: Cortisol levels in pregnancy as a psychobiological predictor for birth weight. Arch Womens Ment Health 2011; 14:33–41.

37 Holsboer F, Lauer CJ, Schreiber W, Krieg JC: Altered hypothalamic-pituitary-adrenocortical regulation in healthy subjects at high familial risk for affective disorders. Neuroendocrinology 1995;62:340–347.

38 López JF, Chalmers DT, Little KY, Watson SJ: A.E. Bennett Research Award. Regulation of serotonin1A, glucocorticoid, and mineralocorticoid receptor in rat and human hippocampus: implications for the neurobiology of depression. Biol Psychiatry 1998;43:547–573.

39 Holson RR, Gough B, Sullivan P, Badger T, Sheehan DM: Prenatal dexamethasone or stress but not ACTH or corticosterone alter sexual behavior in male rats. Neurotoxicol Teratol 1995;17:393–401.

40 Henry C, Kabbaj M, Simon H, Le Moal M, Maccari S: Prenatal stress increases the hypothalamo-pituitary-adrenal axis response in young and adult rats. J Neuroendocrinol 1994;6:341–345.

41 Vallée M, Mayo W, Dellu F, Le Moal M, Simon H, Maccari S: Prenatal stress induces high anxiety and postnatal handling induces low anxiety in adult offspring: correlation with stress-induced corticosterone secretion. J Neurosci 1997;17:2626–2636.

42 Weinstock M: Does prenatal stress impair coping and regulation of hypothalamic-pituitary-adrenal axis? Neurosci Biobehav Rev 1997;21:1–10.

43 Weinstock M, Matlina E, Maor GI, Rosen H, McEwen BS: Prenatal stress selectively alters the reactivity of the hypothalamic-pituitary adrenal system in the female rat. Brain Res 1992;595:195–200.

44 Day JC, Koehl M, Deroche V, Le Moal M, Maccari S: Prenatal stress enhances stress- and corticotropin-releasing factor-induced stimulation of hippocampal acetylcholine release in adult rats. J Neurosci 1998;18:1886–1892.

45 Peters DA: Prenatal stress: effect on development of rat brain adrenergic receptors. Pharmacol Biochem Behav 1984;21:417–422.

46 Peters DA: Maternal stress increases fetal brain and neonatal cerebral cortex 5-hydroxytryptamine synthesis in rats: a possible mechanism by which stress influences brain development. Pharmacol Biochem Behav 1990;35:943–947.

47 Pincus-Knackstedt MK, Joachim RA, Blois SM, Douglas AJ, Orsal AS, Klapp BF, Wahn U, Hamelmann E, Arck PC: Prenatal stress enhances susceptibility of murine adult offspring toward airway inflammation. J Immunol 2006;177:8484–8492.

48 Buske-Kirschbaum A, Krieger S, Wilkes C, Rauh W, Weiss S, Hellhammer DH: Hypothalamic-pituitary-adrenal axis function and the cellular immune response in former preterm children. J Clin Endocrinol Metab 2007;92:3429–3435.

49 Buske-Kirschbaum A, Fischbach S, Rauh W, Hanker J, Hellhammer D: Increased responsiveness of the hypothalamus-pituitary-adrenal (HPA) axis to stress in newborns with atopic disposition. Psychoneuroendocrinology 2004;29:705–711.

50 Joachim R, Zenclussen AC, Polgar B, Douglas AJ, Fest S, Knackstedt M, Klapp BF, Arck PC: The progesterone derivative dydrogesterone abrogates murine stress-triggered abortion by inducing a Th2 biased local immune response. Steroids 2003;68: 931–940.

51 Arck P, Hansen PJ, Mulac Jericevic B, Piccinni MP, Szekeres-Bartho J: Progesterone during pregnancy: endocrine-immune cross talk in mammalian species and the role of stress. Am J Reprod Immunol 2007;58:268–279.

52 Leonhardt A, Glaser A, Wegmann M, Hackenberg R, Nüsing RM: Expression of prostanoid receptors in human lower segment pregnant myometrium. Prostaglandins Leukot Essent Fatty Acids 2003;69: 307–313.

53 Blois SM, Ilarregui JM, Tometten M, Garcia M, Orsal AS, Cordo-Russo R, Toscano MA, Bianco GA, Kobelt P, Handjiski B, Tirado I, Markert UR, Klapp BF, Poirier F, Szekeres-Bartho J, Rabinovich GA, Arck PC: A pivotal role for galectin-1 in fetomaternal tolerance. Nat Med 2007;13:1450–1457.

54 Blois SM, Kammerer U, Alba Soto C, Tometten MC, Shaikly V, Barrientos G, Jurd R, Rukavina D, Thomson AW, Klapp BF, Fernández N, Arck PC: Dendritic cells: key to fetal tolerance? Biol Reprod 2007;77:590–598.

55 Blois SM, Barrientos G, Garcia MG, Orsal AS, Tometten M, Cordo-Russo RI, Klapp BF, Santoni A, Fernández N, Terness P, Arck PC: Interaction between dendritic cells and natural killer cells during pregnancy in mice. J Mol Med (Berl) 2008;86: 837–852.

56 Hanna J, Mandelboim O: When killers become helpers. Trends Immunol 2007;28:201–206.

57 Szekeres-Bartho J, Halasz M, Palkovics T: Progesterone in pregnancy; receptor-ligand interaction and signaling pathways. J Reprod Immunol 2009;83: 60–64.

58 Nepomnaschy PA, Welch K, McConnell D, Strassmann BI, England BG: Stress and female reproductive function: a study of daily variations in cortisol, gonadotrophins, and gonadal steroids in a rural Mayan population. Am J Hum Biol 2004;16: 523–532.

59 Arck PC, Rücke M, Rose M, Szekeres-Bartho J, Douglas AJ, Pritsch M, Blois SM, Pincus MK, Bärenstrauch N, Dudenhausen JW, Nakamura K, Sheps S, Klapp BF: Early risk factors for miscarriage: a prospective cohort study in pregnant women. Reprod Biomed Online 2008;17:101–113.

60 Creel S, Winnie JA Jr, Christianson D: Glucocorticoid stress hormones and the effect of predation risk on elk reproduction. Proc Natl Acad Sci USA 2009;106: 12388–12393.

61 Piasek M, Blanusa M, Kostial K, Laskey JW: Placental cadmium and progesterone concentrations in cigarette smokers. Reprod Toxicol 2001;15: 673–681.

62 Ng SP, Steinetz BG, Lasano SC, Zelikoff JT: Hormonal changes accompanying cigarette smoke-induced preterm births in a mouse model. Exp Biol Med (Maywood) 2006;231:1403–1409.

63 Perry MJ, Ouyang F, Korrick SA, Venners SA, Chen C, Xu X, Lasley BL, Wang X: A prospective study of serum DDT and progesterone and estrogen levels across the menstrual cycle in nulliparous women of reproductive age. Am J Epidemiol 2006;164:1056–1064.

64 Wójtowicz AK, Milewicz T, Gregoraszczuk EŁ: DDT and its metabolite DDE alter steroid hormone secretion in human term placental explants by regulation of aromatase activity. Toxicol Lett 2007;173: 24–30.

65 Windham GC, Lee D, Mitchell P, Anderson M, Petreas M, Lasley B: Exposure to organochlorine compounds and effects on ovarian function. Epidemiology 2005;16:182–190.

66 Schau B: Asthma bronchiale. Monatsschr Kinderheilkd 2010;158:137–141.

67 Holgate ST: Genetic and environmental interaction in allergy and asthma. J Allergy Clin Immunol 1999; 104:1139–1146.

68 Hubscher T: Immune and biochemical mechanisms in the allergic disease of the upper respiratory tract; role of antibodies, target cells, mediators and eosinophils. Ann Allergy 1977;38:83–90.
69 DiIulio NA, Xu H, Fairchild RL: Diversion of CD4+ T cell development from regulatory T helper to effector T helper cells alters the contact hypersensitivity response. Eur J Immunol 1996;26:2606–2612.
70 Akbari O, DeKruyff RH, Umetsu DT: Pulmonary dendritic cells producing IL-10 mediate tolerance induced by respiratory exposure to antigen. Nat Immunol 2001;2:725–731.
71 Hansen G, Yeung VP, Berry G, Umetsu DT, DeKruyff RH: Vaccination with heat-killed Listeria as adjuvant reverses established allergen-induced airway hyperreactivity and inflammation: role of CD8+ T cells and IL-18. J Immunol 2000;164:223–230.
72 Akbari O, Freeman GJ, Meyer EH, Greenfield EA, Chang TT, Sharpe AH, Berry G,DeKruyff RH, Umetsu DT: Antigen-specific regulatory T cells develop via the ICOS-ICOS-ligand pathway and inhibit allergen-induced airway hyperreactivity. Nat Med 2002;8:1024–1032.
73 Pichavant M, Matangkasombut P, Dekruyff RH, Umetsu DT: Natural killer T cells regulate the development of asthma. Expert Rev Clin Immunol 2009;5:251–260.
74 Bullens DM, Truyen E, Coteur L, Dilissen E, Hellings PW, Dupont LJ, Ceuppens JL: IL-17 mRNA in sputum of asthmatic patients: linking T cell driven inflammation and granulocytic influx? Respir Res 2006;7:135.
75 Holloway JA, Warner JO, Vance GH, Diaper ND, Warner JA, Jones CA: Detection of house-dust-mite allergen in amniotic fluid and umbilical-cord blood. Lancet 2000;356:1900–1902.
76 Szépfalusi Z, Pichler J, Elsässer S, van Duren K, Ebner C, Bernaschek G, Urbanek R: Transplacental priming of the human immune system with environmental allergens can occur early in gestation. J Allergy Clin Immunol 2000;106:530–536.
77 Miller RL, Chew GL, Bell CA, Biedermann SA, Aggarwal M, Kinney PL, Tsai WY, Whyatt RM, Perera FP, Ford JG: Prenatal exposure, maternal sensitization, and sensitization in utero to indoor allergens in an inner-city cohort. Am J Respir Crit Care Med 2001;164:995–1001.
78 Szépfalusi Z, Loibichler C, Hänel-Dekan S, Dehlink E, Gerstmayr M, Pichler J, Eiwegger T, Horvat R, Urbanek R: Most of diaplacentally transferred allergen is retained in the placenta. Clin Exp Allergy 2006;36:1130–1137.
79 Mold JE, Michaëlsson J, Burt TD, Muench MO, Beckerman KP, Busch MP, Lee TH, Nixon DF, McCune JM: Maternal alloantigens promote the development of tolerogenic fetal regulatory T cells in utero. Science 2008;322:1562–1565.
80 Uthoff H, Spenner A, Reckelkamm W, Ahrens B, Wölk G, Hackler R, Hardung F, Schaefer J, Scheffold A, Renz H, Herz U: Critical role of preconceptional immunization for protective and nonpathological specific immunity in murine neonates. J Immunol 2003;171:3485–3492.
81 Victor JR Jr, Fusaro AE, Duarte AJ, Sato MN: Preconception maternal immunization to dust mite inhibits the type I hypersensitivity response of offspring. J Allergy Clin Immunol 2003;111:269–277.
82 Leme AS, Hubeau C, Xiang Y, Goldman A, Hamada K, Suzaki Y, Kobzik L: Role of breast milk in a mouse model of maternal transmission of asthma susceptibility. J Immunol 2006;176:762–769.
83 Jutel M, Akdis M, Budak F, Aebischer-Casaulta C, Wrzyszcz M, Blaser K, Akdis CA: IL-10 and TGF-beta cooperate in the regulatory T cell response to mucosal allergens in normal immunity and specific immunotherapy. Eur J Immunol 2003;33:1205–1214.
84 Ling EM, Smith T, Nguyen XD, Pridgeon C, Dallman M, Arbery J, Carr VA, Robinson DS: Relation of CD4+CD25+ regulatory T-cell suppression of allergen-driven T-cell activation to atopic status and expression of allergic disease. Lancet 2004;363:608–615.
85 Grindebacke H, Wing K, Andersson AC, Suri-Payer E, Rak S, Rudin A: Defective suppression of Th2 cytokines by CD4CD25 regulatory T cells in birch allergics during birch pollen season. Clin Exp Allergy 2004;34:1364–1372.
86 Bellinghausen I, Klostermann B, Knop J, Saloga J: Human CD4+CD25+ T cells derived from the majority of atopic donors are able to suppress TH1 and TH2 cytokine production. J Allergy Clin Immunol 2003;111:862–868.
87 Taams LS, Vukmanovic-Stejic M, Smith J, Dunne PJ, Fletcher JM, Plunkett FJ, Ebeling SB, Lombardi G, Rustin MH, Bijlsma JW, Lafeber FP, Salmon M, Akbar AN: Antigen-specific T cell suppression by human CD4+CD25+ regulatory T cells. Eur J Immunol 2002;32:1621–1630.
88 Schaub B, Liu J, Höppler S, Haug S, Sattler C, Lluis A, Illi S, von Mutius E: Impairment of T-regulatory cells in cord blood of atopic mothers. J Allergy Clin Immunol 2008;121:1491–1499.
89 Schaub B, Liu J, Schleich I, Höppler S, Sattler C, von Mutius E: Impairment of T helper and T regulatory cell responses at birth. Allergy 2008;63:1438–1447.

90 Schaub B, Liu J, Höppler S, Schleich I, Huehn J, Olek S, Wieczorek G, Illi S, von Mutius E: Maternal farm exposure modulates neonatal immune mechanisms through regulatory T cells. J Allergy Clin Immunol 2009;123:774–782.
91 Smith M, Tourigny MR, Noakes P, Thornton CA, Tulic MK, Prescott SL: Children with egg allergy have evidence of reduced neonatal CD4(+)CD25(+) CD127(lo/–) regulatory T cell function. J Allergy Clin Immunol 2008;121:1460–1466.
92 Wright RJ, Visness CM, Calatroni A, Grayson MH, Gold DR, Sandel MT, Lee-Parritz A, Wood RA, Kattan M, Bloomberg GR, Burger M, Togias A, Witter FR, Sperling RS, Sadovsky Y, Gern JE: Prenatal maternal stress and cord blood innate and adaptive cytokine responses in an inner-city cohort. Am J Respir Crit Care Med 2010;182:25–33.
93 Cookson H, Granell R, Joinson C, Ben-Shlomo Y, Henderson AJ: Mothers' anxiety during pregnancy is associated with asthma in their children. J Allergy Clin Immunol 2009;123:847–853.
94 Braun-Fahrländer C, Riedler J, Herz U, Eder W, Waser M, Grize L, Maisch S, Carr D, Gerlach F, Bufe A, Lauener RP, Schierl R, Renz H, Nowak D, von Mutius E, Allergy and Endotoxin Study Team: Environmental exposure to endotoxin and its relation to asthma in school-age children. N Engl J Med 2002;347:869–877.
95 Conrad ML, Ferstl R, Teich R, Brand S, Blümer N, Yildirim AO, Patrascan CC, Hanuszkiewicz A, Akira S, Wagner H, Holst O, von Mutius E, Pfefferle PI, Kirschning CJ, Garn H, Renz H: Maternal TLR signaling is required for prenatal asthma protection by the nonpathogenic microbe *Acinetobacter lwoffii* F78. J Exp Med 2009;206:2869–2877.
96 Polansky JK, Kretschmer K, Freyer J, Floess S, Garbe A, Baron U, Olek S, Hamann A, von Boehmer H, Huehn J: DNA methylation controls Foxp3 gene expression. Eur J Immunol 2008;38:1654–1663.
97 Wieczorek G, Asemissen A, Model F, Turbachova I, Floess S, Liebenberg V, Baron U, Stauch D, Kotsch K, Pratschke J, Hamann A, Loddenkemper C, Stein H, Volk HD, Hoffmüller U, Grützkau A, Mustea A, Huehn J, Scheibenbogen C, Olek S: Quantitative DNA methylation analysis of FOXP3 as a new method for counting regulatory T cells in peripheral blood and solid tissue. Cancer Res 2009;69:599–608.
98 Huehn J, Polansky JK, Hamann A: Epigenetic control of FOXP3 expression: the key to a stable regulatory T-cell lineage? Nat Rev Immunol 2009;9: 83–89.
99 Feinberg AP: Epigenomics reveals a functional genome anatomy and a new approach to common disease. Nat Biotechnol 2010;28:1049–1052.
100 Forsythe P, Inman MD, Bienenstock J: Oral treatment with live *Lactobacillus reuteri* inhibits the allergic airway response in mice. Am J Respir Crit Care Med 2007;175:561–569.
101 Blümer N, Sel S, Virna S, Patrascan CC, Zimmermann S, Herz U, Renz H, Garn H: Perinatal maternal application of *Lactobacillus rhamnosus* GG suppresses allergic airway inflammation in mouse offspring. Clin Exp Allergy 2007;37:348–357.
102 Feleszko W, Jaworska J, Rha RD, Steinhausen S, Avagyan A, Jaudszus A, Ahrens B, Groneberg DA, Wahn U, Hamelmann E: Probiotic-induced suppression of allergic sensitization and airway inflammation is associated with an increase of T regulatory-dependent mechanisms in a murine model of asthma. Clin Exp Allergy 2007;37:498–505.
103 Kalliomäki M, Salminen S, Arvilommi H, Kero P, Koskinen P, Isolauri E: Probiotics in primary prevention of atopic disease: a randomized placebo-controlled trial. Lancet 2001;357:1076–1079.
104 Boyle RJ, Ismail IH, Kivivuori S, Licciardi PV, Robins-Browne RM, Mah LJ, Axelrad C, Moore S, Donath S, Carlin JB, Lahtinen SJ, Tang ML: Lactobacillus GG treatment during pregnancy for the prevention of eczema: a randomized controlled trial. Allergy 2011;66:509–616.
105 Nassenstein C, Dawbarn D, Pollock K, Allen SJ, Erpenbeck VJ, Spies E, Krug N, Braun A: Pulmonary distribution, regulation, and functional role of Trk receptors in a murine model of asthma. J Allergy Clin Immunol 2006;118:597–605.
106 Veres TZ, Rochlitzer S, Shevchenko M, Fuchs B, Prenzler F, Nassenstein C, Fischer A, Welker L, Holz O, Müller M, Krug N, Braun A: Spatial interactions between dendritic cells and sensory nerves in allergic airway inflammation. Am J Respir Cell Mol Biol 2007;37:553–561.
107 Nassenstein C, Braun A, Nockher WA, Renz H: Neurotrophin effects on eosinophils in allergic inflammation. Curr Allergy Asthma Rep 2005;5: 204–211.
108 Chen CY, Bonham AC, Plopper CG, Joad JP: Neuroplasticity in nucleus tractus solitarius neurons after episodic ozone exposure in infant primates. J Appl Physiol 2003;94:819–827.
109 Blennerhassett MG, Tomioka M, Bienenstock J: Formation of contacts between mast cells and sympathetic neurons in vitro. Cell Tissue Res 1991;265: 121–128.

110 Quarcoo D, Schulte-Herbrüggen O, Lommatzsch M, Schierhorn K, Hoyle GW, Renz H, Braun A: Nerve growth factor induces increased airway inflammation via a neuropeptide-dependent mechanism in a transgenic animal model of allergic airway inflammation. Clin Exp Allergy 2004;34: 1146–1151.
111 Lommatzsch M, Braun A, Renz H: Neurotrophins in allergic airway dysfunction: what the mouse model is teaching us. Ann NY Acad Sci 2003;992: 241–249.
112 Hu C, Wedde-Beer K, Auais A, Rodriguez MM, Piedimonte G: Nerve growth factor and nerve growth factor receptors in respiratory syncytial virus-infected lungs. Am J Physiol Lung Cell Mol Physiol 2002;283:L494–502.
113 Hoyle GW, Graham RM, Finkelstein JB, Nguyen KP, Gozal D, Friedman M: Hyperinnervation of the airways in transgenic mice overexpressing nerve growth factor. Am J Respir Cell Mol Biol 1998;18: 149–57.
114 Piedimonte G: Contribution of neuroimmune mechanisms to airway inflammation and remodeling during and after respiratory syncytial virus infection. Pediatr Infect Dis J 2003;22(2 suppl): S66–S74.
115 Tortorolo L, Langer A, Polidori G, Vento G, Stampachiacchere B, Aloe L, Piedimonte G: Neurotrophin overexpression in lower airways of infants with respiratory syncytial virus infection. Am J Respir Crit Care Med 2005;172:233–237.
116 Nikolaou KE, Malamitsi-Puchner A, Boutsikou T, Economou E, Boutsikou M, Puchner KP, Baka S, Hassiakos D: The varying patterns of neurotrophin changes in the perinatal period. Ann NY Acad Sci 2006;1092:426–433.
117 Malamitsi-Puchner A, Nikolaou KE, Economou E, Boutsikou M, Boutsikou T, Kyriakakou M, Puchner KP, Hassiakos D: Intrauterine growth restriction and circulating neurotrophin levels at term. Early Hum Dev 2007;83:465–469.
118 Tometten M, Blois S, Arck PC: Nerve growth factor in reproductive biology: link between the immune, endocrine and nervous system? Chem Immunol Allergy 2005;89:135–148.

Dr. Maike Pincus
Charité, University Medicine Berlin, Campus Virchow
Department of Pediatrics, Division of Pneumology and Immunology
Augustenburger Platz 1
DE–13353 Berlin (Germany)
Tel. +49 30 450 566 182, E-Mail maike.pincus@charite.de

Bienenstock J (ed): Allergy and the Nervous System.
Chem Immunol Allergy. Basel, Karger, 2012, vol 98, pp 85–99

Mind-Body Interrelationship in DNA Methylation

Moshe Szyf

Department of Pharmacology and Therapeutics, Sackler Program in Epigenetics and Psychobiology, McGill University, Montreal, Que., Canada

Abstract

DNA methylation is an enzymatic modification of the DNA molecule that confers unique differential identities upon similar DNA sequences. DNA methylation plays a critical role in cellular differentiation by conferring cell-type identity upon differentiated tissues in multicellular organisms by an innate developmentally programmed process. Recent data points to the possibility that DNA methylation plays a role in responding to external cues and conferring environment-context identity to DNA. DNA methylation is implicated in the response to early life social environment and might be playing an important role in setting up stable behavioral phenotypes in response to early-life social environment. The critical question is whether these responses are limited to the brain or involve the immune system as well. Addressing this question has important implications on understanding the mechanisms involved in DNA methylation mediated responses to the environment and how they impact the phenotype as well as on the possibility of studying the associations between DNA methylation and behavior and behavioral pathologies in living humans. A model is presented suggesting that DNA methylation acts as a mechanism of genome adaptation to the environment that is genomewide and systemwide. New data suggesting associations between DNA methylation patterns in white blood cells and the social environment will be discussed.

DNA Methylation

DNA methylation is a covalent modification of DNA [1] that is catalyzed by DNA methyltransferase enzymes (DNMT) which transfer a methyl moiety from the methyl donor S-adenosyl methionine (SAM) to the 5′ position on cytosine bases in DNA in most plans and animals [2, 3]. 6-Methyl adenine is found in bacteria [4] and certain lower eukaryotes [5, 6].

A high fraction of CG dinucleotide sequences in the genome is methylated [7]. There is evidence from genomic sequencing [8] and other specific gene studies [9] that other cytosines are methylated as well. However, the fraction of cytosines in non-

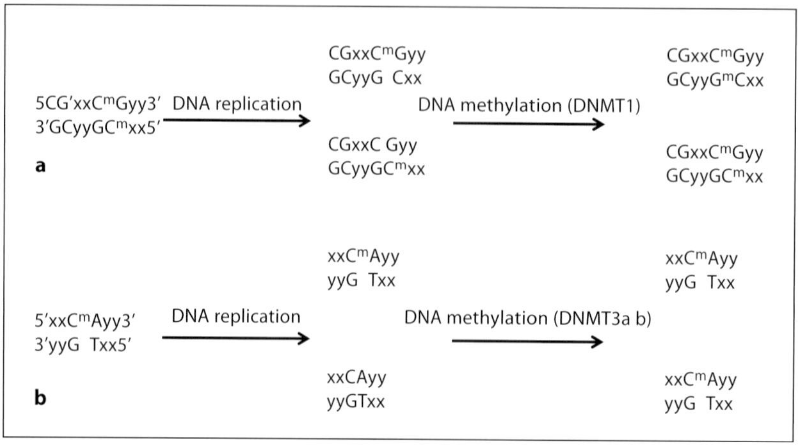

Fig. 1. Inheritance of DNA methylation during DNA replication. **a** Hemimethylated CG dinucleotide sequences are generated during DNA replication. These are preferentially recognized by the maintenance DNA methyltransferase DNMT1. The methylation state of the parental strand will be copied by the enzyme to the daughter strand. If the parental strand is unmethylated, a fully unmethylated strand is generated during cell division that is not methylated by the maintenance DNA methyltransferase. **b** A newly generated CA dinucleotide sequence does not have a guide in the template strand as the complementary dinucleotide sequence is GT. This site is de novo methylated by either DNMT3a or DNMT3b. It is unclear how the methylation state of these sites is memorized during DNA replication.

CG sequences that are methylated is significantly low. CG methylation is the only cytosine methylation that is found in a palindromic sequence; across a CG on the template strand there will be a CG on the complementary strand. This is therefore the only sequence where DNA methylation in one strand could be copied to the other by semiconservative DNA methyltransferases (fig. 1). It was demonstrated that DNMT1 could accurately copy DNA methylation from a template strand to the complementary unmethylated strand since it preferentially recognizes a hemimethylated substrate; a hemimethylated CG substrate is generated during DNA synthesis when a methylated CG is copied as a new unmethylated CG dinucleotide sequence [10]. Razin and Riggs [3] have suggested that this could explain the mitotic inheritance of DNA methylation. Thus, one of the properties of DNA methylation is that it is potentially heritable (fig. 1). An unanswered question is how are non-CG methylated sites replicated during cell division. Methylation of newly synthesized non-CG sites could not be determined by the state of methylation of the template strand since newly synthesized CC CA or CT sites are complemented by GG GT and GA on the template (fig. 1). Other mechanisms must exist that allow copying of the DNA methylation in non-CG sites [11]. It has been suggested that de novo DNMT3a or 3b which methylate unmethylated DNA substrates as efficiently as hemi-methylated substrates [12] are responsible for methylating non-CG as well as CG sites [13]; however, it is unclear how these enzymes could act to conserve DNA methylation patterns upon cell division.

Methyl moieties on DNA could be further modified by hydroxylation [14], formylation and carboxylation [15]. This modification of 5-methylcytosines is catalyzed by the TET enzymes (Ten Eleven Translocation Enzymes) [16]. The role that these modified methyl cytosines are playing in controlling gene expression is unclear. Several studies proposed that modified methylcytosines are intermediates in active demethylation pathways [15, 17, 18] but data suggest that, at least in some tissues, 5-hydroxymethylcytosine (5hmC) is maintained stably in the genome and might play a functional role in regulating genome function [14, 19]. Genomewide mapping of 5hmC in the brain suggests that 5hmC is mostly found in genes and is enriched at the promoters and in the intragenic regions (gene bodies). The presence of 5hmC in the gene bodies was positively correlated with gene expression [20]. Genomewide mapping of 5-hmC and TET1, showed association with both active or inactive chromatin marks [21, 22]. There is good reason to suspect that modification of methylated cytosines further refines the gene silencing signal of 5-methylcytosine.

DNA Methylation Confers Cell Type Identity on Identical DNA Sequences

One of the most important questions in embryology was understanding how could one genome express the stable multiple phenotypes required for the functioning of a multicellular organism? Waddington coined the term epigenetics more than half a century ago to indicate that the genome is canalized during gestation to acquire different epigenetic landscapes. There are several reasons why DNA methylation could act as a central component of the 'epigenetic' mechanism that stably marks DNA and confers upon identical genetic material cell-type-specific identities (fig. 2).

First, cell-specific DNA methylation patterns that are formed during cellular differentiation by innate developmental programs were described almost two decades ago [23, 24] and were recently confirmed by whole genome methylome mapping [8] (fig. 2). Second, differentiated cell types are stable phenotypes that need to be maintained for a lifetime. DNA methylation patterns at the palindromic CG dinucleotides could be accurately copied and therefore there is a mechanism for maintaining DNA methylation patterns through numerous cell divisions (fig. 1). Third, there is strong evidence that DNA methylation in regulatory sequences can silence gene expression. In vitro methylation of promoters results in silencing of gene expression in reporter assays [25]. Pharmacological inhibition of DNA methylation [26] or depletion of DNMT1 [27] results in induction of gene expression and a change in cell identity. Fourth, there is an inverse correlation between gene expression and promoter DNA methylation. This has been proposed three decades ago [23] and was confirmed by recent genome wide studies [28]. Genomewide studies show that promoters are devoid of DNA methylation and that that the same is true for certain regulatory regions [8]. Fifth, differentiation of cells in vitro is associated with changes in DNA methylation

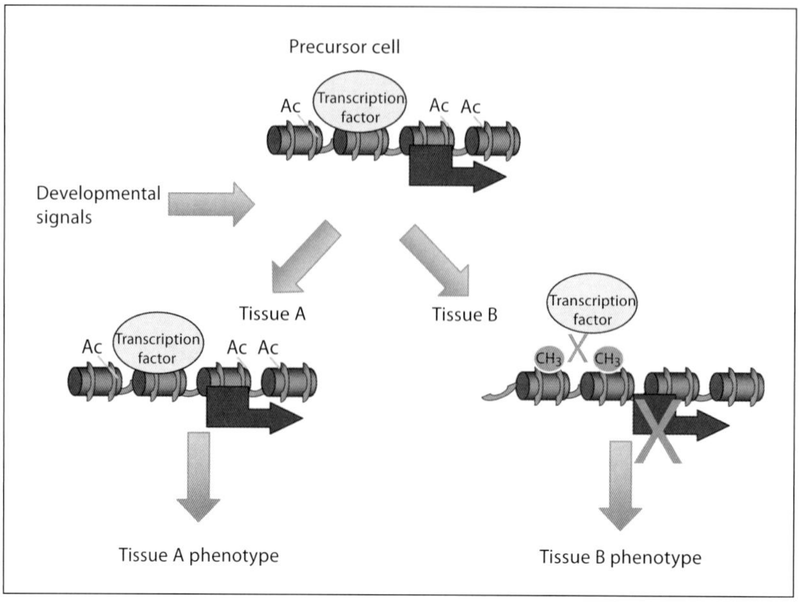

Fig. 2. DNA methylation confers upon identical sequences cell type identity. Although the DNA sequence is identical in different tissues, the state of DNA methylation is different. Methylation of the same gene in tissue B results in its silencing while its unmethylated state in tissue A enables expression. This allows for phenotypic diversity in spite of genetic identity. Ac = Histone acetylation; CH_3 = methylation; horizontal arrow = transcription; X = inhibition.

[29]. This was reconfirmed recently using next generation sequencing of bisulfite converted human embryonal stem cells and fetal fibroblast DNA [8]. Inhibitors of DNA methylation [30] as well as depletion of DNMT1 trigger cellular differentiation [27]. DNMT1 knockout mice are embryonal lethal and exhibit deficiencies in embryonal development [31].

DNA methylation is tightly correlated with other chromatin modifications such as histone acetylation and DNA methylation (for review of this interrelationship, see [32]).

The fact that DNA methylation is so critical for cell fate and cellular differentiation implies that DNA methylation in differentiated cells should remain stable. This was believed to be defined by the biochemical characteristics of DNA methylation reactions in differentiated cells. Maintenance DNMT1 copies accurately the DNA methylation pattern in dividing cells and there must be absence of enzymes that either add (de novo DNMTs) or remove (demethylase) methyl groups from DNA [3]. This model has precluded considering DNA methylation as a mechanism for adaptation of gene expression after birth. However, there is data to suggest that the model could be modified to accommodate the possibility of DNA methylation changes in response to external environmental triggers.

DNA Methylation as a Mechanism of Genomewide and Systemwide Genome Adaptation

It stands to reason that environmental exposures play a critical role in modulating the phenotype. It is also clear that external social exposures play a critical role in brain and behavioral development during childhood. The critical question is whether DNA methylation plays a role in these processes. Does DNA methylation change in response to external signals coming from the social and other environments as it does in response to the innate signals of embryonal development?

The role of DNA methylation in cellular differentiation has taught us that DNA methylation could act as a mechanism for conferring differential chemical identities to identical DNA sequences. During cellular differentiation such a mechanism can explain how one genome expresses multiple phenotypes in a multicellular organism. This is the question that Waddington and his colleagues had struggled with [33]. We suggest that the same mechanism can be at work in other instances where identical DNA sequences need to adapt different stable genome expression programs (fig. 3).

Based on these and other observations that will be discussed below we hypothesized that DNA methylation could act as a genome adaptation mechanism at multiple time scales from evolutionary time scales to proximal physiological time scales. At critical time points in life, such as early life, DNA methylation could serve as a genome adaptation mechanism to anticipated life-long environments based on cues derived from the early environment [34]. It is also proposed that since the environments that mammals and humans are exposed to early in life and later in life are complex involving interacting social, biological and physical spheres, the adaptation to early environment would involve multiple genes and functional gene networks and multiple systems including both the central nervous system ('mind') and the immune system ('body'). We therefore hypothesize that DNA methylation is tightly involved in mind-body integrated responses to the environment.

DNA Methylation Alterations in Response to Early Life Adversity during Gestation

An example of the long-term phenotypic effects of adverse external conditions during gestation is the impact of maternal diet during pregnancy on offspring metabolic health [35]. It was hypothesized that DNA methylation alterations are involved in this response. The Jirtle group has shown in the agouti (A(vy)) mouse model that maternal dietary methyl content supplementation affected the coat color of her offspring through DNA methylation changes [36–39]. In addition, nutritional manipulation is known to affect DNA methylation states in primates [40] and rodents [41]. In rodents, a protein-restricted diet results in an altered metabolic phenotype in the offspring that can be passed to the next generation and this involves significant

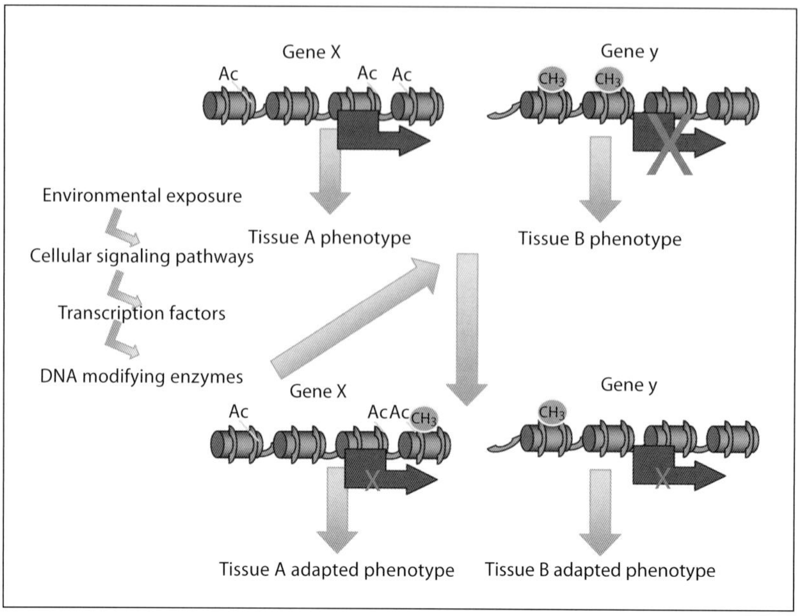

Fig. 3. DNA methylation adapts the state of gene expression in response to external signals, a model. Differential methylation of identical genes in different individuals that had different early life experiences, such as differences in maternal care, confer environmental context identity to similar DNA sequences creating phenotypic diversity in spite of genetic identity. A mechanism for this adaptation is proposed that is based on our studies of the effects of maternal care in rodents. Behavioral experiences trigger a signaling pathway that activates transcription factors that deliver DNA and chromatin-modifying enzymes to several genes in multiple tissues resulting in genomewide and systemwide alterations in DNA methylation. This alteration in DNA methylation occurs on the background of tissue specific DNA methylation patterns that were generated by innate developmental processes.

changes in DNA methylation in PPARalpha and GR promoters [41]. In a rat model of maternal high-fat (MHF) nutrition, the offspring develop a postnatal phenotype that closely resembles that of the human metabolic syndrome. In this model changes in DNA methylation and expression of the hepatic cell cycle inhibitor *Cdkn1a* were observed [42].

These results could invoke two alternative hypotheses. A rather simple and somewhat trivial hypothesis is that intervention with nutrients during pregnancy results in chemical imbalance that stochastically affects the generation of DNA methylation patterns during critical stages in development. Such a hypothesis is consistent with the idea that DNA methylation patterns are defined exclusively by innate developmental programs that could be disrupted by chemical imbalance. An alternative hypothesis is that nutritional imbalance delivers an adversity signal that is interpreted by the DNA methylation machinery as such and that DNA methylation states are programmed to respond to external signals as well as innate signals. If this is the case, then DNA methylation is a mechanism for genome adaptation to early life adversity. It is difficult to resolve this question using gestational nutritional models. These models are also unable to address the question of whether DNA methylation serves as a genome adaptation process after birth and during childhood, a period in life when external social, physical and biological environments are known to have a profound impact on the phenotype.

DNA Methylation Responses to Social Adversity after Birth

The main question is whether DNA methylation is reversible after birth [43]? Is the pattern of DNA methylation that is fashioned by innate developmental processes a final state or is it in a dynamic state which is responsive to external signals?

Although there was resistance in the field to accept the possibility of a reversible DNA methylation in postmitotic tissues, there is significant evidence for this hypothesis [44–48]. It has been shown that brain extracts are capable of demethylating 'naked' DNA substrate in vitro [49–51]. The strongest evidence for dynamic methylation-demethylation comes from several studies showing active demethylation in postmitotic neurons [52–55]. Conditional knock out of DNMT1 in postmitotic neurons results in DNA demethylation suggesting the presence of demethylation activity in nondividing neurons which is critical for a dynamic methylation pattern in the brain [56].

In order for DNA methylation to be maintained dynamically throughout life it is essential for the DNA methylation reaction to be reversible [43, 57]. Bhattacharya et al have proposed an active direct DNA demethylation that removes the methyl group from DNA catalyzed by the protein MBD2b [43, 57], this however was later contested [58]. A mechanism for active demethylation by MBD2b was proposed by Hamm et al. [59]. There has been a longstanding resistance in the field to accept that DNA methylation is reversible in differentiated tissues but this is essential if external signals derived from the environment could affect DNA methylation states after birth and later in life. Several indirect mechanisms of DNA demethylation have been proposed. First, DNMTs were proposed to deaminate the methyl cytosine to thymidine creating a C/T mismatch, which is then corrected by a mismatch-repair mechanism [60]. Second, Growth arrest and DNA-damage-inducible, alpha (GADD45A), a DNA repair protein was proposed to participate in catalysis of active DNA demethylation by an unknown DNA repair based mechanism [61]. Other studies have suggested involvement of GADD45B in demethylation in the brain [62]. Third, a complex sequence of coupled enzymatic reactions of deamination and mismatch repair were shown to be involved in demethylation in zebrafish: activation-induced cytidine deaminase (AID, which converts 5-meC to thymine), a G:T mismatch-specific thymine glycosylase methyl-CpG-binding domain protein 4 (MBD4) and repair promoted by GADD45A [63]. AID has been implicated in the global demethylation in mouse primordial germ cells as well [64]. An open question is the role of the newly discovered modification 5-hydroxymethylcytosine as a potential intermediate in the DNA demethylation reaction [14]. Recent data suggest that TET1 the enzyme that catalyzes the hydroxylation of 5-methylcytosine is present and required for stem cell maintenance of inner cell mass specification [16] and for activity-driven demethylation in neurons [17]. 5-Hydroxymethylation catalyzed by TET1 is followed by deamination of the 5-hydroxymethylated base by AID/APOBEC (apolipoprotein B mRNA-editing enzyme complex) family of cytidine deaminases and base excision repair enzymes replace the deaminated base with an unmethylated cytosine (BER) [17]. More recently, it has been proposed that 5-hydoxymethylcytosine is further carboxylated and this serves as a substrate for yet unknown decarboxylases that release the entire modified methyl moiety [15]. However, recent data show that loss of 5-hydroxymethylcytosine in the paternal genome during preimplantation occurs through a passive process that involves rounds of replication in absence of methylation and hydroxylation rather than an active removal by glycosylases such as TDG (thymidine deglycosylase) or decarboxylases [65]. Moreover, in myeloid cancers with mutant TET2 and deficient 5-hydroxymethylation activity DNA is hypomethylated rather than hypermethylated as would be expected if TET2 is involved in DNA demethylation [66]. These data are inconsistent with the hypothesis that TET2 is involved in DNA demethylation.

Notwithstanding the precise biochemistry, the fact that DNA methylation is reversible even in postmitotic tissue provides justification for examining the possibility that DNA methylation patterns are adapted to environmental signals including social signals in early life.

The clearest evidence that DNA methylation states can respond to external signals and that these signals are not limited to gestation comes from studies examining the impact of early life social environments on rodents DNA methylation patterns. Experiments by Weaver et al. [52] have demonstrated that differences in maternal care result in differences in DNA methylation transcription factor binding and histone acetylation in the hippocampus of the offspring. This epigenetic difference was maintained in the rats into adulthood. This study illustrated for the first time how an external behavioral signal such as intensity of maternal care could result in a change in chemical modification of DNA by methylation in the brain. The epigenetic response was mediated by activation of a serotoninergic signaling pathway that involved activation of protein kinase A and activation of a transcription factor NGFIA that delivered DNA and chromatin modifying enzymes to the NR3C1 gene [67]. This study charts a plausible pathway for external environmental social signals to target the DNA and alter states of DNA methylation and chromatin modification.

The DNA methylation state that is programmed by maternal care is stable throughout life but is nevertheless amenable to pharmacological methylation later in life in both directions towards increased or decreased DNA methylation [68, 69]. This suggests that DNA methylation states that are adapted to the environment early in life are dynamically maintained throughout life. This illustrates the unique properties and therapeutic potential of DNA methylation and epigenetic adaptations.

Early studies addressing the question of whether DNA methylation might act as a mechanism that programs gene expression in response to social adversity used a candidate gene approach and focused on the brain as an obvious target tissue. For example, exposure of infant rats to stressed caretakers that displayed abusive behavior produced persisting changes in methylation of BDNF gene promoter in the adult prefrontal cortex [70]. Early-life stress (ELS) in mice caused sustained DNA hypomethylation of an important regulatory region of the arginine vasopressin (AVP) gene [71].

Broad Response of the DNA Methylation State to Early Life Adversity

Although candidate gene approaches that show gene- and site-specific changes in DNA methylation in response to early life adversity are intellectually pleasing, it is nevertheless evident that the phenotypes described to be associated with early life adversity involve multiple gene functions and multiple systems in the body. If DNA methylation acts as a true genome adaptation mechanism it cannot be limited to several candidate genes. There is evidence supporting the hypothesis that the DNA methylation response to early life adversity leaves a broad mark in the genome. First, a family of ribosomal RNA promoters (rRNA) was shown to be differentially methylated in a cohort of suicide victims who were abused as children. rRNA genes are not considered to be a typical candidate gene in human behavioral pathologies [72]. More recently, we analyzed a 7-million-basepair region of chromosome 18 containing the NR3C1 gene in the hippocampus of adult rats [73]. A multidimensional epigenetic analysis of mRNA expression, histone acetylation and DNA methylation revealed coordinate clustered epigenetic changes associated with maternal behavior in the genome of their offspring across broad areas in the genome. Interestingly, the chromosomal region containing the *protocadherin-alpha, protocadherin-beta*, and *protocadherin-gamma (Pcdh)* gene families implicated in synaptogenesis show the highest differential response to maternal care [73]. This study illustrates that the response to early life adversity in the epigenome is widespread. Interestingly, similar broad differences in a syntenic genomic region spanning six and half million basepairs centered at the NR3C1 gene in the hippocampus was observed between humans who experienced abuse as children and non-abused controls [Suderman et al., unpubl. data]. This study illustrates evolutionary conservation of a broad DNA methylation response to child adversity. This is consistent with the hypothesis that DNA methylation is a mechanism of genome-adaptation to early life adversity.

The DNA Methylation Response to Early Life Social Adversity Is Not Limited to the Brain and Includes the Immune System as Well

A cardinal question is whether the DNA methylation changes that respond to early life adversity are limited to the brain or whether they occur in other physiological systems as well. There are several reasons to hypothesize that the DNA methylation response would be systemwide. First, early life environments are not isolated, they are usually coordinated. A long line of data have established that the physiological response to early life socioeconomic adversity is not limited to the brain [74–76]. Bio adversity, physical adversity and social adversity tend to cluster. It is possible therefore that a coordinated response in several tissues would react to these complex environments. Second, it stands to reason that there is a tight interrelationship between behavior, the regulation of metabolic states and the immune system. The best-studied example is the bilateral relationship between the HPA axis and the immune system. The HPA axis is a critical component of the bidirectional communication between immune and neuroendocrine systems. It is well known that increase in glucocorticoids in response to activation of the HPA axis results in silencing of gene expression of pro-inflammatory proteins and cytokines [77] and cytokines are known to affect the HPA axis [78–80]. Inflammatory cytokines have systemic effects far beyond the canonical immune response such as the classical 'sickness behavior' symptoms [81–83], which are similar to those of major depression and are induced by interferon alpha. Cytokine aberrations were suggested to be associated with various behavioral disorders such as anxiety disorder, depression, suicide, childhood mood disorder and post-traumatic stress disorder (PTSD) [84–91]. Early life social class can affect the expression of genes bearing response elements to CREB/ATF, NFKB and the glucocorticoid receptor (GR) in white blood cells [92].

It is therefore plausible that DNA methylation adaptations that are responsive to social behavior involve both the brain and the peripheral immune system as components of an integrated evolutionary conserved response that adapts the entire organism to anticipated life-long environments. However, different gene pathways are anticipated to be modified in different tissues since they evidently have different physiological roles in body-wide adaptations. As DNA methylation patterns are tissue specific as discussed above [23], it is not anticipated that the same DNA methylation changes would necessarily occur in both brain and peripheral tissues. It is hypothesized that several changes in DNA methylation in each tissue would target distinct gene pathways that are critical for the relevant physiological tasks of the tissue. However, it is possible that there are other genes that share common roles in several tissues and that the DNA methylation state of these genes will be modified similarly in different tissues in response to external cues.

Data are emerging to support this hypothesis. First, a recent study in differentially reared rhesus monkeys revealed changes in DNA methylation associated with rearing that are widespread in DNA derived from both T cells and prefrontal cortex [Provencal, Tremblay, Suomi et al., submitted 2011]. Second, we have initiated a study of the impact of socioeconomic positioning on DNA methylation that examined blood DNA from the British birth cohort of 1958. This study detected a signature of DNA methylation that was associated with early life adversity [93]. The DNA methylation changes that were associated with early life adversity clustered in large DNA segments across the genome supporting the hypothesis that social environment DNA methylation signatures are found systemwide and could be examined in peripheral blood cells. Third, post-traumatic stress was recently shown to be associated with DNA methylation changes in blood cells in genes that were involved in immune function [94].

Several candidate genes were found to be altered in peripheral blood cells in association with behavioral exposures and phenotypes. For example, the NR3C1 promoter was more methylated in lymphocytes in newborns exposed prenatally to maternal depression than control newborns [95]. Pituitary adenylate cyclase-activating polypeptide (PACAP), a protein known to be involved in the stress response in the pituitary, was found to be differentially methylated in peripheral blood cells in humans with post-traumatic stress syndrome [96]. A study that illustrated a peripheral response in DNA to social adversity early in life showed telomere lengths differences between orphans in the Bucharest Early Intervention Project who were placed under high-quality foster care compared with those subjected to continued care in institutions [97]. Although this study did not examine the role of DNA methylation in telomere length, it illustrated the intimate relationship between social exposure and DNA function in peripheral white blood cells.

The emerging realization that DNA methylation programming that is relevant to behavior might have peripheral manifestations has important mechanistic, therapeutic and diagnostic implications. If this is true, it will allow a better understanding of the intimate bilateral relationship of the brain and the immune system and how this interrelationship affects life-long adaptations of physiology and behaviors. Moreover, it will allow us to study epigenetic processes that are relevant to the brain in living humans.

Conclusions

DNA methylation is a mechanism that confers different identities upon identical sequences. This is important in cellular differentiation when one genome has to perform a vast variety of different programs in the different tissues of a multicellular organism. Innate and predictable developmental processes dictate this differentiation of DNA methylation patterns. What is emerging, however, is that the same mechanism can act in conferring 'environmental-context' identities on DNA in response to external signals before and after birth. The DNA methylation pattern adaptations in response to environmental signals affect several functional gene pathways and are clustered in long-range genomic regions. The response is not limited to the brain and affects the immune system as well. This is consistent with an intimate relationship between the immune system and the brain in coordinating a life-long response to early life signals. A great challenge will be to decipher the functional relationship between the gene pathways whose DNA methylation state is altered in response to early life experience in both immune cells and the brain and the long-term changes in behavioral and physical phenotypes. Identification of functional gene pathways that exhibit differential DNA methylation in response to behavioral signals might provide a clue as to the intimate interrelationships between mind and body in shaping life-long phenotypes.

Acknowledgements

The work from the M.S. laboratory described in this chapter is funded by grants from the Canadian Institute for Advanced Research, Canadian Institute for Health Research, The National Cancer Institute of Canada, the Sackler program in Epigenetics and Psychobiology at McGill University. M.S. is supported by a GSK/CIHR professorship.

References

1 Hotchkiss RD: The quantitative separation of purines, pyrimidines, and nucleosides by paper chromatography. J Biol Chem 1948;175:315–332.
2 Jeltsch A: Reading and writing DNA methylation. Nat Struct Mol Biol 2008;15:1003–1004.
3 Razin A, Riggs AD: DNA methylation and gene function. Science 1980;210:604–610.
4 Theil EC, Zamenhof S: Studies on 6-methylaminopurine (6-methyladenine) in bacterial deoxyribonucleic acid. J Biol Chem 1963;238:3058–3064.
5 Gorovsky MA: Genome organization and reorganization in *Tetrahymena*. Annu Rev Genet 1980;14:203–239.
6 Karrer KM, Vannuland TA: Methylation of adenine in the nuclear DNA of Tetrahymena is internucleosomal and independent of histone H1. Nucleic Acids Res 2002;30:1364–1370.
7 Gruenbaum Y, Stein R, Cedar H, Razin A: Methylation of CpG sequences in eukaryotic DNA. FEBS Lett 1981;124:67–71.
8 Lister R, Pelizzola M, Dowen RH, et al: Human DNA methylomes at base resolution show widespread epigenomic differences. Nature 2009;462:315–322.
9 Fuso A, Ferraguti G, Grandoni F, et al: Early demethylation of non-CpG, CpC-rich, elements in the myogenin 5′-flanking region: a priming effect on the spreading of active demethylation. Cell Cycle 2010;9:3965–3976.
10 Gruenbaum Y, Cedar H, Razin A: Substrate and sequence specificity of a eukaryotic DNA methylase. Nature 1982;295:620–622.
11 Szyf M: A dynamic methylome; implications of non-CG methylation/demethylation. Cell Cycle 2010;9:3846–3847.
12 Okano M, Bell DW, Haber DA, Li E: DNA methyltransferases Dnmt3a and Dnmt3b are essential for de novo methylation and mammalian development. Cell 1999;99:247–257.
13 Jurkowska RZ, Jurkowski TP, Jeltsch A: Structure and function of mammalian DNA methyltransferases. Chembiochem 2011;12:206–222.
14 Kriaucionis S, Heintz N: The nuclear DNA base 5-hydroxymethylcytosine is present in Purkinje neurons and the brain. Science 2009;324:929–930.
15 Ito S, Shen L, Dai Q, et al: Tet proteins can convert 5-methylcytosine to 5-formylcytosine and 5-carboxylcytosine. Science 2011;333:1300–1303.

16 Ito S, D'alessio AC, Taranova OV, Hong K, Sowers LC, Zhang Y: Role of Tet proteins in 5mC to 5hmC conversion, ES-cell self-renewal and inner cell mass specification. Nature 2010;466:1129–1133.
17 Guo JU, Su Y, Zhong C, Ming Gl, Song H: Hydroxylation of 5-methylcytosine by TET1 promotes active DNA demethylation in the adult brain. Cell 2011;145:423–434.
18 He YF, Li BZ, Li Z, et al: Tet-mediated formation of 5-carboxylcytosine and its excision by TDG in mammalian DNA. Science 2011;333:1303–1307.
19 Pastor WA, Pape UJ, Huang Y, et al: Genome-wide mapping of 5-hydroxymethylcytosine in embryonic stem cells. Nature 2011;473:394–397.
20 Jin SG, Wu X, Li AX, Pfeifer GP: Genomic mapping of 5-hydroxymethylcytosine in the human brain. Nucleic Acids Res 2011;39:5015–5024.
21 Wu H, D'alessio AC, Ito S, et al: Genome-wide analysis of 5-hydroxymethylcytosine distribution reveals its dual function in transcriptional regulation in mouse embryonic stem cells. Genes Dev 2011;25: 679–684.
22 Wu H, Zhang Y: Tet1 and 5-hydroxymethylation: a genome-wide view in mouse embryonic stem cells. Cell Cycle 2011;10:2428–2436.
23 Razin A, Szyf M: DNA methylation patterns. Formation and function. Biochim Biophys Acta 1984;782:331–342.
24 Benvenisty N, Szyf M, Mencher D, Razin A, Reshef L: Tissue-specific hypomethylation and expression of rat phosphoenolpyruvate carboxykinase gene induced by in vivo treatment of fetuses and neonates with 5-azacytidine. Biochemistry 1985;24: 5015–5019.
25 Stein R, Razin A, Cedar H: In vitro methylation of the hamster adenine phosphoribosyltransferase gene inhibits its expression in mouse L cells. Proc Natl Acad Sci USA 1982;79:3418–3422.
26 Jones PA: Altering gene expression with 5-azacytidine. Cell 1985;40:485–486.
27 Szyf M, Rouleau J, Theberge J, Bozovic V: Induction of myogenic differentiation by an expression vector encoding the DNA methyltransferase cDNA sequence in the antisense orientation. J Biol Chem 1992;267:12831–12836.
28 Rauch TA, Wu X, Zhong X, Riggs AD, Pfeifer GP: A human B cell methylome at 100-base pair resolution. Proc Natl Acad Sci USA 2009;106:671–678.
29 Razin A, Webb C, Szyf M, et al: Variations in DNA methylation during mouse cell differentiation in vivo and in vitro. Proc Natl Acad Sci USA 1984; 81:2275–2279.
30 Taylor SM, Constantinides Pα, Jones PA: 5-Azacytidine, DNA methylation, and differentiation. Curr Top Microbiol Immunol 1984;108:115–127.
31 Li E, Bestor TH, Jaenisch R: Targeted mutation of the DNA methyltransferase gene results in embryonic lethality. Cell 1992;69:915–926.
32 D'alessio AC, Szyf M: Epigenetic tête-à-tête: the bilateral relationship between chromatin modifications and DNA methylation. Biochem Cell Biol 2006;84:463–476.
33 Van Speybroeck L: From epigenesis to epigenetics: the case of C.H. Waddington. Ann NY Acad Sci 2002;981:61–81.
34 Szyf M: The early life social environment and DNA methylation; DNA methylation mediating the long-term impact of social environments early in life. Epigenetics 2011;6:971–978.
35 Hanson MA, Gluckman PD: Developmental origins of health and disease: new insights. Basic Clin Pharmacol Toxicol 2008;102:90–93.
36 Waterland RA, Jirtle Rl: Transposable elements: targets for early nutritional effects on epigenetic gene regulation. Mol Cell Biol 2003;23:5293–5300.
37 Dolinoy DC, Das R, Weidman JR, Jirtle Rl: Metastable epialleles, imprinting, and the fetal origins of adult diseases. Pediatr Res 2007;61:30R–37R.
38 Dolinoy DC, Weidman JR, Waterland RA, Jirtle Rl: Maternal genistein alters coat color and protects Avy mouse offspring from obesity by modifying the fetal epigenome. Environ Health Perspect 2006;114: 567–572.
39 Jirtle Rl, Skinner MK: Environmental epigenomics and disease susceptibility. Nat Rev Genet 2007;8: 253–262.
40 Unterberger A, Szyf M, Nathanielsz PW, Cox LA: Organ and gestational age effects of maternal nutrient restriction on global methylation in fetal baboons. J Med Primatol 2009;38:219–227.
41 Burdge GC, Slater-Jefferies J, Torrens C, Phillips ES, Hanson MA, Lillycrop KA: Dietary protein restriction of pregnant rats in the F0 generation induces altered methylation of hepatic gene promoters in the adult male offspring in the F1 and F2 generations. Br J Nutr 2007;97:435–439.
42 Dudley KJ, Sloboda DM, Connor Kl, Beltrand J, Vickers MH: Offspring of mothers fed a high fat diet display hepatic cell cycle inhibition and associated changes in gene expression and DNA methylation. PLoS One 2011;6:e21662.
43 Ramchandani S, Bhattacharya SK, Cervoni N, Szyf M: DNA methylation is a reversible biological signal. Proc Natl Acad Sci USA 1999;96:6107–6112.
44 Oswald J, Engemann S, Lane N, et al: Active demethylation of the paternal genome in the mouse zygote. Curr Biol 2000;10:475–478.

45 Lucarelli M, Fuso A, Strom R, Scarpa S: The dynamics of myogenin site-specific demethylation is strongly correlated with its expression and with muscle differentiation. J Biol Chem 2001;276:7500–7506.
46 Bruniquel D, Schwartz RH: Selective, stable demethylation of the interleukin-2 gene enhances transcription by an active process. Nat Immunol 2003;4:235–240.
47 Wilks A, Seldran M, Jost JP: An estrogen-dependent demethylation at the 5′ end of the chicken vitellogenin gene is independent of DNA synthesis. Nucleic Acids Res 1984;12:1163–1177.
48 Szyf M, Theberge J, Bozovic V: Ras induces a general DNA demethylation activity in mouse embryonal P19 cells. J Biol Chem 1995;270:12690–12696.
49 Mastronardi FG, Noor A, Wood DD, Paton T, Moscarello MA: Peptidyl argininedeiminase 2 CpG island in multiple sclerosis white matter is hypomethylated. J Neurosci Res 2007;85:2006–2016.
50 Dong E, Nelson M, Grayson DR, Costa E, Guidotti A: Clozapine and sulpiride but not haloperidol or olanzapine activate brain DNA demethylation. Proc Natl Acad Sci USA 2008;105:13614–13619.
51 Fuso A, Nicolia V, Cavallaro RA, Scarpa S: DNA methylase and demethylase activities are modulated by one-carbon metabolism in Alzheimer's disease models. J Nutr Biochem 2011;22:242–251.
52 Weaver IC, Cervoni N, Champagne FA, et al: Epigenetic programming by maternal behavior. Nat Neurosci 2004;7:847–854.
53 Feng J, Zhou Y, Campbell Sl, et al: Dnmt1 and Dnmt3a maintain DNA methylation and regulate synaptic function in adult forebrain neurons. Nat Neurosci 2010;13:423–430.
54 Levenson JM, Roth Tl, Lubin FD, et al: Evidence that DNA (cytosine-5) methyltransferase regulates synaptic plasticity in the hippocampus. J Biol Chem 2006;281:15763–15773.
55 Miller CA, Sweatt JD: Covalent modification of DNA regulates memory formation. Neuron 2007;53: 857–869.
56 Feng J, Fan G: The role of DNA methylation in the central nervous system and neuropsychiatric disorders. Int Rev Neurobiol 2009;89:67–84.
57 Bhattacharya SK, Ramchandani S, Cervoni N, Szyf M: A mammalian protein with specific demethylase activity for mCpG DNA. Nature 1999;397:579–583.
58 Hendrich B, Guy J, Ramsahoye B, Wilson VA, Bird A: Closely related proteins MBD2 and MBD3 play distinctive but interacting roles in mouse development. Genes Dev 2001;15:710–723.
59 Hamm S, Just G, Lacoste N, Moitessier N, Szyf M, Mamer O: On the mechanism of demethylation of 5-methylcytosine in DNA. Bioorg Med Chem Lett 2008;18:1046–1049.
60 Kangaspeska S, Stride B, Metivier R, et al: Transient cyclical methylation of promoter DNA. Nature 2008;452:112–115.
61 Barreto G, Schafer A, Marhold J, et al: Gadd45a promotes epigenetic gene activation by repair-mediated DNA demethylation. Nature 2007;445:671–675.
62 Ma DK, Jang MH, Guo JU, et al: Neuronal activity-induced Gadd45b promotes epigenetic DNA demethylation and adult neurogenesis. Science 2009;323: 1074–1077.
63 Rai K, Huggins IJ, James SR, Karpf AR, Jones DA, Cairns BR: DNA demethylation in zebrafish involves the coupling of a deaminase, a glycosylase, and gadd45. Cell 2008;135:1201–1212.
64 Popp C, Dean W, Feng S, et al: Genome-wide erasure of DNA methylation in mouse primordial germ cells is affected by AID deficiency. Nature 2010; 463:1101–1105.
65 Inoue A, Zhang Y: Replication-dependent loss of 5-hydroxymethylcytosine in mouse preimplantation embryos. Science 2011;334:194.
66 Ko M, Huang Y, Jankowska AM, et al: Impaired hydroxylation of 5-methylcytosine in myeloid cancers with mutant TET2. Nature 2010;468:839–843.
67 Weaver IC, D'alessio AC, Brown SE, et al: The transcription factor nerve growth factor-inducible protein a mediates epigenetic programming: altering epigenetic marks by immediate-early genes. J Neurosci 2077;27:1756–1768.
68 Weaver IC, Champagne FA, Brown SE, et al: Reversal of maternal programming of stress responses in adult offspring through methyl supplementation: altering epigenetic marking later in life. J Neurosci 2005;25:11045–11054.
69 Weaver IC, Meaney MJ, Szyf M: Maternal care effects on the hippocampal transcriptome and anxiety-mediated behaviors in the offspring that are reversible in adulthood. Proc Natl Acad Sci USA 2006;103:3480–3485.
70 Roth Tl, Lubin FD, Funk AJ, Sweatt JD: Lasting epigenetic influence of early-life adversity on the BDNF gene. Biol Psychiatry 2009;65:760–769.
71 Murgatroyd C, Patchev AV, Wu Y, et al: Dynamic DNA methylation programs persistent adverse effects of early-life stress. Nat Neurosci 2009;12: 1559–1566.
72 Mcgowan PO, Sasaki A, Huang TC, et al: Promoter-wide hypermethylation of the ribosomal RNA gene promoter in the suicide brain. PLoS ONE 2008;3: e2085.
73 Mcgowan PO, Suderman M, Sasaki A, et al: Broad epigenetic signature of maternal care in the brain of adult rats. PLoS One 2011;6:e14739.
74 Cunha F, Heckman JJ: The economics and psychology of inequality and human development. J Eur Econ Assoc 2009;7:320–364.

75 Power C, Hertzman C, Matthews S, Manor O: Social differences in health: life-cycle effects between ages 23 and 33 in the 1958 British birth cohort. Am J Public Health 1997;87:1499–1503.
76 Power C, Atherton K, Strachan DP, et al: Life-course influences on health in British adults: effects of socio-economic position in childhood and adulthood. Int J Epidemiol 2007;36:532–539.
77 Turnbull AV, Rivier Cl: Regulation of the hypothalamic-pituitary-adrenal axis by cytokines: actions and mechanisms of action. Physiol Revs 1999;79: 1–71.
78 Mastorakos G, Ilias I: Interleukin-6: a cytokine and/or a major modulator of the response to somatic stress. Ann NY Acad Sci 2006;1088:373–381.
79 Pace TW, Hu F, Miller AH: Cytokine-effects on glucocorticoid receptor function: relevance to glucocorticoid resistance and the pathophysiology and treatment of major depression. Brain Behav Immun 2007;21:9–19.
80 Turnbull AV, Rivier C: Regulation of the HPA axis by cytokines. Brain Behav Immun 1995;9:253–275.
81 Kronfol Z, Remick DG: Cytokines and the brain: implications for clinical psychiatry. Am J Psychiatry 2000;157:683–694.
82 Capuron L, Gumnick JF, Musselman Dl, et al: Neurobehavioral effects of interferon-alpha in cancer patients: phenomenology and paroxetine responsiveness of symptom dimensions. Neuropsychopharmacology 2002;26:643–652.
83 Schiepers OJ, Wichers MC, Maes M: Cytokines and major depression. Prog Neuropsychopharmacol Biol Psychiatry 2005;29:201–217.
84 Dowlati Y, Herrmann N, Swardfager W, et al: A meta-analysis of cytokines in major depression. Biol Psychiatry 2010;67:446–457.
85 Groer MW, Morgan K: Immune, health and endocrine characteristics of depressed postpartum mothers. Psychoneuroendocrinology 2007;32:133–139.
86 Hoge EA, Brandstetter K, Moshier S, Pollack MH, Wong KK, Simon NM: Broad spectrum of cytokine abnormalities in panic disorder and posttraumatic stress disorder. Depress Anxiety 2009;26:447–455.
87 Hallberg L, Janelidze S, Engstrom G, Wisen AG, Westrin A, Brundin L: Exercise-induced release of cytokines in patients with major depressive disorder. J Affect Disord 2010;126:262–267.
88 Janelidze S, Mattei D, Westrin A, Traskman-Bendz L, Brundin L: Cytokine levels in the blood may distinguish suicide attempters from depressed patients. Brain Behav Immun 2011;25:335–339.
89 Kawamura N, Kim Y, Asukai N: Suppression of cellular immunity in men with a past history of posttraumatic stress disorder. Am J Psychiatry 2001;158: 484–486.
90 Koo JW, Duman RS: IL-1beta is an essential mediator of the antineurogenic and anhedonic effects of stress. Proc Natl Acad Sci USA 2008;105:751–756.
91 O'Brien SM, Scott LV, Dinan TG: Cytokines: abnormalities in major depression and implications for pharmacological treatment. Hum Psychopharmacol 2004;19:397–403.
92 Miller GE, Chen E, Fok AK, et al: Low early-life social class leaves a biological residue manifested by decreased glucocorticoid and increased proinflammatory signaling. Proc Natl Acad Sci USA 2009; 106:14716–14721.
93 Borghol N, Suderman M, Mcardle W, et al: Associations with early-life socio-economic position in adult DNA methylation. Int J Epidemiol 2012;41:62–74.
94 Uddin M, Aiello AE, Wildman DE, et al: Epigenetic and immune function profiles associated with posttraumatic stress disorder. Proc Natl Acad Sci USA 2010;107:9470–9475
95 Oberlander TF, Weinberg J, Papsdorf M, Grunau R, Misri S, Devlin AM: Prenatal exposure to maternal depression, neonatal methylation of human glucocorticoid receptor gene (NR3C1) and infant cortisol stress responses. Epigenetics 2008;3:97–106.
96 Ressler KJ, Mercer KB, Bradley B, et al: Posttraumatic stress disorder is associated with PACAP and the PAC1 receptor. Nature 2011;470:492–497.
97 Drury SS, Theall K, Gleason MM, et al: Telomere length and early severe social deprivation: linking early adversity and cellular aging. Mol Psychiatry 2011 May 17. [Epub ahead of print].

Dr. Moshe Szyf
Department of Pharmacology and Therapeutics
Sackler Program in Epigenetics and Psychobiology, McGill University
3655 Sir William Osler Promenade
Montreal, QC H3G 1Y3 (Canada)
Tel. +1 514 398 4400, E-Mail moshe.szyf@mcgill.ca

Bienenstock J (ed): Allergy and the Nervous System.
Chem Immunol Allergy. Basel, Karger, 2012, vol 98, pp 100–117

Neurotrophins in Chronic Allergic Airway Inflammation and Remodeling

Harald Renz · Ayşe Kılıç

Institute of Laboratory Medicine and Pathobiochemistry, Molecular Diagnostics, Philipps University Marburg, Marburg, Germany

Abstract

Allergic asthma is a chronic inflammatory disease characterized by the production of allergen-specific IgE antibodies, TH2 inflammation, airway hyperresponsiveness and airway remodeling. Airway remodeling represents the disease-limiting stage during disease progression, and the underlying cellular molecular network resulting in airway remodeling are still poorly defined. In addition to the well-established TH2-dependent inflammatory response, several lines of investigation reveal that this regulation in the peripheral central nervous system contributes to disease development, exacerbation and progression. Several members of the neurotrophin family (e.g. nerve growth factor, brain-derived neurotrophic factor) are important transmitters of signals between the immune and the nervous system. Recent data indicate that NGF contributes to the development of airway remodeling in an inflammation and TGF-independent manner. These and other data open the opportunity to therapeutically interfere also on this level of regulation as a novel approach.

Neurotrophins (NTs) comprise a family of homologous proteins, showing similarities in receptor utilization and activity. Initially identified for their critical role in promoting neuronal growth, survival and differentiation [1], there is growing evidence for an eminent role of NTs exceeding the nervous system. NTs, which are elevated systemically and locally in the lung during allergic asthma, serve as 'trophic' factors for different immune cells, including cells of the innate and adaptive immune system. They promote survival, proliferation and differentiation as well as mediator release by immune cells. Beyond this immunomodulatory role of NTs, a direct role in controlling structural cell activity during inflammation and repair process has been established. These findings implicate a critical role for NTs in deregulated and chronic inflammatory processes, which finally lead to tissue remodeling in allergic asthma. This chapter summarizes the knowledge of NTs in allergic asthma and remodeling processes in the chronic inflamed lung.

Neurotrophins: Family Members and Synthesis

Classically, the NT family comprises four proteins, all similar in structure and function: nerve growth factor (NGF), brain-derived neurotrophic factor (BDNF), NT-3 and NT4/NT5.

NTs are synthesized as preproprotein precursors of ~27 kDa, which are cleaved intracellularly by furin or pro-hormone convertases to form pro-NTs [2]. These pro-NTs are either packed into constitutive vesicles in the case of pro-NGF, pro-NT3 and pro-NT4/NT5, or pro-BDNF is loaded into regulated secretory vesicles for secretion. Extracellularly, these pro-NTs are further processed by plasmin or the matrix metalloproteinases (MMP) 3 and 7 to release the mature NTs with a molecular weight of ~13–15 kDa. Mature NTs BDNF, NT3 and NT4 share approximately 50% sequence identity with NGF and all show a high degree of homology across species (90–100%).

Neurotrophin Receptors and Basics of Neurotrophin Signaling

NTs exert their divergent biological effects by utilizing two structurally unrelated receptor systems: the tropomyosin-related tyrosin kinases (Trk) and the 'pan-neurotrophin' receptor of 75 kDa ($p75^{NTR}$) (Fig. 1).

Trk receptors, with molecular weights of 140–145 kDa, are preferentially activated by the binding of mature NT dimers (dissociation constant [K_d] 10^{-11} M) for which they show ligand specificity. The TrkA receptor preferentially binds NGF, while TrkB interacts with BDNF and NT4/NT5 and the TrkC receptor is activated by binding of NT3 [3, 4]. These receptors are expressed in both full-length and truncated isoforms [3]. Although the expression of truncated receptor isoforms is documented, their functional role remains unclear. Biological activity of NTs requires binding to full-length Trk receptors.

Binding of an NT dimer leads to dimerization of two receptor chains and subsequent auto-phosphorylation. Intracellularly, three main pathways are activated: phospholipase C γ (PLCγ), phosphatidyl-inositol 3-kinase (PI3K) and the mitogen-activated protein kinsases (MAPK), extracellular regulated kinase (ERK) and p38MAPK [5]. Signaling via Trk receptors induces activation, migration and survival in the target cell.

The $p75^{NTR}$ belongs to the tumor necrosis factor (TNF) receptor/Fas/CD40 superfamily. It binds all four NTs, preferably the pro-NTs, with the same affinity (K_d 10^{-9} M). Binding of NTs leads to trimerization of the receptor chains and subsequent activation of intracellular pathways, which evoke two different effects in the signal perceiving cells. Activation of c-jun terminal kinase (JNK) and subsequent phosphorylation of pro-apoptotic proteins, including Bad, p53 and Bax, induces cytochrome c release from mitochondria. This further leads to caspase-3 and caspase-9

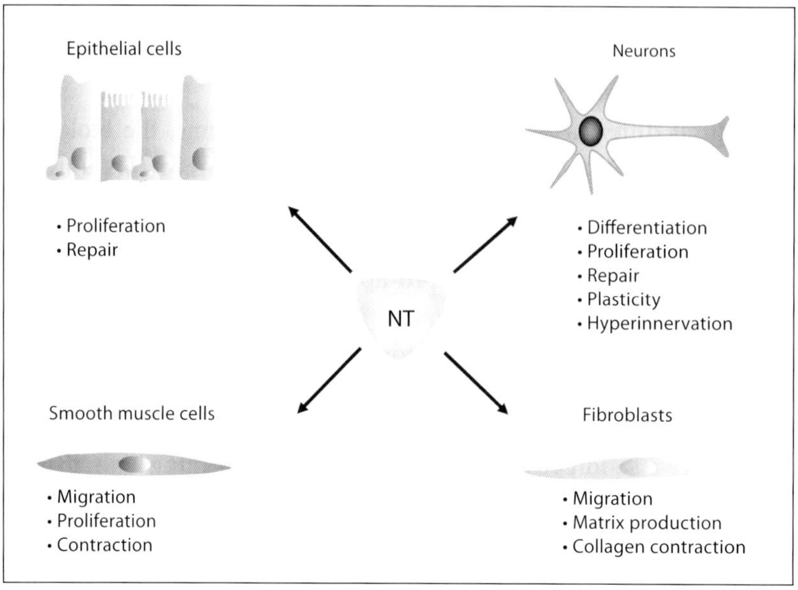

Fig. 2. Sources and targets of NT in the allergic inflamed lung: structural cells.

on proliferating epithelial cells [13]. In the presence of an inflammatory stimulus, provided by TNF-α and IL-1β [14], an augmented expression of epithelial NT was observed in vitro. These findings indicate that NGF signaling is active in the injured epithelium and silenced in the normal lung.

Beneath the airway epithelium, a thin layer of pulmonary fibroblasts resides. Using human bronchial biopsy sections NT expression by these cells was shown. Although the functions of NT in lung fibroblasts are still being explored, there is evidence for a prominent role of NGF. The expression of NGF as well as its receptors TrkA and $p75^{NTR}$ could be confirmed in cultured human and murine pulmonary fibroblasts [15, 16].

Besides the above-mentioned structural cells, there is evidence for NT production by smooth muscle cells as well. In lung sections of nonasthmatic human subjects, constitutive expression of the ligands NGF, BDNF and NT3 by airway smooth muscle cells (ASM) was detected [12]. While expression of TrkB could be confirmed by immunocytochemistry, $p75^{NTR}$ was not. Yet, more recent studies performed on isolated human bronchial smooth muscle cells, show the expression of BDNF, NT-3 and NT-4 as well as the receptors TrkB, TrkC and $p75^{NTR}$ [17, 18]. In the presence of an inflammatory response, when cytokines like IL-1β and TNF-α are present, ASM strongly upregulate the expression of NT. Using the model of isolated bronchial ASM, IL-1β induced expression of NGF and BDNF, as well as TNF-α increased BDNF and NT-3 levels are documented. In contrast, the proinflammatory cytokine interferon (IFN)-γ selectively increases NGF-levels while decreasing BDNF expression [19,

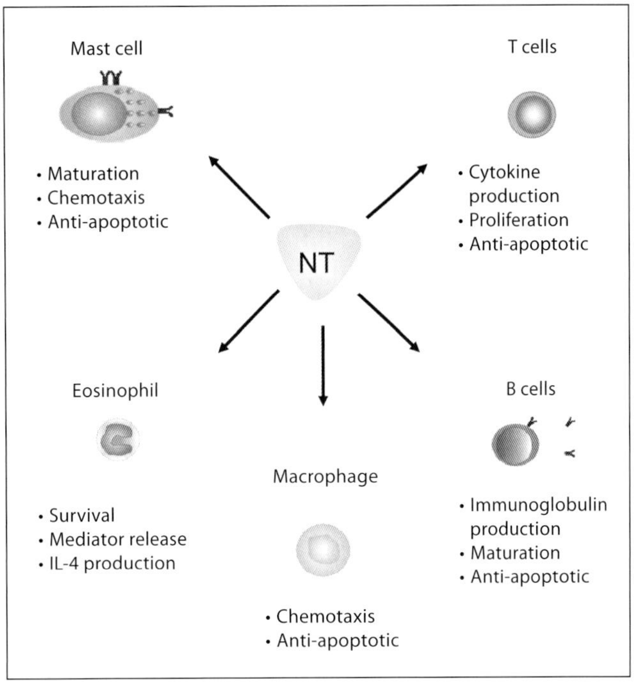

Fig. 3. Sources and targets of NT in the allergic inflamed lung: inflammatory cells.

20]. In contrast to NT function in bronchial ASM, the role of NT in vascular smooth muscle cell biology is less well defined. Thus far, the expression of NGF and $p75^{NTR}$ were identified.

Neurotrophin Expression in the Immune System

Allergic diseases are characterized by a unique activation pattern of innate and adaptive immune cells resulting in cellular and humoral immune responses such as eosinophilia and production of immunoglobulin (Ig) E antibodies.

Although NTs were discovered and described as neuronal growth factors, the expression of NTs and NT receptors has been reported in various cell types. Especially immune cells are capable of expressing the ligands and several NT receptors depending on the developmental and activation state (Fig. 3).

Lymphocytes. Based on cognate and noncognate signals naïve CD4+ T cells perceive during sensitization to an allergen, their differentiation T helper type 2 (TH2) cells occurs. By secreting characteristic soluble mediators, these cells shape and orchestrate the subsequent inflammatory response, inducing IgE production in B cells, maturation of eosinophils in the bone marrow and differentiation of epithelial cells into mucus-producing cells. The expression of NGF and TrkA but not

$p75^{NTR}$ is documented in TH2 cells. In contrast to TH2 cells, in TH1 cells as another inflammatory subset neither the expression ligands nor receptors could be confirmed, linking NT to helper type 2-mediated diseases. Same as TH2 cells, B cells are not only producers [21, 22] but also responders to NT signaling. For B cells, the expression of ligands as well as both NGF receptors, Trks and $p75^{NTR}$, is documented [23]. Yet the expression pattern of the receptors seems to be restricted to different developmental and differentiation stages. While the expression of BDNF and its receptor TrKB is linked to proper development of B lymphocytes, mature and finally differentiated CD138+ plasma cells rather express NGF and TrkA as wells NT3 and TrkC [21].

Mast cells, as resident tissue cells, are critical effector cells in allergic diseases. Upon binding of allergens to membrane bound IgE receptors, these cells become activated and release a plethora of soluble mediators, directly contributing to immediate hypersensitivity reactions. Mast cells express NGF, BDNF and NT3 as well as their corresponding receptors TrkA, TrkB and TrkC [24]. Besides being a target cell population for NTs, mast cells produce NGF, BDNF and NT3. Upon IgE cross-linking triggered release of NGF occurs [25], suggesting that allergens induce NT release in diseases such as asthma.

Eosinophils represent the major cell population infiltrating allergic inflamed airways. They differentiate from precursors in the bone marrow and, after short systemic circulation, home to the inflamed tissue. Depending on the organ compartment, maturation and activation state, eosinophils are able to express all NT receptors. In bone marrow, the expression of TrkB and TrkC, but not TrkA and $p75^{NTR}$, is documented [26]. The expression of NT receptors in peripheral blood eosinophils is controversially discussed. While one study was able to show the expression of all receptors on peripheral blood eosinophils showing varying levels of Trk- mRNA and protein levels among patients [27]. Another study was not able to detect these receptors in eosinophils recovered from allergic patients. In contrast, eosinophils recovered from bronchoalveolar lavage (BAL) after allergen provocation of allergic asthmatics express all NT receptors. Besides representing a target cell population for NTs, eosinophils are possible cellular sources for these soluble mediators [28].

Monocytes and macrophages were identified as strong producers of NGF and BDNF in humans and animals. Human peripheral blood monocytes constitutively express BDNF [29] and NGF [30]. In allergic patients, the cellular content as well as the release of NGF was found to be significantly enhanced compared to healthy donors. Whereas BDNF and NT3 levels did not differ among both groups [31]. For alveolar macrophages capable of producing cytokines critically involved in the induction and propagation of an allergic immune response [32], an elevated expression of NGF and BDNF is documented after allergen challenge in a murine model of allergic airway inflammation [33, 34]. Pro-inflammatory cytokines, including IL-6 and TNF-α, which are released after monocytes/macrophage activation, induce the secretion of BDNF by these cells [35].

While these data clearly identify immune cells as major sources for NT production during allergic inflammation, the affected target cell populations, either other immune or resident structural cells, are still under investigation. It is very likely that NTs modulate the expression of cytokines and receptors in immune cells, making these cells more susceptible to the surrounding milieu and therefore shaping or shifting the pattern of inflammation. Evidence for such an effect is reported in dendritic cells (DC). Depending on the atopic state of a subject, NTs exert opposing effects on TrkA and TrkB expressing DCs. Upon NGF and BDNF treatment, dendritic cells from healthy subjects produce anti-inflammatory IL-10, while DCs from allergic patients secrete pro-inflammatory IL-6 [36].

The diverse expression pattern of NT and their receptor systems combined with the versatile functions elicited in different cell populations implicates a key role for NT in complex inflammatory diseases. In chronic inflammatory diseases both immune as well as structural cells are constantly activated and, with the release of a variety of soluble mediators, control the ongoing immune response which finally affects organ function.

Neurotrophins in Atopic Diseases

NT levels are low under physiologic conditions; however, their levels increase significantly in allergic diseases. In bronchial asthma, high levels of systemic NGF, BDNF and NT3 [37] as well as enhanced local expression of NGF and BDNF are detectable in BAL fluid [38]. Local expression of these NTs is further augmented by allergen provocation in both human and mouse [38], suggesting that allergen challenge represents a strong trigger for NT production in the airways. In other atopic diseases, including allergic rhinitis and atopic dermatitis, elevated levels of peripheral blood and local, including nasal lavage and skin, NGF and BDNF are reported [39]. In atopic dermatitis, these increased NT levels show a positive correlation with severity of the disease. Although, these data show a clear association between allergic diseases and NTs, the sources of NTs as well as target cell populations and functional consequences in target cells are still being defined.

Neurotrophins in Chronic Allergic Airway Inflammation and Remodeling

During the ongoing allergic immune response, infiltrating immune cells secrete a plethora of toxic metabolites, growth factors and cytokines, which induce proliferation of resident structural and neuronal cells resulting in morphological and functional changes of the lung tissue. A consequence of this augmented release of inflammatory mediators is neuronal dysfunction. Yet, there is growing evidence that neurons and activated resident structural cells not only represent target cell population, but are capable of influencing the immune response by secreting cytokines and soluble mediators. In this context, NTs have gained great attention. They represent signaling molecules, exerting bidirectional activity, regulating inflammatory interactions between neuronal, immune and structural cells. This section summarizes the knowledge of NT function in chronic allergic airway inflammation and remodeling.

Neurotrophins and Airway Hyperresponsiveness

Airway hyperresponsiveness, as a characteristic feature of bronchial asthma, consists of an increased sensitivity of the airways, in particular neuronal cells, to an inhaled constrictor agonist. Allergic airway inflammation affects neuronal activity at both the function of afferent sensory nerves and synaptic transmission within autonomic ganglia. Sensory nerve endings become exposed as a consequence of epithelial cell shedding in allergic airway inflammation. This elicits activation of these cells and triggers an axonal response. This immediate response provides a protective mucosal defense mechanism, resulting in coughing and sneezing. These physiologic reactions serve to clear the upper and lower airways from irritant agents. Changes in sensory innervation of asthmatic airways are regulated by mediators released during allergic inflammation. The mechanism of NT-mediated airway hyperreactivity (AHR) has been elucidated using animal models of allergic airway inflammation, in which sensory airway reactivity was measured using the vanilloid receptor agonist capsaicin.

Transgenic overexpression of NGF in murine airway epithelial cells (NGF-Tg mice) results in an increase of tachykinin-containing sensory fibers in airways and an augmented reactivity to capsaicin [40]. Vice versa, sensory reactivity is almost abolished in transgenic mice lacking functional $p75^{NTR}$ expression, which is possibly due to reduced amounts of substance P in the lungs of these mice [41]. Although, sensory nerves innervating the airways express NT receptors [42], the contribution of NTs to airway hyperresponsiveness is mediated by the induction of neuropeptide synthesis and release. Neuropeptides of the tachykinin family, including substance P and neurokinins A and B, are the main neurotransmitters of the excitatory sensory nervous system. An increase of substance P-immunoreactive nodose neurons is observed in allergen-challenged animals. Intratracheal application of NGF causes the same effect. NGF induces neuropeptide expression [43] and a phenotypic switch in sensory airway innervation. This switch is inducing de novo synthesis of substance P and therefore allowing more sensory neurons to become part of the tachykinergic lung innervation [44]. Using the model of isolated tracheal rings, NGF was shown to increase airway reactivity by inducing the release of stored substance P from sensory nerve endings, independently of neuropeptide synthesis in soma [45].

Although, a direct role of NTs on sensory neurons is documented, cholinergic neurons, regulating airway smooth muscle tone and contractility, do not represent a direct target cell population for NTs. However, an indirect regulation of cholinergic neurons is provided by directly altering the local axonal reflex circuit. Irritation of sensory neurons triggers airway smooth muscle contractility through activation of cholinergic receptors. Therefore, NT-mediated alterations in sensory innervation subsequently modulate bonchoconstrictor pathways [46].

Although NGF does not activate cholinergic neurons, in vitro data provide evidence that direct activation of smooth muscle cells via Trk receptors may occur in chronic allergic airways disease. Activation of ASM through Trk receptors may provide a further mechanism for rapid $[Ca^{2+}]_i$ mobilization contributing to increased smooth muscle contractility and therefore bronchocontriction.

Neurotrophins and Allergic Airway Inflammation

The airway epithelium, serving as the first line of defense to inhaled allergens and infectious agents, becomes activated when coming into contact with enzymatically active allergens. This activation initiates a cascade of events which result in recruitment of different immune cells aiming to clear the invading agent. The inflammatory response is controlled by the release of epithelial factors either recruiting immune cells or ensuring their survival at the site of inflammation. Once the foreign agent is removed, levels of epithelium derived factors decrease and terminate the immune response. Therefore, factors which are actively secreted by airway epithelial cells following allergen provocation regulate the subsequent inflammatory response. NT serve as such epithelium derived factors, able to affect the activity of infiltrating immune cells. Epithelial-derived NGF and BDNF levels are increased in humans and mouse models of allergic asthma after allergen provocation. In vitro experiments, performed on human airway epithelial cells, suggest an induction of NT expression by proinflammatory cytokines such as TNF-α and IL-1β [14].

Allergic inflammation is controlled by the activity of TH2 cells. A functional role for NTs in regulating the activity of this cell population, central to allergic diseases, has been established by showing TrkA and NGF but not $p75^{NTR}$ expression. TrkA activation in TH2 cells is associated with the induction of proliferation as well as modulation of TH2-dependent immunoglobulin synthesis. Activation of the transcription factor c-fos by NGF and TrkA signaling increases the synthesis of IL-4 and IL-10 in TH2 cells [33]. This finding implicates, that especially NGF modulates the severity of allergic airway inflammation. The role of NTs in TH2-related diseases is further highlighted by the finding that TrkA expression is restricted to TH2 cells and could not be confirmed on TH1 cells. One downstream event of TH2 activation is the production of IgE antibodies by B cells. Same as TH2 cells, B cells are not only producers but also responders to NT signaling. For B cells, the expression of ligands as well as NT receptors is documented. In mature B cells, NGF induces proliferation and differentiation events and further augments immunoglobulin expression. NGF not only affects short-term events in B cells, but also promotes survival of memory B cells [23]. This effect is mediated by downstream activation of p38 MAPK in these cells, inducing anti-apoptotic protein expression and activation of the NFκB pathway. In terminally differentiated plasma cells, which not only home to primary and secondary lymphoid organs, but also reside within the inflamed tissue, NGF together with NT3 exerts anti-apoptotic activity [21]. Therefore, NTs are critically involved in regulating the atopic state of an individual and promote IgE-dependent inflammatory responses.

Mast cells represent a subset of effector cells, which is activated by IgE. In allergic inflamed tissues mast cell numbers are increased. Soluble factors are thought to regulate their infiltration into and residency at the inflamed tissue. Especially NGF was shown to regulate number and activity of mast cell in allergic inflamed airways. In asthmatic airways, increased mast cells numbers go in line with elevated NGF levels in BAL fluid [47]. The functional relevance of NGF in mast cells activity was analyzed in a murine model of allergic airway inflammation. In this, blockade of NGF signaling, by intranasal application of a neutralizing antibody, was shown to prevent the allergen induced early phase reaction, which is initiated by mast cell degranulation [48, 49]. A converse approach, using transgenic overexpression of NGF in murine airway epithelial cells (NGF-Tg mice), showed an augmented early phase reaction, measured by allergen-induced bronchoconstriction and serotonin release [49]. These observed effects were further characterized on the molecular level in various studies. In these, NGF was shown to regulate process like homing, survival and differentiation of mast cells. NGF acts as a chemoattractant [50] and as a cofactor for stem cell factor in preventing apoptosis of these cells [51]. NGF itself, as well as a combination of NGF and stem cell factor, induces and increases the expression of mast cell markers, including IgE-receptor type I (FcεRI), chymase and mast cell-specific tryptase [52]. Furthermore, NGF modulates the expression of inflammatory cytokines in these cells, e.g. induction of IL-6 [53] and reduction of TNF-α [54] expression. NGF not only acts on mast cells but is also released by IgE crosslinking. NGF could therefore modulate airway inflammation by acting in an autocrine manner regulating mast cell activity, or by exerting its effect in a paracrine fashion affecting resident or recruited cells.

In the late phase of the allergic immune response large numbers of eosinophils are recruited to the inflamed lung. These cells become activated in the lung and secrete a plethora of toxic metabolites, e.g. eosinophilic peroxidase (EPO) and eosinophil cationic protein (ECP), and substantially contribute to tissue destruction. Although these cells are programmed to die within a short time, factors, which promote survival of these cells in the tissue, critically regulate the severity of tissue destruction. Although data on tissue eosinophils are not available, studies performed on BAL eosinophils of asthmatics hint towards a function of NT in these cells. This effect was delineated, when BAL eosinophils were cultured in the presence of NTs. After observing prolonged survival of these cells in the presence of NTs, their role as survival factors for BAL eosinophils was established [55]. Studies performed in mice further strengthened this observation. NGF-Tg mice showed a significantly enhanced recruitment of eosinophils to the allergic inflamed airways compared to WT littermates. This phenomenon was proven to be attributable to increased NGF levels in the airways, by using a function blocking anti-NGF antibody in a mouse model of allergic airway inflammation. In this study a clear reduction of eosinophil numbers in the airways was observed [49]. In line with the latter observation, studies conducted in $p75^{NTR}$-deficient mice show decreased numbers of eosinophils in allergic inflamed lung tissue as well [56].

Taking into consideration that the above-mentioned sequence of processes is repetitively initiated upon allergen contact, it is justifiable to conclude that especially NGF is critically involved in the initiation and progression of allergic airway inflammation. NGF is secreted in high levels by the activated airway epithelium and augments the activity and survival of all immune cells vigorously participating in the allergic reaction. The fact, that these immune cells not only respond to NGF, but secrete NGF upon activation as well, implicate that the behavior of these cells is not only regulated in an autocrine but also paracrine manner by each other. Such regulation leads to the formation of a vicious cycle, in which NGF amplifies the allergic immune response by augmenting the activity and survival of immune cells (Fig. 4). This causes further tissue destruction and results in even higher levels of NGF, paving the way for yet another round of inflammation and tissue destruction.

Neurotrophins and Airway Remodeling

A consequence of recurring allergen contact is the destruction of the lung tissue. The injured airways react with the initiation of repair mechanisms aiming tissue integrity. The process of tissue repair comprises three distinct phases: (1) transient inflammation for the clearance of injured and apoptotic cells, (2) matrix production and proliferation of resident epithelial cells and fibroblasts for the reconstitution of the epithelial lining, and (3) the remodeling phase in which the aberrantly produced matrix is degraded. In order to assure proper repair of the tissue, these three phases are tightly controlled and occur sequentially. Yet, as a result of a repetitive allergen contact, the inflammatory as well as repair machinery becomes activated at parallel sites in the tissue. Due to overlap of these distinct steps, deregulation of the repair process occurs, leading to structural changes in the asthmatic airways. These alterations include epithelial shedding and the occurrence of mucus-producing goblet cells in the epithelium, thickening of the reticular basement membrane, comprising excessively produced matrix proteins like collagens, and thickening of the smooth muscle layer.

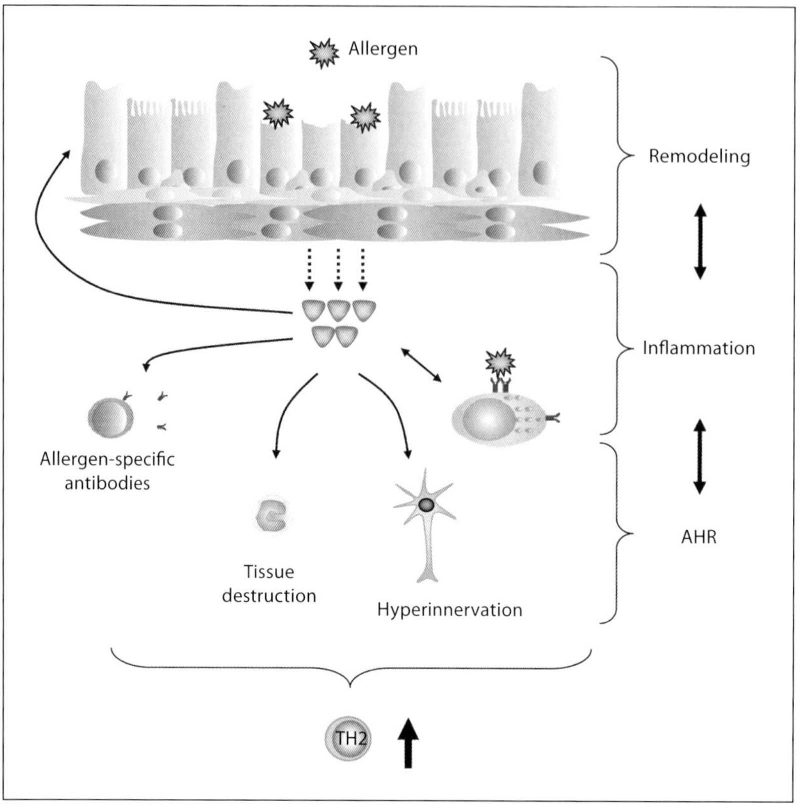

Fig. 4. NTs in chronic allergic airway inflammation and remodeling. NTs are released upon tissue damage by airway structural cells, including the epithelium, fibroblasts and smooth muscle cells. This could serve as an initial signal for the upregulation of NT receptors on incoming inflammatory cells and structural cells in an autocrine and/or paracrine manner. NT-induced survival and activation of inflammatory cells leads to augmented tissue destruction and in turn to higher NT production. This allows NT to modulate many processes, including hyperinnervation, AHR, airway remodeling and an increased TH2 phenotype, exacerbating the symptoms of asthma.

A role for epithelial NT expression in modulating lung structure and function was established in in vitro experiments and mouse models of epithelial damage. Using the in vitro model of RSV infection of cultured human bronchial epithelial cells, Othumpangat et al. [11] were able to show the importance of NGF for epithelial survival. In this study, enhanced epithelial apoptosis was observed in the absence of NGF. Using a mouse model of naphthalene-induced depletion of Clara cells as well as in vitro experiments performed on airway epithelial cells, our group was able to show that NGF enhances Clara cell proliferation. In these studies, blockade of NGF activity with a neutralizing antibody resulted in delayed wound closure. Conversely, epithelial repair was accelerated in the presence of high NGF in murine airways and therefore showing the reparative activity of NGF in lungs [13].

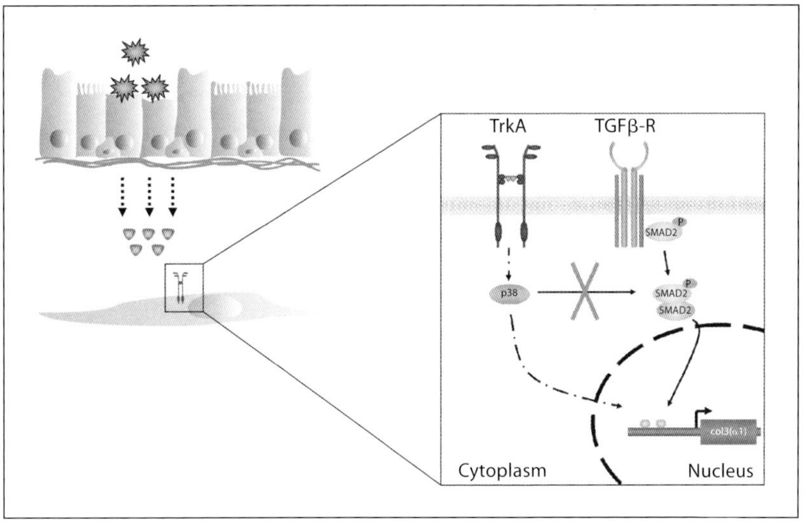

Fig. 5. NGF induces airway fibrosis. NGF, secreted by injured airway epithelial cells, can bind to TrkA receptors on lung fibroblasts. Activation of downstream p38 MAPK, independently of the TGFβ/SMAD pathway, induces type III collagen expression and contributes to augmented deposition of collagen fibers in asthmatic airways.

Yet, for proper repair a close interaction of epithelial cells and fibroblasts is important. Therefore, epithelial repair strongly depends on and at the same time, by secreting soluble mediators, controls fibroblast activity. A misbalance in this interaction, e.g. overproduction of epithelial factors, can easily lead to aberrant activation of fibroblasts and result in organ fibrosis. Several in vitro results show responsiveness of fibroblasts to NGF signaling. Migration as well as contraction of these cells was shown to be influenced by NGF. Studies of our own group could further elucidate an important role for NGF in matrix production. Using a mouse model for chronic allergic airway inflammation, we could show that aberrant NGF production contributes to subepithelial airway fibrosis by directly affecting collagen deposition in inflamed airways. By functionally blocking NGF activity during the course of this model with an antibody, alleviated levels of collagen productions was observed. Conversely, NGF-Tg mice already show increased amounts of collagen in the airways in the absence of an inflammatory response. Using the in vitro system of cultured mouse lung fibroblasts, we were able to detect a NGF-dependent induction of type III collagen expression (Fig. 5). Further studies revealed that this effect was mediated via the NGF receptor TrkA and downstream p38 MAPK activation, independently of the TGFβ/SMAD pathway. Although cultured mouse lung fibroblasts express $p75^{NTR}$ as well, we could not confirm a functional role of this receptor system in mediating matrix expression induced by NGF, neither in vitro nor in vivo [15]. Yet, these data implicate that NGF levels need to be tightly controlled in the lung in order to prevent pathological changes. Combined with the above mentioned functions of NGF in airway epithelial cells, NGF might act either in an autocrine or a paracrine fashion on these cell types.

Whether NGF affects smooth muscle hypertrophy in chronic allergic airways is not well understood. In vitro studies performed on isolated human bronchial smooth muscle cells helped to define the role of single NT and receptor systems on ASM function. In this regard, BDNF and NT4 were shown to enhance $[Ca^{2+}]_i$ and force responses of ASM to agonists like acetylcholine (ACh). In contrast, NT-3 seems to counteract these two NT by blunting the $[Ca^{2+}]_i$ response. These data indicate a modulatory role of NT in terms of controlling ASM contractility, regardless of their cellular source. Besides regulating this rapid response in SMC, BDNF was shown to regulate proliferation of these cells. By activating proliferation-specific pathways like ERK1/2 and PI3K/Akt1, BDNF was shown to enhance human ASM cell proliferation [57] and could therefore affect ASM hypertrophy in asthmatic airways.

This far, NGF as well as $p75^{NTR}$ were identified to impact vascular smooth muscle cell functions. By activating similar pathways like platelet-derived growth factor -BB, NGF induces migration, but not proliferation, of these cells [58]. Activation of $p75^{NTR}$, by a not yet defined specific NT, elicits apoptotic responses in vascular smooth muscle cells [59].

Concluding Remarks

NTs, initially described as growth and differentiation factors for neuronal cells, are now recognized as central players in complex immunological diseases like bronchial asthma. NT levels, which are elevated locally in asthmatic subjects, control the activity of various immune cells actively participating in the allergic response. The growing knowledge on NT effects on structural cells in the allergic inflamed lung, combined with the immunomodulatory activity of NT, puts these molecules into focus of orchestrating bidirectional interactions of these cells in complex inflammatory diseases.

Taken together, there is overwhelming evidence for an important role of NGF (and also other NTs) in the pathogenesis of chronic inflammatory conditions. This has been exemplified in the case of asthma in this article. Based on the role of NT in amplifying the TH2-driven immune response, augmenting airway hyperresponsiveness, promoting airway remodeling and misguiding repair mechanism on airway epithelium, NGF seems a novel relevant target for therapeutic intervention in asthma. To our knowledge, however, we are not aware about currently ongoing clinical trials investigating this concept. NGF could be targeted by (monoclonal) antibodies, small molecules, aptamers as well as by oligonucleotides on the level of mRNA expression.

References

1 Levi-Montalcini R: The nerve growth factor 35 years later. Science 1987;237:1154–1162.

2 Lessmann V, Gottmann K, Malcangio M: Neurotrophin secretion: current facts and future prospects. Prog Neurobiol 2003;69:341–374.

3 Lu B, Pang PT, Woo NH: The yin and yang of neurotrophin action. Nat Rev Neurosci 2005;6:603–614.

4 Teng KK, Hempstead BL: Neurotrophins and their receptors: signaling trios in complex biological systems. Cell Mol Life Sci 2004;61:35–48.

5 Reichardt LF: Neurotrophin-regulated signalling pathways. Philos Trans R Soc Lond B Biol Sci 2006;361:1545–1564.

6 Blochl A, Blochl R: A cell-biological model of $p75^{NTR}$ signaling. J Neurochem 2007;102:289–305.

7 Kanning KC, Hudson M, Amieux PS, Wiley JC, Bothwell M, Schecterson LC: Proteolytic processing of the p75 neurotrophin receptor and two homologs generates C-terminal fragments with signaling capability. J Neurosci 2003;23:5425–5436.

8 Garcia-Suarez O, Perez-Pinera P, Laura R, Germana A, Esteban I, Cabo R, Silos-Santiago I, Cobo JL, Vega JA: TrkB is necessary for the normal development of the lung. Respir Physiol Neurobiol 2009;167:281–291.

9 Lommatzsch M, Braun A, Mannsfeldt A, Botchkarev VA, Botchkareva NV, Paus R, Fischer A, Lewin GR, Renz H: Abundant production of brain-derived neurotrophic factor by adult visceral epithelia. Implications for paracrine and target-derived neurotrophic functions. Am J Pathol 1999;155:1183–1193.

10 Hahn C, Islamian AP, Renz H, Nockher WA: Airway epithelial cells produce neurotrophins and promote the survival of eosinophils during allergic airway inflammation. J Allergy Clin Immunol 2006;117:787–794.

11 Othumpangat S, Gibson LF, Samsell L, Piedimonte G: NGF is an essential survival factor for bronchial epithelial cells during respiratory syncytial virus infection. PLoS One 2009;4:e6444.

12 Ricci A, Felici L, Mariotta S, Mannino F, Schmid G, Terzano C, Cardillo G, Amenta F, Bronzetti E: Neurotrophin and neurotrophin receptor protein expression in the human lung. Am J Respir Cell Mol Biol 2004;30:12–19.

13 Sonar SS, Schwinge D, Kilic A, Yildirim AO, Conrad ML, Seidler K, Muller B, Renz H, Nockher WA: Nerve growth factor enhances Clara cell proliferation after lung injury. Eur Respir J 2010;36:105–115.

14 Fox AJ, Patel HJ, Barnes PJ, Belvisi MG: Release of nerve growth factor by human pulmonary epithelial cells: role in airway inflammatory diseases. Eur J Pharmacol 2001;424:159–162.

15 Kilic A, Sonar SS, Yildirim AO, Fehrenbach H, Nockher WA, Renz H: Nerve growth factor induces type III collagen production in chronic allergic airway inflammation. J Allergy Clin Immunol 2011;128:1058–1066.

16 Micera A, Vigneti E, Pickholtz D, Reich R, Pappo O, Bonini S, Maquart FX, Aloe L, Levi-Schaffer F: Nerve growth factor displays stimulatory effects on human skin and lung fibroblasts, demonstrating a direct role for this factor in tissue repair. Proc Natl Acad Sci USA 2001;98:6162–6167.

17 Prakash YS, Iyanoye A, Ay B, Mantilla CB, Pabelick CM: Neurotrophin effects on intracellular Ca^{2+} and force in airway smooth muscle. Am J Physiol Lung Cell Mol. Physiol 2006;291:L447–L456.

18 Prakash YS, Thompson MA, Pabelick CM: Brain-derived neurotrophic factor in TNF-alpha modulation of Ca^{2+} in human airway smooth muscle. Am J Respir Cell Mol Biol 2009;41:603–611.

19 Hamid Q, Tulic M: Immunobiology of asthma. Annu Rev Physiol 2009;71:489–507.

20 Kemi C, Grunewald J, Eklund A, Hoglund CO: Differential regulation of neurotrophin expression in human bronchial smooth muscle cells. Respir Res 2006;7:18.

21 Abram M, Wegmann M, Fokuhl V, Sonar S, Luger EO, Kerzel S, Radbruch A, Renz H, Zemlin M. Nerve growth factor and neurotrophin-3 mediate survival of pulmonary plasma cells during the allergic airway inflammation. J Immunol 2009;182:4705–4712.

22 Santambrogio L, Benedetti M, Chao MV, Muzaffar R, Kulig K, Gabellini N, Hochwald G: Nerve growth factor production by lymphocytes. J Immunol 1994;153:4488–4495.

23 Torcia M, De Chiara G, Nencioni L, Ammendola S, Labardi D, Lucibello M, Rosini P, Marlier LN, Bonini P, Dello SP, Palamara AT, Zambrano N, Russo T, Garaci E, Cozzolino F: Nerve growth factor inhibits apoptosis in memory B lymphocytes via inactivation of p38 MAPK, prevention of Bcl-2 phosphorylation, and cytochrome C release. J Biol Chem 2001;276:39027–39036.

24 Tam SY, Tsai M, Yamaguchi M, Yano K, Butterfield JH, Galli SJ: Expression of functional TrkA receptor tyrosine kinase in the HMC-1 human mast cell line and in human mast cells. Blood 1997;90:1807–1820.

25 Xiang Z, Nilsson G: IgE receptor-mediated release of nerve growth factor by mast cells. Clin Exp Allergy 2000;30:1379–1386.
26 Labouyrie E, Dubus P, Groppi A, Mahon FX, Ferrer J, Parrens M, Reiffers J, de Mascarel A, Merlio JP: Expression of neurotrophins and their receptors in human bone marrow. Am J Pathol 1999;154:405–415.
27 Noga O, Englmann C, Hanf G, Grutzkau A, Guhl S, Kunkel G: Activation of the specific neurotrophin receptors TrkA, TrkB and TrkC influences the function of eosinophils. Clin Exp Allergy 2002;32:1348–1354.
28 Solomon A, Aloe L, Pe'er J, Frucht-Pery J, Bonini S, Bonini S, Levi-Schaffer F: Nerve growth factor is performed in and activates human peripheral blood eosinophils. J Allergy Clin Immunol 1998;102:454–460.
29 Kerschensteiner M, Gallmeier E, Behrens L, Leal VV, Misgeld T, Klinkert WE, Kolbeck R, Hoppe E, Oropeza-Wekerle RL, Bartke I, Stadelmann C, Lassmann H, Wekerle H, Hohlfeld R: Activated human T cells, B cells, and monocytes produce brain-derived neurotrophic factor in vitro and in inflammatory brain lesions: a neuroprotective role of inflammation? J Exp Med 1999;189:865–870.
30 Caroleo MC, Costa N, Bracci-Laudiero L, Aloe L: Human monocyte/macrophages activate by exposure to LPS overexpress NGF and NGF receptors. J Neuroimmunol 2001;113:193–201.
31 Rost B, Hanf G, Ohnemus U, Otto-Knapp R, Groneberg DA, Kunkel G, Noga O: Monocytes of allergics and non-allergics produce, store and release the neurotrophins NGF, BDNF and NT-3. Regul Pept 2005;124:19–25.
32 Pouliot P, Turmel V, Gelinas E, Laviolette M, Bissonnette EY: Interleukin-4 production by human alveolar macrophages. Clin Exp Allergy 2005;35:804–810.
33 Braun A, Appel E, Baruch R, Herz U, Botchkarev V, Paus R, Brodie C, Renz H: Role of nerve growth factor in a mouse model of allergic airway inflammation and asthma. Eur J Immunol 1998;28:3240–3251.
34 Braun A, Lommatzsch M, Mannsfeldt A, Neuhaus-Steinmetz U, Fischer A, Schnoy N, Lewin GR, Renz H: Cellular sources of enhanced brain-derived neurotrophic factor production in a mouse model of allergic inflammation. Am J Respir Cell Mol Biol 1999;21:537–546.
35 Schulte-Herbruggen O, Nassenstein C, Lommatzsch M, Quarcoo D, Renz H, Braun A: Tumor necrosis factor-alpha and interleukin-6 regulate secretion of brain-derived neurotrophic factor in human monocytes. J Neuroimmunol 2005;160:204–209.
36 Noga O, Peiser M, Altenahr M, Knieling H, Wanner R, Hanf G, Grosse R, Suttorp N: Differential activation of dendritic cells by nerve growth factor and brain-derived neurotrophic factor. Clin Exp Allergy 2007;37:1701–1708.
37 Virchow JC, Julius P, Lommatzsch M, Luttmann W, Renz H, Braun A: Neurotrophins are increased in bronchoalveolar lavage fluid after segmental allergen provocation. Am J Respir Crit Care Med 1998; 158:2002–2005.
38 Rochlitzer S, Nassenstein C, Braun A: The contribution of neurotrophins to the pathogenesis of allergic asthma. Biochem Soc Trans 2006;34:594–599.
39 Raap U, Braunstahl GJ: The role of neurotrophins in the pathophysiology of allergic rhinitis. Curr Opin Allergy Clin Immunol 2010;10:8–13.
40 Hoyle GW, Graham RM, Finkelstein JB, Nguyen KP, Gozal D, Friedman M: Hyperinnervation of the airways in transgenic mice overexpressing nerve growth factor. Am J Respir Cell Mol Biol 1998; 18:149–157.
41 Graham RM, Friedman M, Hoyle GW: Sensory nerves promote ozone-induced lung inflammation in mice. Am J Respir Crit Care Med 2001;164: 307–313.
42 Lieu T, Kollarik M, Myers AC, Undem BJ: Neurotrophin and GDNF family ligand receptor expression in vagal sensory nerve subtypes innervating the adult guinea pig respiratory tract. Am J Physiol Lung Cell Mol Physiol 2011;300: L790–L798.
43 De Vries A, Dessing MC, Engels F, Henricks PA, Nijkamp FP: Nerve growth factor induces a neurokinin-1 receptor- mediated airway hyperresponsiveness in guinea pigs. Am J Respir Crit Care Med 1999;159:1541–1544.
44 Hunter DD, Myers AC, Undem BJ: Nerve growth factor-induced phenotypic switch in guinea pig airway sensory neurons. Am J Respir Crit Care Med 2000;161:1985–1990.
45 De Vries A, van Rijnsoever C, Engels F, Henricks PA, Nijkamp FP: The role of sensory nerve endings in nerve growth factor-induced airway hyperresponsiveness to histamine in guinea-pigs. Br J Pharmacol 2001;134:771–776.
46 Bachar O, Adner M, Uddman R, Cardell LO: Nerve growth factor enhances cholinergic innervation and contractile response to electric field stimulation in a murine in vitro model of chronic asthma. Clin Exp Allergy 2004;34:1137–1145.

47 Kassel O, de Blay F, Duvernelle C, Olgart C, Israel-Biet D, Krieger P, Moreau L, Muller C, Pauli G, Frossard N: Local increase in the number of mast cells and expression of nerve growth factor in the bronchus of asthmatic patients after repeated inhalation of allergen at low-dose. Clin Exp Allergy 2001;31:1432–1440.

48 De Vries A, Engels F, Henricks PA, Leusink-Muis T, Fischer A, Nijkamp FP: Antibodies directed against nerve growth factor inhibit the acute bronchoconstriction due to allergen challenge in guinea-pigs. Clin Exp Allergy 2002;32:325–328.

49 Path G, Braun A, Meents N, Kerzel S, Quarcoo D, Raap U, Hoyle GW, Nockher WA, Renz H: Augmentation of allergic early-phase reaction by nerve growth factor. Am J Respir Crit Care Med 2002;166:818–826.

50 Sawada J, Itakura A, Tanaka A, Furusaka T, Matsuda H: Nerve growth factor functions as a chemoattractant for mast cells through both mitogen-activated protein kinase and phosphatidylinositol 3-kinase signaling pathways. Blood 2000;95:2052–2058.

51 Kanbe N, Kurosawa M, Miyachi Y, Kanbe M, Saitoh H, Matsuda H: Nerve growth factor prevents apoptosis of cord blood-derived human cultured mast cells synergistically with stem cell factor. Clin Exp Allergy 2000;30:1113–1120.

52 Welker P, Grabbe J, Gibbs B, Zuberbier T, Henz BM: Nerve growth factor-beta induces mast-cell marker expression during in vitro culture of human umbilical cord blood cells. Immunology 2000;99:418–426.

53 Horigome K, Pryor JC, Bullock ED, Johnson EM Jr: Mediator release from mast cells by nerve growth factor. Neurotrophin specificity and receptor mediation. J Biol Chem 1993;268:14881–14887.

54 Marshall JS, Gomi K, Blennerhassett MG, Bienenstock J: Nerve growth factor modifies the expression of inflammatory cytokines by mast cells via a prostanoid-dependent mechanism. J Immunol 1999;162:4271–4276.

55 Nassenstein C, Braun A, Erpenbeck VJ, Lommatzsch M, Schmidt S, Krug N, Luttmann W, Renz H, Virchow JC Jr: The neurotrophins nerve growth factor, brain-derived neurotrophic factor, neurotrophin-3, and neurotrophin-4 are survival and activation factors for eosinophils in patients with allergic bronchial asthma. J Exp Med 2003;198:455–467.

56 Kerzel S, Path G, Nockher WA, Quarcoo D, Raap U, Groneberg DA, Dinh QT, Fischer A, Braun A, Renz H: Pan-neurotrophin receptor p75 contributes to neuronal hyperreactivity and airway inflammation in a murine model of experimental asthma. Am J Respir Cell Mol Biol 2003;28:170–178.

57 Aravamudan B, Thompson M, Pabelick C, Prakash YS: Brain derived neurotrophic factor induces proliferation of human airway smooth muscle cells. J Cell Mol Med 2011 Jun 9. doi: 10.1111/j.1582-4934.2011.01356.x [Epub ahead of print].

58 Kraemer R, Nguyen H, March KL, Hempstead B: NGF activates similar intracellular signaling pathways in vascular smooth muscle cells as PDGF-BB but elicits different biological responses. Arterioscler Thromb Vasc Biol 1999;19:1041–1050.

59 Wang S, Bray P, McCaffrey T, March K, Hempstead BL, Kraemer R: p75(NTR) mediates neurotrophin-induced apoptosis of vascular smooth muscle cells. Am J Pathol 2000;157:1247–1258.

Prof. Harald Renz
Institute of Laboratory Medicine and Pathobiochemistry
Molecular Diagnostics, Philipps University Marburg
Baldingerstrasse
DE–35043 Marburg (Germany)
Tel. +49 6421 58 66234, E-Mail renzh@med.uni-marburg.de

Bienenstock J (ed): Allergy and the Nervous System.
Chem Immunol Allergy. Basel, Karger, 2012, vol 98, pp 118–141

Pathways Underlying Afferent Signaling of Bronchopulmonary Immune Activation to the Central Nervous System

Matthew W. Hale[a,b] · Graham A.W. Rook[c] · Christopher A. Lowry[a,d]

[a]Department of Integrative Physiology and Center for Neuroscience, University of Colorado Boulder, Boulder, Colo., USA; [b]School of Psychological Science, La Trobe University, Melbourne, Australia; [c]Centre for Clinical Microbiology, Department of Infection, University College London (UCL), London, and [d]Henry Wellcome Laboratories for Integrative Neuroscience and Endocrinology, University of Bristol, Bristol, UK

Abstract

Bronchopulmonary inflammation, such as that associated with asthma, activates afferent neural pathways. We recently demonstrated that localized inflammation in the lungs, induced by intratracheal administration of ovalbumin in ovalbumin-preimmunized mice (an animal model of asthma) results in activation of the dorsolateral part of the nucleus of the solitary tract, a major target of vagal afferent fibers innervating the lungs and airways. Activation of the nucleus of the solitary tract was evident in the absence of activation of the area postrema, a circumventricular organ, consistent with the hypothesis that localized inflammation in the bronchopulmonary system can signal to the central nervous system via specific neural pathways, in the absence of circulating proinflammatory mediators. The pattern of brain activation in ovalbumin-challenged mice differs from the pattern of activation in mice challenged with heat-killed *Mycobacterium vaccae*, suggesting that qualitative aspects of bronchopulmonary inflammation determine the overall pattern of brain activation. The mechanisms through which localized bronchopulmonary inflammation signals to the central nervous system is poorly understood, but appears to involve both vagal and spinal afferent pathways. In this chapter, we review our current understanding of the anatomical pathways through which localized inflammation in the bronchopulmonary system influences central nervous system function.

In this review, we focus on the relatively unexplored question of how localized bronchopulmonary immune activation and disease may signal to the central nervous system (CNS), with a focus on afferent vagal and spinal signaling pathways. It is hoped that this will provide insights into new avenues of research that may contribute to our understanding of the interface between pulmonary disease, including asthma, and central nervous system (CNS) function. From a clinical point of view, there are

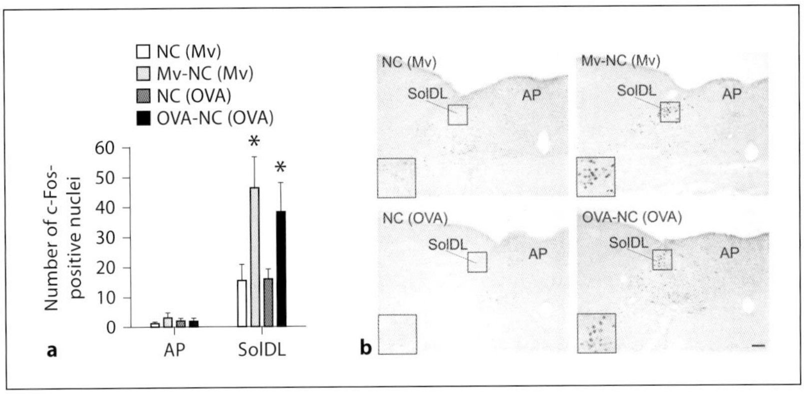

Fig. 1. Both intratracheal (i.t.) injection of ovalbumin (OVA) coupled to nitrocellulose beads (OVA-NC) and *Mycobacterium vaccae* (Mv) coupled to nitrocellulose beads (MV-NC) induce c-Fos expression in the nucleus of the solitary tract (nTS) but not in the area postrema (AP). Adapted with permission from Lowry et al. [5]. **a** Bar graphs illustrate the mean number (± SEM) of c-Fos-immunoreactive (ir) nuclei in the AP and solitary nucleus, dorsolateral part (SolDL). **b** Photomicrographs illustrate c-Fos responses to Mv-NC in *M. vaccae*–preimmunized mice or to OVA-NC in OVA/alum-preimmunized mice in the SolDL and AP. Small black boxes indicate regions shown at higher magnification in insets. Scale bar = 100 μm; insets = 50 μm. Mv = Preimmunization with s.c. injections of *M. vaccae*; Mv-NC, i.t. challenge with *M. vaccae*-NC; OVA = preimmunization with s.c. injections of OVA/alum; OVA-NC = i.t. challenge with OVA-NC. * $p < 0.05$, compared with the appropriate *M. vaccae*- or OVA/alum-preimmunized, vehicle-injected control group, Fisher's protected least significant difference test. For full experimental details, see Lowry et al. [5].

two crucial issues that involve lung-CNS communication. First, why does major depressive disorder occur in approximately half of all patients with asthma [1], or sarcoidosis [2], and in a quarter of all patients with chronic obstructive pulmonary disease (COPD) [3]? Secondly, why do psychosocial stressors precipitate or exacerbate asthma attacks [4]? We will focus on the former question, exploring pathways through which bronchopulmonary inflammation affects brain function, and implications for mental health.

We have found that localized, bronchopulmonary immune activation using intratracheal (i.t.) administration of ovalbumin in ovalbumin-sensitized mice (an animal model of asthma) activates specific subsets of neurons in the nucleus of the solitary tract (nTS) in the brainstem (fig. 1; also see Lowry et al. [5]). In these studies, ovalbumin was coupled to nitrocellulose beads, which bind tightly to proteins and prevent the antigen from entering the systemic circulation. Using this approach, i.t. injection of ovalbumin increased expression of c-Fos, the protein product of the immediate-early gene, *c-fos*, a marker of neuronal activation, in the solitary nucleus, dorsolateral part (SolDL) but not in the adjacent area postrema. The absence of activation of the area postrema, a circumventricular organ, suggests that i.t. ovalbumin activated neurons in the SolDL through activation of vagal afferent fibers, as i.v. injections of proinflammatory mediators such as interleukin-1β (IL-1β) strongly activate the area postrema [6, 7].

In separate studies, we have shown that activation of cardiopulmonary serotonin type 3 (5-HT_3) receptors following intra-atrial injections of the 5-HT_3 receptor agonist, phenylbiguanide results in a similar pattern of activation within the nucleus of the solitary tract [8]. Intra-atrial injections of phenylbiguanide selectively activate cardiopulmonary afferent vagal and spinal C fibers, suggesting that activation of afferent vagal C fibers could account for the pattern of activation observed following i.t. injections of ovalbumin. Intra-atrial injections of phenylbiguanide result in rapid, pronounced bradycardia, a decrease in blood pressure and a decrease in the rate and depth of respiration [9], the so-called Bezold-Jarisch reflex. Thus, activation of bronchopulmonary or cardiopulmonary afferents, including C fibers, selectively activates the SolDL region of the nTS, which is likely to play an important role in cardiorespiratory reflexes in asthma. These data also suggest that peripheral serotonergic systems play an important role in relaying signals of inflammation from the bronchopulmonary system to the brain. Toward the end of this chapter, we will consider in detail potential mechanisms through which serotonergic systems in the airways may relay signals of bronchopulmonary inflammation to the CNS.

Intratracheal injection of heat-killed, sonicated preparations of the nonpathogenic saprophytic bacterium, *Mycobacterium vaccae*, in *M. vaccae*-preimmunized mice also activates neurons in the SolDL, suggesting that qualitatively different types of bronchopulmonary immune activation can activate vagal afferent fibers innervating the nTS [5]. However, i.t. injections of *M. vaccae* activate a subset of midbrain serotonergic neurons in the interfascicular part of the dorsal raphe nucleus (DRI), an effect that is associated with antidepressant-like behavioral responses, whereas i.t. injections of ovalbumin or intra-atrial administration of phenylbiguanide do not [5], suggesting that qualitatively different type of bronchopulmonary immune activation differentially affect CNS function. These findings lead to the question of how bronchopulmonary inflammation signals to the CNS, and how qualitatively different types of immune activation differentially signal to the CNS. In this chapter, we review the current understanding of afferent innervation of the lungs and airways, and potential mechanisms underlying the effects of bronchopulmonary immune activation on CNS function.

Multiple Pathways May Signal Peripheral Immune Activation to the CNS

Multiple hypotheses have been proposed to account for how peripheral inflammation alters CNS function: (1) proinflammatory cytokines, e.g. IL-1, cross the blood-brain barrier using specific transporter mechanisms and act directly on target cells [10], (2) proinflammatory cytokines enter the CNS at circumventricular organs, which have a reduced blood-brain barrier [11], (3) proinflammatory cytokines act via receptors on endothelial cells of the blood-brain barrier to yield secondary paracrine signals that diffuse into the brain [12–15], and (4) proinflammatory cytokines act locally in peripheral organs or organ systems to induce neural signals that are relayed to the CNS by cranial, visceral, or spinal primary afferent neurons [16–21]. In the current chapter, we will focus on the fourth hypothesis – examining the hypothesis that afferent vagal and spinal neurons relay signals of bronchopulmonary inflammation to the CNS.

We have found that bronchopulmonary inflammation and activation of the CNS can persist in the absence of measureable increases in plasma cytokines including IL-1β, IL-6, and tumor necrosis factor-α (TNF-α) [5]. In contrast, local expression of IL-1β messenger RNA (following i.t. injections of *M. vaccae* antigen coupled to nitrocellulose beads) or IL-6 messenger RNA (following i.t. injections of ovalbumin coupled to nitrocellulose beads) within bronchopulmonary tissue is dramatically elevated with a time course paralleling CNS activation [5]. These preliminary findings suggest that under some conditions, particularly in the presence of localized inflammation, stimulation of neural pathways may be the primary driving force for activation of the CNS in response to bronchopulmonary inflammation.

Afferent Innervation of the Lungs and Airways

Below, we consider the sources of afferent fibers innervating the bronchopulmonary system; we outline the types of afferent fibers that may be involved, their topographical projections to the CNS, and potential mechanisms for local cytokine signaling to sensory nerve endings.

The lungs and airways are richly innervated by sensory, sympathetic and parasympathetic systems [22–26]. There is a dual afferent innervation of the lung consisting of (1) afferent projections traveling in the sympathetic nerve branches to the spinal cord, and (2) myelinated and nonmyelinated fibers traveling in the vagus nerve to the nTS in the medulla.

Types of Afferent Fibers Transmitting Signals of Bronchopulmonary Inflammation to the CNS

Afferent fibers innervating the lung and airways are of at least two major types, C fibers and Aδ-fibers (table 1).

Of particular interest with respect to the potential influences of bronchopulmonary disease on CNS function, for reasons specified below, are the nonmyelinated fibers (C fibers) traveling in the vagus nerve [for review, see 24]. Approximately four-fifths of the vagal afferent fibers innervating the airways and lungs are of this type. These fibers arise from both the lower airways and lungs; terminal enlargements of sensory

Table 1. Types of afferent fibers in the airways and lungs

Fibre type	Conduction velocity ms^{-1}	Other characteristics	References
C-fibers	<6	unmyelinated	Coleridge and Coleridge, 1984 [24]; see also Riccio et al., 1996 [39]; Stansfeld and Wallis, 1985 [175]; Undem and Weinreich, 1993 [176]
Aδ-fibers	>6	myelinated	Stansfeld and Wallis, 1985 [177]

appearance are regularly present in alveolar walls, alveolar ducts, and between epithelial cells of the tracheal mucosa. There are strong similarities between these sensory nerve endings and the cutaneous C fibers that mediate sensations of itch and burning pain in inflammation of the skin. Afferent vagal C fibers give rise to low amplitude potentials in small multi-fiber bundles, have slow conduction velocities, and are responsive to noxious stimuli such as congestion, embolism, edema, and inflammation [for review, see 24].

The vagus nerve includes two ganglia that give rise to afferent innervation of the bronchopulmonary system, the nodose and jugular ganglia. Support for the hypothesis that afferent C fibers originating in the nodose ganglia transmit signals of inflammation to the CNS is derived from studies of neuropeptide expression in afferent C fibers innervating peripheral organs. The peripheral terminals of the C fibers are complex organelle structures, each containing vesicularly packaged neuropeptides including calcitonin gene-related peptide (CGRP) and tachykinins, including substance P (SP) and neurokinin A [NKA; 27, 28]. These peptides are synthesized in vagal afferent ganglia (nodose and jugular ganglia) and transported peripherally to the nerve terminals [29]. Activation of these terminals may result in local release of terminal contents via an axon reflex mechanism – independent of classical reflex pathways passing through the CNS [30–32].

Although global destruction of C fiber afferents by repeated systemic treatment during adulthood with capsaicin can reduce CNS activation [33], the hypothesis that C fibers are solely responsible for vagally mediated signaling of peripheral inflammation to the CNS has been strongly disputed [34]. Nonetheless, local inflammatory signals produced in the lung almost certainly activate afferent vagal C fibers under pathophysiological conditions. Endogenous chemicals involved in inflammatory responses, for example prostaglandins (prostaglandin E_1 (PGE_1), PGE_2, $PGF_{2\alpha}$, and prostacyclin (PGI_2)) [35], as well as histamine, serotonin, and bradykinin are known to activate pulmonary vagal C fibers [24; reviewed by 25]. Among other roles in inflammatory responses, PGE_2, histamine, and bradykinin increase vascular permeability and thus these agents may contribute to coordinated vascular and neural responses during inflammatory responses [36].

Evidence suggests that the activity of afferent C fibers plays little or no part in the control of normal breathing pattern [37]. In contrast, they play a major part in the control of tachypnea (rapid, shallow breathing) occurring in certain pathological diseases of the lung including patchy areas of collapse, hemorrhage, edema, infarction, microembolism, and experimental pneumonia [37, 38]. The tachypnea is not due to hypoxemia, or pain [38] and therefore must be derived from an alternative stimulus. Whereas afferent vagal C fibers usually have a slow, regular firing pattern, conspicuous trains of impulses have been observed during inflation in afferent C fibers supplying regions of lung with inflammation [24]. These data imply neural afferents – including pulmonary C fibers in the vagus – signal the presence of bronchopulmonary inflammation to the CNS. It is equally possible that other types of afferent fibers, for example, small myelinated (Aδ) fibers conducting at intermediate velocities, are also involved (table 1). The majority of tracheal and bronchopulmonary afferent Aδ-fibers arise from the nodose ganglia [23, 39].

Location of Neuronal Cell Bodies Providing Afferent Innervation of the Airways and Lungs

Afferent innervation of the airways and lungs originates in the jugular and nodose vagal ganglia and also in upper thoracic dorsal root ganglia (T1–T6, fig. 2). Sensory fibers projecting from the nodose and jugular ganglia represent functionally and neurochemically distinct phenotypes [40, 41], consistent with the observation that these ganglia have different embryonic origins [42]. Therefore, based on unique developmental and anatomical characteristics, these ganglia may be differentially involved in transmitting signals of inflammation from the airways and lungs to the CNS.

Which Afferent Fiber Pathways Transmit Signals of Inflammation from the Lungs to the CNS?

In the trachea, the predominant afferent supply appears to be vagal, in that neuronal cell bodies of afferent fibers innervating the trachea are predominantly located bilaterally in the nodose ganglia (but also in the jugular ganglia and, rarely, in the spinal ganglia) [23, 43–47]. In contrast, in the lung the afferent supply is derived from both vagal and spinal (predominantly T1-T6) sources [23, 43, 48]. The observation that morphologically, neurochemically and functionally distinct populations of afferent fibers exist in the nodose vagal ganglia, jugular vagal ganglia, and dorsal root ganglia (T1-T6) [40, 41] suggests the intriguing possibility that different inflammatory stimuli may affect CNS function through different neurochemical mechanisms and/or neuroanatomical pathways.

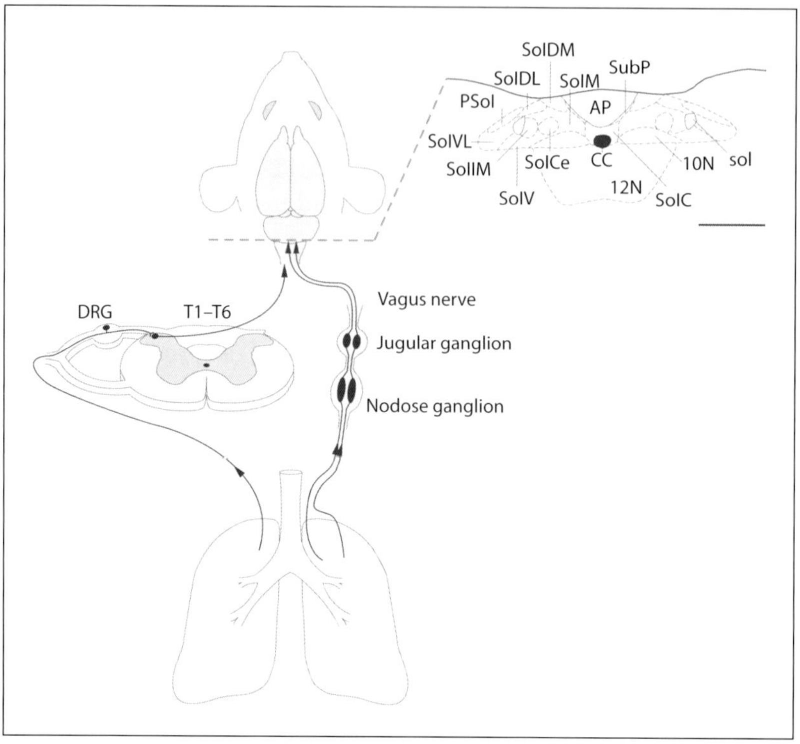

Fig. 2. Schematic diagram showing the afferent innervation of the bronchopulmonary system. Afferent fibers originating in the vagal ganglia innervate primarily ipsilateral targets but also cross over in the pulmonary plexus to reach contralateral targets. Neuronal cell bodies providing afferent innervation of the respiratory tract are located in the jugular, nodose, and dorsal root ganglia (DRG) at thoracic levels (T1-T6). Vagal afferent fibers from the bronchopulmonary system innervate topographically organized regions of the nucleus of the solitary tract (see text for details). The brain targets of bronchopulmonary spinal afferents are not known. The diagram in the top right corner illustrates subregions of the nucleus of the solitary tract and surrounding nuclei in the mouse brain at –7.48 mm bregma and is adapted from a standard stereotaxic atlas of the mouse brain [177]. 10N = Dorsal motor nucleus of the vagus; 12N = hypoglossal nucleus; AP = area postrema; CC = central canal; DRG = dorsal root ganglion; PSol = parasolitary tract; sol = solitary tract; SolC = solitary nucleus, commissural part; SolCe = solitary nucleus, central part; SolDL = solitary nucleus, dorsolateral part; SolDM = solitary nucleus, dorsomedial part; SolIM = solitary nucleus, intermediate part; SolM = solitary nucleus, medial part; SolV = solitary nucleus, ventral part; SolVL = solitary nucleus, ventrolateral part; SubP = subpostrema area. Scale bar = 500 μm.

Support for a Role for Afferent Fibers Originating in the Vagal Nodose Ganglia in Mediating Signals of Bronchopulmonary Inflammation

The most compelling evidence to date argues for a preferential role for afferent C fibers in the nodose ganglia in relaying signals of inflammation from the bronchopulmonary system to the CNS. This is the case in spite of the fact that the majority of tracheal and bronchopulmonary afferent C fibers arise from the jugular ganglia [23, 39, 48].

Evidence suggests that biosynthesis and axonal transport of sensory neuropeptides may be induced in sensory neurons in the nodose ganglia under some pulmonary inflammatory conditions. Although the nodose ganglia contain mainly thin, myelinated (Aδ) fibers innervating the airways and lungs [41], a small percentage (~1%) of nodose fibers innervating the airways and lungs are CGRP/SP-immunoreactive afferent C fibers [23, 48]. Bronchopulmonary inflammation results in a 3- to 4-fold increase of CGRP, SP, and NKA in the airways 24 h following allergen challenge in ovalbumin-sensitized and challenged guinea pigs [49]. Also, 24 h after challenge, the number of tachykinin-immunoreactive nodose ganglion neurons increases by 25%. These changes are associated with a de novo increase in the number of cells expressing preprotachykinin A mRNA (encoding SP and NKA) in the nodose ganglia at 12 h (but not 24 h). These changes are believed to be due to an upregulation of neuropeptide synthesis in the nodose vagal ganglia and neuropeptide transport to afferent nerve terminals in the airways and lungs. Changes in other sensory ganglia innervating the airways were not observed. Physiologic studies suggest that CGRP – NKA – SP release from afferent C fiber terminals may play an important role in mediating the immediate hypersensitivity (allergic) response in the airways [27, 50–56]. For example, Ellis and Undem [56] demonstrated that in animals sensitized to ovalbumin, the addition of antigen markedly increased electrical field stimulation of tracheal smooth muscle contractions in vitro (approximately 3- to 6-fold). Electrical field stimulation of tracheal smooth muscle contractions were tetrodotoxin-sensitive (indicating that they were due to a neuronal response) and abolished by pretreatment with capsaicin or by a combination of neurokinin $(NK)_1$ and NK_2 receptor antagonists, indicating that they were mediated by afferent C fibers containing tachykinins. Together, the observations described above suggest that afferent C fibers arising from the nodose ganglia are potential candidates for transmitting signals of allergic and inflammatory responses from the airways and lungs to the CNS.

The above studies focused on transport of inflammatory neuropeptides from the nodose ganglia to the airways and lungs. It is also possible that, during inflammation, these sensory neuropeptides are simultaneously transported from the perikarya in the nodose ganglia along the branch of the neuron directed toward the CNS. Consequently, these neurons may simultaneously alter peptidergic neuronal signaling in the airways and lungs and peptidergic neuronal signaling in the CNS, i.e. the nTS and its multisynaptic connections in the brain (see below).

As mentioned above, the nodose ganglia contain mainly thin, myelinated (Aδ) fibers innervating the airways and lungs [41]. Evidence suggests that – in addition to afferent C fibers – afferent Aδ-fibers may transmit signals of inflammation from the lungs and airways to the CNS. Studies using several animal models have shown that the rapidly adapting mechanosensitive Aδ-fibers in the large airways can initiate defensive reflexes including cough and bronchoconstriction. Riccio et al. [39] were the first to directly investigate the influence of allergic inflammation on the excitability of bronchopulmonary vagal afferent fibers. These studies used an isolated in vitro preparation – including trachea, larynx and main bronchi with the right vagus and nodose ganglion – from guinea pigs passively immunized 24 h previously with serum containing anti-ovalbumin antibody. The mechanical sensitivity of small, rapidly adapting pulmonary stretch receptor (RAR), myelinated Aδ afferent fibers from immunized guinea pigs (but not nonimmunized control guinea pigs) was increased over 4-fold following airway exposure to antigen. The neurochemical or immune mediators of this increased sensitivity are unknown, although tachykinins do not appear to be essential. In summary, evidence suggests that both thin, unmyelinated, slow-conducting afferent C fibers – some of which contain tachykinins – and thin, myelinated, faster-conducting, afferent Aδ-fibers derived from the nodose ganglia may contribute to signaling of bronchopulmonary inflammation to the CNS.

Support for a Role for Afferent Fibers Originating in the Vagal Jugular Ganglia in Mediating Signals of Bronchopulmonary Inflammation

Based solely on the hypothesis that afferent C fibers may be involved in transmitting signals of inflammation to the CNS (see above), the vagal jugular ganglia are potential candidates for transmitting signals of inflammation from the airways and lungs to the CNS. Electrophysiological and anatomic studies indicate that the jugular ganglia contain equal numbers of C fiber and thin myelinated (Aδ) fiber tracheal afferent somata [39, 41]. Appropriately, afferent neurons within the jugular ganglia are frequently CGRP-/SP-immunoreactive [23, 42, 48, 57]. Compared to the nodose ganglia, very few functional studies of the jugular ganglia have been conducted.

Support for a Role for Afferent Fibers Originating in the Dorsal Root Ganglia (T1-T6), 'Sympathetic Afferents' in Mediating Signals of Inflammation

Anatomical [48] and functional [58, 59] studies support the existence of afferent innervation of the bronchopulmonary system derived from spinal sources. This may account for the proportion (about 40%) of the capsaicin-sensitive SP-immunoreactive afferent fibers in the lung that have a nonvagal origin [60]. Virtually nothing is known about the functional properties of afferent C fibers (principally derived from T1-T6 thoracic dorsal root ganglia) arising from the airways and lungs [24]. However, the proposal that these primary sympathetic afferents are involved in modulating or mediating signals of inflammation is consistent with the observation that inhaled irritants alter neuronal afferent activity in the thoracic spinal cord (T2-T4) – even in the presence of vagal blockade [61]. Thus, like the jugular and nodose vagal ganglia, afferent C fibers traveling within sympathetic branches to T1-T6 dorsal root ganglia (especially T2-T3 levels) [43] remain candidates for modulating or transmitting signals of inflammation from the airways and lungs to the CNS.

Table 2. Central sensory connections of respiratory structures determined using anterograde and transganglionic transport of horseradish peroxidase in cats

Brainstem region	Larynx	Extrathoracic trachea	Intrathoracic trachea	Right main bronchus	Right upper lobe of lung	Presumed fiber type(s)
ap	–	–	–	+	+	C-fibers
dmnX	–	–	+	–	–	
Subnuclei of the NTS						
dlnTS	++	++	+++	+	+++	Aδ-fibers (RAR)
dnTS	+	++	++	+	+	Aδ-fibers (RAR), C-fibers
mnTS	+	++	+	+	+	Aδ-fibers (RAR), C-fibers
ncom	++	++	++	+	++	Aδ-fibers (RAR), C-fibers
ni	+++	++	–	++	+	Aδ-fibers (SAR)
nI	–	+	+	++	+	Aδ-fibers (RAR), Aδ-fibers (SAR)
sg	–	+	+	–	–	C-fibers
vlnTS	++	+++	++	+++	+++	Aδ-fibers (SAR)
vnTS	+	+	+	+	–	

Adapted with permission from Kalia and Mesulam [62], license #2737910347294. +++ = Heavy projection; ++ = moderate projection; + = light projection.
For references, see text. ap = Area postrema; dmnX = dorsal motor nucleus of the vagus; dlnTS = dorsolateral subnucleus of the nucleus of the solitary tract; dnTS = dorsal subnucleus of the nucleus of the solitary tract; mnTS = medial subnucleus of the solitary tract; ncom = subcommissural nucleus, "commissural nucleus" (ganglion) of Cajal – a subnucleus of the nucleus of the solitary tract; ni = interstitial subnucleus of the nucleus of the solitary tract; nI = intermediate subnucleus of the nucleus of the solitary tract; sg = subnucleus gelatinosus of the nucleus of the solitary tract; vlnTS = ventrolateral subnucleus of the nucleus of the solitary tract; vnTS = ventral subnucleus of the nucleus of the solitary tract.

Central Projections of Vagal Afferent Neuronal Fibers

The central projections of vagal afferent neuronal fibers innervating the tracheal and bronchopulmonary systems have been studied previously in cats [62, 63], rats [64], and mice [65]. The most detailed studies have been conducted in cats; anterograde and transganglionic transport of horseradish peroxidase has been used to study the central sensory connections of the laryngeal, tracheobronchial, and pulmonary branches of the vagus nerve in the cat [62]. The specific afferent projections identified in this study are illustrated in table 2. To summarize, although afferent projections are widely distributed throughout different subdivisions of the nTS, the strongest projections from the extrathoracic trachea, intrathoracic trachea, main bronchus, and lung are directed to the dorsolateral and ventrolateral subdivisions of the nTS as well as, more caudally, the subcommissural nucleus.

This pattern of innervation of the nTS by bronchopulmonary afferents is different from the pattern of neuronal activation observed after intraperitoneal [66] or intravenous [17] injection of IL-1β, where neuronal activation is primarily observed in the medial and commissural subnuclei of the nTS. These observations suggest that peripheral inflammation arising from different organ systems may transmit signals of inflammation to different neural substrates at the level of the nTS.

Functionally Distinct Vagal Afferent Fibers Have Topographically Organized Projections to the nTS

Electrophysiological and neuroanatomical tracing studies suggest that functionally different vagal afferent fibers innervate different targets within the CNS. For example, slowly adapting pulmonary stretch receptors (SAR) give rise to myelinated afferents that join the vagus nerve and terminate in the nTS. SAR are activated by airway distension and transmit information related to lung volume to neurons in the nTS that control inspiratory and expiratory duration [44]. Target regions for these neurons are located ipsilaterally within and just dorsal to the ventrolateral nTS, the interstitial nucleus of the nTS, and the intermediate nucleus of the nTS, principally in rostral regions of the nTS [67, 68]. RAR also give rise to myelinated afferents that join the vagus nerve and terminate in the nTS. RAR are stimulated during hyperpnea, pneumothorax and anaphylaxis, and by a variety of noxious agents [69]. Target regions for these neurons are located almost exclusively in the medial and caudal portions of the ipsi- and contralateral nTS including the caudal portions of the medial and intermediate subnuclei, the dorsal and dorsolateral subnuclei, and the commissural subnucleus of the nTS [70, 71]. In contrast to SAR afferents, no RAR innervation of the ventral and ventrolateral nuclei of the nTS was found. The critical finding from these studies is that SAR and RAR fibers innervate separate targets within the nTS – with the SAR innervating more rostral and ventral regions and the RAR more dorsal and caudal regions [67, 68, 70, 71].

Functional studies suggest that pulmonary C fibers mediating the pulmonary C fiber reflex – consisting of rapid shallow breathing (which may be preceded by apnea), bradycardia, and hypotension – act on yet another population of target neurons. Based on functional studies, some of these target neurons are located in a discrete region caudal to the obex within the dorsomedial aspect of the commissural nucleus of the nTS [72, 73]. Antidromic mapping studies in cats suggest that bronchial and pulmonary C fibers also innervate a region rostral to the obex in the medial portions of the nTS and area postrema, with dense innervation of the borders of the gelatinosus nucleus (sg) (or parvicellular nucleus) throughout its rostrocaudal extent [73]. Careful anatomical studies indicate further that – in addition to the medial, gelatinosus, and commissural nuclei – unmyelinated C fibers project to the dorsal subnucleus [74]. In contrast to SAR fibers, no bronchopulmonary C fiber projections have been observed in the intermediate or the ventrolateral subnuclei, consistent with the observation that neurons excited by electrical stimulation of nonmyelinated pulmonary vagal fibers are restricted to medial regions of the nTS [75]. Collectively, these studies have led to the proposal of a 'modality-specific (and thus functional) organization of the vagal primary afferent projections to the nTS' [73].

The projections of SAR [67, 76–78], RAR [70, 71], and bronchopulmonary C fibers show some overlap but clearly have unique projection patterns within subnuclei of the nTS (table 2). Projections of anatomically and functionally distinct pulmonary afferent neurons to topographically defined regions of the nTS provide an opportunity to gain insight into the specific neuronal pathways and specific types of afferent fibers involved in mediating signals of inflammation from the lungs to the CNS.

Afferent Projections of the Nodose and Jugular Ganglia Are Topographically Distinct

A single study has specifically identified the afferent terminal projections of the cat jugular ganglia [79]. The central projections of the jugular ganglia were found to be far more restricted than those derived from the nodose ganglion and the vagus in general (see above). Following selective labeling of afferents arising from the jugular ganglia, terminal labeling was observed in (1) the dorsal lateral subnucleus of the nTS (corresponding to RAR afferent targets, see above); (2) the nucleus interpolaris and nucleus caudalis of spinal V; (3) the ventrolateral aspect of the cuneate nucleus, and (4) the superficial laminae (I, II) of the rostral C_1-dorsal horn. Of these, only the projections to the dorsal lateral subnucleus of the nTS are believed to arise from bronchopulmonary sources [62]. The projections descending in the dorsal aspect of the spinal trigeminal tract to the trigeminal brainstem nuclear complex, cuneate nucleus, and upper cervical dorsal horn [79] may be derived from cutaneous fibers contained in the auricular branch of the vagus nerve [reviewed in 63]. Thus, in summary, the main medullary target of bronchopulmonary neurons with cell bodies situated in the jugular ganglion appears to be the dorsal lateral subnucleus of the nTS. This is in clear contrast to the more widespread medullary targets of bronchopulmonary afferent neurons as a whole [62, 72–74].

Functional Properties of the Dorsal Lateral Subnucleus of the nTS

In addition to receiving afferent bronchopulmonary fibers derived from neurons with cell bodies in the jugular ganglia [79], the dorsal lateral subnucleus of the nTS is known to relay baro- and chemoreceptive information from the aortic arch [80]. This region also corresponds well with a region previously shown to be associated with cardiovascular neuronal activity [81]. The overlapping afferent terminals from cardiovascular and bronchopulmonary sources may provide an anatomical substrate for central integration of respiratory and cardiovascular function. Since the jugular ganglion has a large proportion of neurons that give rise to afferent C fibers, these neurons projecting to the dorsal lateral subnucleus of the nTS may participate in the 'pulmonary chemoreflexes' evoked by activation of bronchopulmonary C fibers by lung autocoids such as serotonin [8, 24].

Functional Properties of the Area Postrema, Medial and Commissural Subnuclei of the nTS

Afferent C-fibers mediating pulmonary defensive reflexes preferentially innervate medial and caudal regions of the nTS, especially the commissural subnucleus of the nTS [24, 68, 70–73]. The commissural subnucleus of the nTS (COM) receives afferent input from both pulmonary RAR (also known as lung irritant receptors) [70, 82] and bronchopulmonary C fibers [73]. A large number of cells within the COM are believed to be second-order neurons activated by pulmonary RAR [83]. Rapidly adapting receptors are involved in respiratory reflexes resulting in changes in respiratory timing and tidal volume, mucus secretion, bronchoconstriction, and coughing [46, 84, 85]. Neuroanatomical tracing studies suggest that the COM is important in both respiratory and autonomic reflex arcs.

Potential Mechanisms for Activation of Bronchopulmonary Afferent Neurons by Local Inflammatory Stimuli

Recent studies have found that while abdominal vagal afferents do not appear to contain IL-1 receptors, abdominal paraganglia, which are functionally linked to vagal fibers, can specifically bind IL-1 receptor antagonist [86]. In addition, macrophages aggregate near vagal fibers and paraganglia after treatment with lipopolysaccharide [87]. These observations suggest close functional relationships among cytokine-producing cell types, paraganglia, IL-1 receptors, and abdominal vagal afferents. Here, we consider the possibility that paraganglia, microparaganglia or the diffuse neuroendocrine system of the lung (neuroepithelial endocrine cells and neuroepithelial bodies) may be involved in signaling inflammation to bronchopulmonary afferent neurons.

Aorticopulmonary Bodies ('Paraganglia')

Paraganglia are widely distributed, morphologically similar neuroendocrine structures that may function as an integrated system sensitive to decreasing pO_2, increasing CO_2, and acidity [88]. Paraganglia have been described in the adventitial connective tissue of major thoracic blood vessels. For example, paraganglia have been observed at the dorsal aspect of the pulmonal bifurcation (the glomus pulmonale, also called the middle aorticopulmonary body, middle aortico-pulmonary glomus, intermediate aorticopulmonary glomus, mittleres paraganglion or paraganglio aortico-polmonare medio; for terminology and review, see ref. [88]). Several additional paraganglia have been described and classified generally as aorticopulmonary bodies; these receive afferent innervation from both vagal and sympathetic sources [see table 25 in ref. 88]. Perikarya of afferent neurons innervating aorticopulmonary bodies are located in the nodose ganglion [89, 90]. Cells in aorticopulmonary bodies contain biogenic amines [91, 92] and may be responsive to hypoxia, hypercapnia and acidemia (functionally resembling the carotid body; reviewed in ref. [88]). Paraganglionic tissue has also been observed embedded in the nodose ganglion or its connective tissue capsule, the vagal glomus or intravagal glomus [93]. Although binding of the IL-1 receptor antagonist to the abdominal paraganglia has been described, involvement of the aorticopulmonary paraganglia, the vagal glomus, or other paraganglia in the thoracic and neck region in transmitting signals of inflammation to the CNS has not been addressed. If such a role is played by these or other paraganglia in the adventitial connective tissue of major thoracic blood vessels, it would most likely be limited to blood-borne stimuli derived from minute branches of the thoracic arteries including the pulmonary artery, bronchial arteries, and possibly the coronary system.

Intrapulmonary Peribronchial Ganglia ('Microparaganglia')

Several studies have identified solitary and groups of potential neuroendocrine cells – containing biogenic amine histofluorescence – associated with the intrapulmonary peribronchial ganglia or 'microparaganglia' that lie in association with large peribronchial nerve trunks [88, 94–102]. Scheuermann et al. [102] suggest that in addition to a vascular chemosensory role, amine-containing microparaganglia cells may act as endocrine or paracrine cells, releasing amines into the local capillary networks or – via a nonsynaptic mechanism – into the extracellular ganglionic tissues, to modulate the activity of ganglionic neurons and nearby trabecular smooth muscle cells. Developmentally, these tissues are derived from the neural crest and belong to the sympathetic nervous system. Biogenic amine-containing cells within these microparaganglia can be present as solitary cells or in clusters and are variously referred to as paraganglionic cells, granule-containing cells, or small intensely fluorescent (SIF) cells. Granule-containing cells are most frequently found in close association with fenestrated blood capillaries [102], which possibly belong to an intraganglionic portal capillary system [103, 104]. They can be distinguished from principal ganglionic neurons at the light and electron microscopic level [102]. Most peribronchial ganglia are located between large bronchi and the accompanying pulmonary arteries, and have close associations with bronchial capillaries [88, 100]. It is clear that paraganglionic cells in the lung can contain dopamine [102] or serotonin [105], although the presence of serotonin immunoreactivity may be dependent upon developmental stage [105]. At the electron-microscopic level, synaptic contact can be observed between multiple types of efferent terminals, including cholinergic type synapses [102], and granule-containing cells [100]. Since IL-1 receptors have previously been associated with paraganglia structures [86], these biogenic amine-containing cells in intrapulmonary ganglia of the lung may be good candidates for transmitting sensory signals of cytokines to afferent fibers. However, no paraganglia are found in the periphery of the lung [88]; therefore, local inflammation in distal regions of the lung is most likely signaled to the CNS via other mechanisms.

Diffuse Neuroendocrine System of the Lung (Neuroepithelial Endocrine Cells and Neuroepithelial Bodies)

The term 'neuroepithelial bodies' was first used by Lauweryns et al. [106] to reflect the prominent nerve supply of epithelial, sensory organ-like structures in the lung. Several excellent reviews of the structural and functional properties of neuroepithelial endocrine cells (NECs) and neuroepithelial bodies (NEBs) have been published [107, 108]. Neuroepithelial endocrine cells and NEBs share identical ultrastructural and neurochemical properties; both are found in close association with unmyelinated afferent axons [reviewed in 108]. A small part of the apical cytoplasm of individual cells often reaches the airway lumen, suggesting a sensory function. These cells show argent affinity (due to innate silver reduction properties of serotonin), serotonin histofluorescence [106, 109–112], and serotonin-like immunoreactivity [105, 113, 114]. Ultrastructural studies indicate that serotonin-containing dense-core granules are most abundant in the cytoplasm facing the basal lamina, suggesting that serotonin is released in proximity to basal structures including capillaries, smooth muscle cells, mucosal glands, adjacent NECs, as well as efferent pulmonary neuronal fibers, and afferent neuronal C fibers [106, 115–121]. Cell bodies for afferent neurons innervating NEBs are located in the nodose ganglia [118]. Studies using cervical vagotomy confirm that the innervation of NEBs is in part vagal [122]. Some NECs have efferent innervation [109] which suggests that signals from the CNS may regulate secretory mechanisms. In addition, reciprocal synapses (that is synaptic contacts in both directions) have been observed between serotonergic NECs and afferent fibers [reviewed in 108]. This relationship may participate in the axon reflex mechanism resulting in local release of afferent terminal contents independent of classical reflex pathways passing through the CNS [30–32, 116].

Neuroepithelial bodies act as pulmonary chemoreceptors [109] and exert their effects by releasing amines and peptides under various conditions, including hypoxia, which stimulates degranulation of NECs in vivo [123]. Prolonged hypoxia appears to cause NEC hyperplasia [124, 125]. Bronchopulmonary irritants also can result in hyperplasia of NECs. In rats chronically exposed to asbestos fibers, there is an increased bombesin-like immunoreactivity and an increase in the number of large and irregular clusters of NECs [126–128]. Similar effects have been observed in an animal model following exposure to cigarette smoke [129], nicotine [130], or nitrosamines [131, 132].

The presence of NECs and NEBs throughout the lung provides an anatomical substrate for local regulation of ventilation, perfusion, or neuronal signaling to the CNS under normal and pathological conditions. Neuroepithelial bodies are most prevalent at points of division of the bronchioles [115, 121, 133, 134]. Early studies [reviewed in 107] suggested that NEBs were more prevalent in fetal and neonatal organisms than in adults. Technical advances allowing whole-mount immunohistochemical demonstration of the distribution of NEBs within the lung suggest that this is not the case [134]. Rather, it seems that the apparent paucity of NEB structures in adults is an artifact due to a constant number of NEBs in rapidly expanding airways. Thus, NEBs may have important regulatory roles in fetal, neonatal, and adult organisms. Due to the presence of reciprocal synapses identified using the electron microscope, NECs and NEBs are ideally situated to signal to afferent fibers [reviewed in 108], especially unmyelinated C fibers in humans [106] and other vertebrate species [101, 109, 110, 115, 135]. These anatomical observations are consistent with the ability of serotonin to stimulate afferent vagal C fibers [24], possibly via activation of 5-HT_3 receptors [8]. The close association between vagal afferent fibers and NEBs is further emphasized by the observation that supranodose vagotomy results in degeneration of ipsilateral axon endings in the NEBs [116, 118]. Of particular note is that in neonatal and adult rats, NEBs are preferentially located at the bifurcation ridges of airways [133, 134, 136–138]. This observation is consistent with morphological studies showing that airway bifurcations have a particularly dense sensory innervation [139–142]. As pointed out by Avadhanam et al. [134], due to airflow dynamics this location is likely to be associated with increased interception and deposition of inhaled irritants or particles and can be conjectured as an ideal location for intrapulmonary chemoreceptors, or, possibly, immunoregulatory sites. Neuroepithelial endocrine cells and NEBs are likely to play a role in signaling of bronchopulmonary inflammation to the CNS and are potential targets for development of novel therapeutic strategies for treatment of symptoms of bronchopulmonary disease.

NECs and NEBs and 'Neurogenic Inflammation'

Neuroepithelial endocrine cells and NEBs are ideally situated to mediate the effects of vagal stimulation, 'neurogenic inflammation', on structures below the epithelial basement membrane, including capillaries, venules and smooth muscle cells. Nerve endings were first observed in close contact with the basal cytoplasm of both solitary and groups of pulmonary NECs by Fröhlich [143] and this observation has been made repeatedly since [101, 102, 106, 109, 110, 121, 122, 135, 144–158]. Detailed studies using serial sections suggest that a single nerve fiber may innervate multiple NECs via bulbous and basket endings after branching or by fusiform 'en passant' varicosities [159].

Vascular Changes Associated with 'Neurogenic Inflammation' May Increase the Accessibility of the Lung and Airways Compartments to Leukocytes

Stress stimuli can exacerbate asthma symptoms [160]. Neurogenic inflammation may play a key role in allergic diseases, such as asthma, and particularly in stress-induced asthma [161]. Neurogenic inflammation induced by stimulation of the vagus nerve is sudden, transient, restricted to venules [162], and the magnitude of the response is dependent upon prior infectious history [163]. As mentioned above, NEBs are preferentially located at the bifurcation ridges of airways [133, 134, 136–138]. Interestingly, within bronchi, neurogenic inflammation induced by electrical stimulation of the vagus nerve results in extravasation of postcapillary venules and collecting venules preferentially near ridges of bronchial bifurcations compared to other regions in the same bronchi [see fig. 2, 5 in 164].

Beyond the bronchial bifurcations discussed above, it was noted that in rats neurogenic inflammation induced by electrical stimulation of the vagus nerve results in a more extensive and diffuse extravasation of postcapillary venules in the anterior membrane, relative to the posterior membrane, especially in the intrathoracic portion of the trachea. In contrast, the posterior membrane of the intrathoracic trachea was nearly devoid of extravasation, except for a distinctive patch of intense extravasation at the carina – the bifurcation of the trachea to form the bronchi [164]. Postcapillary venules are abundant in the posterior membrane, they are simply not involved in the extravasation response [164]. This pattern mirrors the distribution of NECs first observed by Dey and colleagues [165], a pattern subsequently revealed in guinea pigs [157, 166] and in rats [131]. In these species the anterior mucosa of the trachea reveals more NECs than the posterior mucosa, and the greatest concentration of cells can be found in the cranial, extrathoracic segment. In addition to the trachea [165, 167–169], NECs are found distributed throughout the bronchi and terminal bronchioles [106, 158, 170–173]. In rats, the cells are most predominant in the trachea and gradually decrease in density toward more distal regions [131, 143]. Thus, the pattern of plasma extravasation during neurogenic inflammation matches very well the overall distribution of NECs and NEBs. Given that these cells are closely apposed to capillaries [reviewed in 108], it seems possible that the pattern of plasma extravasation observed during neurogenic inflammation is principally due to neuropeptide or neurotransmitter release from the basal pole of NECs and NEBs. Consequently, the NECs and NEBs may form a functionally related, diffuse system orchestrating a coordinated, neurally mediated vascular response (extravasation), followed by immune infiltration. Evidence suggests that these effects would be in part dependent upon release of SP from afferent nerve endings [162, 164].

If the pattern of plasma extravasation does reflect vagal innervation of NECs and NEBs, this may provide a hypothetical framework for (1) how exposure to a multitude of different stressors, leading to the acute alarm-reaction, can lead to congestion, edema, dilation of the perivascular lymphatic spaces and plasma-transudation into lung compartments [174], (2) how immune cells are recruited to specific lung compartments, and (3) how prior immunological history can lead to dynamic changes in subsequent immune response.

Conclusions

Bronchopulmonary inflammation, such as that associated with i.t. administration of ovalbumin coupled to nitrocellulose beads in ovalbumin-preimmunized mice (an animal model of asthma), activates vagal afferent fibers, and presumably afferent spinal fibers, that lead to specific patterns of CNS activation. These effects are likely to involve afferent signaling from serotonergic NECs and NEBs lining the airways. Further studies are likely to lead to a greater understanding of neural mechanisms underlying the effects of bronchopulmonary inflammation on CNS-dependent functions, including anxiety and affect.

Acknowledgements

This work was supported by an NSF CAREER Award to C.A.L. by the National Science Foundation (Grant No. 0845550). Any opinions, findings, and conclusions or recommendations expressed in this material are those of the author(s) and do not necessarily reflect the views of the National Science Foundation.

References

1 Van Lieshout RJ, Bienenstock J, MacQueen GM: A review of candidate pathways underlying the association between asthma and major depressive disorder. Psychosom Med 2009;71:187–195.

2 Chang B, Steimel J, Moller DR, et al: Depression in sarcoidosis. Am J Respir Crit Care Med 2001;163:329–334.

3 Hanania NA, Mullerova H, Locantore NW, et al: Determinants of depression in the ECLIPSE chronic obstructive pulmonary disease cohort. Am J Respir Crit Care Med 2011;183:604–611.

4 Haczku A, Panettieri RA Jr: Social stress and asthma: the role of corticosteroid insensitivity. J Allergy Clin Immunol 2010;125:550–558.

5 Lowry CA, Hollis JH, Pan B, et al: Identification of an immune-responsive mesolimbocortical serotonergic system: potential role in regulation of emotional behavior. Neuroscience 2007;146:756–772.

6 Buller KM, Xu Y, Day TA: Indomethacin attenuates oxytocin and hypothalamic-pituitary-adrenal axis responses to systemic interleukin-1 beta. J Neuroendocrinol 1998;10:519–528.

7 Ericsson A, Liu C, Hart RP, Sawchenko PE: Type-1 interleukin-1 receptor in the rat-brain – distribution, regulation, and relationship to sites of IL-1-induced cellular activation. J Comp Neurol 1995;361:681–698.

8 de Vries A, Paton JF, Lightman SL, Lowry CA: Characterisation of c-Fos expression in the central nervous system of mice following right atrial injections of the 5-HT(3) receptor agonist phenylbiguanide. Auton Neurosci 2005;123:62–75.

9 Paton JFR: Pattern of cardiorespiratory afferent convergence to solitary tract neurons driven by pulmonary vagal C-fiber stimulation in the mouse. J Neurophysiol 1998;79:2365–2373.

10 Banks WA, Ortiz L, Plotkin SR, Kastin AJ: Human interleukin (IL) 1 alpha, murine IL-1 alpha and murine IL-1 beta are transported from blood to brain in the mouse by a shared saturable mechanism. J Pharmacol Exp Ther 1991;259:988–996.
11 Broadwell RD, Brightman MW: Entry of peroxidase into neurons of the central and peripheral nervous systems from extracerebral and cerebral blood. J Comp Neurol 1976;166:257–283.
12 Katsuura G, Arimura A, Koves K, Gottschall PE: Involvement of organum vasculosum of lamina terminalis and preoptic area in interleukin 1 beta-induced ACTH release. Am J Physiol 1990;258(1 Pt 1): E163–E171.
13 Stitt JT: Passage of immunomodulators across the blood-brain barrier. Yale J Biol Med 1990;63:121–131.
14 Cunningham ET Jr, Wada E, Carter DB, Tracey DE, Battey JF, De Souza EB: In situ histochemical localization of type I interleukin-1 receptor messenger RNA in the central nervous system, pituitary, and adrenal gland of the mouse. J Neurosci 1992;12: 1101–1114.
15 Yabuuchi K, Minami M, Katsumata S, Satoh M: Localization of type I interleukin-1 receptor mRNA in the rat brain. Brain Res Mol Brain Res 1994;27: 27–36.
16 Nijima A: The afferent discharges from sensors for interleukin 1ß in the hepato-portal system in the rat. J Physiol (Lond) 1992;446:236P.
17 Ericsson A, Kovacs KJ, Sawchenko PE: A functional anatomical analysis of central pathways subserving the effects of interleukin-1 on stress-related neuroendocrine neurons. J Neurosci 1994;14:897–913.
18 Wan W, Westmore L, Sorensen CM, Greenberg AH, Nance DM: Neural and biochemical mediators of endotoxin- and stress-induced *c-fos* expression in the rat brain. Brain Res Bull 1994;34:7–15.
19 Nijima A: The afferent discharges from sensors for interleukin 1 beta in the hepatoportal system in the anesthetized rat. J Auton Nerv Syst 1996;61:287–291.
20 Layé S, Bluthe RM, Kent S, et al: Subdiaphragmatic vagotomy blocks induction of IL-1ß mRNA in mice brain in response to peripheral LPS. Am J Physiol 1995;268:R1327–R1331.
21 Watkins LR, Maier SF, Goehler LE: Cytokine-to-brain communication: a review and analysis of alternative mechanisms. Life Sci 1995;57:1011–1026.
22 Fryer AD, Costello RW, Yost BL, et al: Antibody to VLA-4, but not to L-selectin, protects neuronal M2 muscarinic receptors in antigen-challenged guinea pig airways. J Clin Invest 1997;99:2036–2044.
23 Kummer W, Fischer A, Kurkowski R, Heym C: The sensory and sympathetic innervation of guinea-pig lung and trachea as studied by retrograde neuronal tracing and double-labelling immunohistochemistry. Neuroscience 1992;49:715–737.
24 Coleridge JCG, Coleridge HM: Afferent vagal C fibre innervation of the lungs and airways and its functional significance. Rev Physiol Biochem Pharmacol 1984;99:1–110.
25 Coleridge HM, Coleridge JC: Pulmonary reflexes: neural mechanisms of pulmonary defense. Annu Rev Physiol 1994;56:69–91.
26 Belvisi MG: Sensory nerves and airway inflammation: role of A delta and C-fibres. Pulm Pharmacol Therapeut 2003;16:1–7.
27 Lundberg JM, Lundblad L, Martling CR, Saria A, Stjarne P, Anggard A: Coexistence of multiple peptides and classic transmitters in airway neurons: functional and pathophysiologic aspects. Am Rev Respir Dis 1987;136:S16–S22.
28 Holzer P: Local effector functions of capsaicin-sensitive sensory nerve endings: involvement of tachykinins, calcitonin gene-related peptide and other neuropeptides. Neuroscience 1988;24:739–768.
29 Zhuo H, Ichikawa H, Helke CJ: Neurochemistry of the nodose ganglion. Prog Neurobiol 1997;52: 79–107.
30 Jancso N, Jancso-Gabor A, Szolcsanyi J: Direct evidence for neurogenic inflammation and its prevention by denervation and by pretreatment with capsaicin. Br J Pharmacol Chemother 1967;31:138–151.
31 Maggi CA: The pharmacology of the efferent function of sensory nerves. J Auton Pharmacol 1991; 11:173–208.
32 Pisarri TE, Coleridge JC, Coleridge HM: Capsaicin-induced bronchial vasodilation in dogs: central and peripheral neural mechanisms. J Appl Physiol 1993; 74:259–266.
33 Watanabe T, Morimoto A, Tan N, et al: ACTH response induced in capsaicin-desensitized rats by intravenous injection of interleukin-1 or prostaglandin E. J Physiol 1994;475:139–145.
34 Bret-Dibat JL, Creminon C, Couraud JY, Kelley KW, Dantzer R, Kent S: Systemic capsaicin pretreatment fails to block the decrease in food-motivated behavior induced by lipopolysaccharide and interleukin-1beta. Brain Res Bull 1997;42:443–449.
35 Hua XY, Jinno S, Back SM, Tam EK, Yaksh TL: Multiple mechanisms for the effects of capsaicin, bradykinin and nicotine on CGRP release from tracheal afferent nerves: role of prostaglandins, sympathetic nerves and mast cells. Neuropharmacology 1994;33:1147–1154.

36 Paul WE: Fundamental Immunology, ed 6. Philadelphia, Wolters Kluwer/Lippincott Williams & Wilkins, 2008.
37 Guz A, Trenchard DW: The role of non-myelinated vagal afferent fibres from the lungs in the genesis of tachypnoea in the rabbit. J Physiol 1971;213:345–371.
38 Trenchard D, Gardner D, Guz A: Role of pulmonary vagal afferent nerve fibres in the development of rapid shallow breathing in lung inflammation. Clin Sci 1972;42:251–263.
39 Riccio MM, Myers AC, Undem BJ: Immunomodulation of afferent neurons in guinea-pig isolated airway. J Physiol 1996;491:499–509.
40 Pedersen KE, Meeker SN, Riccio MM, Undem BJ: Selective stimulation of jugular ganglion afferent neurons in guinea pig airways by hypertonic saline. J Appl Physiol 1998;84:499–506.
41 Riccio MM, Kummer W, Biglari B, Myers AC, Undem BJ: Interganglionic segregation of distinct vagal afferent fibre phenotypes in guinea-pig airways. J Physiol 1996;496:521–530.
42 Ayer-LeLievre CS, Seiger A: Development of substance P-immunoreactive neurons in cranial sensory ganglia of the rat. Int J Dev Neurosci 1984; 2:451–463.
43 Dalsgaard CJ, Lundberg JM: Evidence for a spinal afferent innervation of the guinea pig lower respiratory tract as studied by the horseradish peroxidase technique. Neurosci Lett 1984;45:117–122.
44 Paintal AS: Vagal sensory receptors and their reflex effects. Physiol Rev 1973;53:159–227.
45 Richardson JB: Nerve supply to the lungs. Am Rev Respir Dis 1979;119:785–802.
46 Sant'Ambrogio G: Information arising from the tracheobronchial tree of mammals. Physiol Rev 1982; 62:531–569.
47 Widdicombe JG: Nervous receptors in the respiratory tract and lungs; in Hornbein T (ed.): Lung Biology in Health and Disease, vol 17, part 1: Regulation of Breathing. New York, Marcel Dekker, 1981, pp 429–472.
48 Springall DR, Cadieux A, Oliveira H, Su H, Royston D, Margaret Polak J: Retrograde tracing shows that CGRP-immunoreactive nerves of rat trachea and lung originate from vagal and dorsal root ganglia. J Autonom Nerv Syst 1987;20:155–166.
49 Fischer A, McGregor GP, Saria A, Philippin B, Kummer W: Induction of tachykinin gene and peptide expression in guinea pig nodose primary afferent neurons by allergic airway inflammation. J Clin Invest 1996;98:2284–2291.
50 Saria A, Lundberg JM, Skofitsch G, Lembeck F: Vascular protein linkage in various tissue induced by substance P, capsaicin, bradykinin, serotonin, histamine and by antigen challenge. Naunyn Schmiedebergs Arch Pharmacol 1983;324:212–218.
51 Manzini S, Maggi CA, Geppetti P, Bacciarelli C: Capsaicin desensitization protects from antigen-induced bronchospasm in conscious guinea-pigs. Eur J Pharmacol 1987;138:307–308.
52 Schreiber J, Slapke J, Nieber K, Oehme P: Influence of capsaicin on the reagibility of the isolated guinea pig trachea. Biomed Biochim Acta 1990;49:97–101.
53 Sestini P, Bienenstock J, Crowe SE, et al: Ion transport in rat tracheal epithelium in vitro. Role of capsaicin-sensitive nerves in allergic reactions. Am Rev Respir Dis 1990;141:393–397.
54 Solway J, Leff AR: Sensory neuropeptides and airway function. J Appl Physiol 1991;71:2077–2087.
55 Barnes PJ: Neurogenic inflammation and asthma. J Asthma 1992;29:165–180.
56 Ellis JL, Undem BJ: Antigen-induced enhancement of noncholinergic contractile responses to vagus nerve and electrical field stimulation in guinea pig isolated trachea. J Pharmacol Exp Ther 1992;262:646–653.
57 Katz DM, Karten HJ: Substance P in the vagal sensory ganglia: localization in cell bodies and pericellular arborizations. J Comp Neurol 1980;193:549–564.
58 Holmes R, Torrance RW: Afferent fibres of the stellate ganglion. Q J Exp Physiol Cogn Med Sci 1959;44:271–281.
59 Kostreva DR, Zuperku EJ, Hess GL, Coon RL, Kampine JP: Pulmonary afferent activity recorded from sympathetic nerves. J Appl Physiol 1975;39:37–40.
60 Lundberg JM, Brodin E, Saria A: Effects and distribution of vagal capsaicin-sensitive substance P neurons with special reference to the trachea and lungs. Acta Physiol Scand 1983;119:243–252.
61 Hummel T, Sengupta JN, Meller ST, Gebhart GF: Responses of T2–4 spinal cord neurons to irritation of the lower airways in the rat. Am J Physiol 1997;273:R1147–R1157.
62 Kalia M, Mesulam MM: Brain stem projections of sensory and motor components of the vagus complex in the cat. II. Laryngeal, tracheobronchial, pulmonary, cardiac, and gastrointestinal branches. J Comp Neurol 1980;193:467–508.
63 Kalia M, Mesulam MM: Intramedullary course of afferent and efferent fibers of the vagus nerve: a study using the tetramethyl benzidine reaction for horseradish peroxidase; in von Euler C, Lagercrantz H (eds): Central Nervous Control Mechanisms in Breathing: Physiological and Clinical Aspects of Regular, Periodic and Irregular Breathing in Adults and in the Perinatal Period. Oxford, Pergamon, 1979, pp 273–285.

64 Kalia M, Sullivan JM: Brainstem projections of sensory and motor components of the vagus nerve in the rat. J Comp Neurol 1982;211:248–265.
65 Funakoshi K, Kusakabe T, Kadota T, Goris RC, Kishida R: Substance P immunoreactivity in the vagal nerve of mice. Neurosci Res 1989;7:235–248.
66 Day HE, Akil H: Differential pattern of c-fos mRNA in rat brain following central and systemic administration of interleukin-1-beta: implications for mechanism of action. Neuroendocrinology 1996;63: 207–218.
67 Kalia M, Richter D: Morphology of physiologically identified slowly adapting lung stretch receptor afferents stained with intra-axonal horseradish peroxidase in the nucleus of the tractus solitarius of the cat. I. A light microscopic analysis. J Comp Neurol 1985;241:503–520.
68 Bonham AC, McCrimmon DR: Neurones in a discrete region of the nucleus tractus solitarius are required for the Breuer-Hering reflex in rat. J Physiol 1990;427:261–280.
69 Pack AI: Sensory inputs to the medulla. Annu Rev Physiol 1981;43:73–90.
70 Davies RO, Kubin L: Projection of pulmonary rapidly adapting receptors to the medulla of the cat: an antidromic mapping study. J Physiol 1986;373: 63–86.
71 Kalia M, Richter D: Rapidly adapting pulmonary receptor afferents. I. Arborization in the nucleus of the tractus solitarius. J Comp Neurol 1988;274: 560–573.
72 Bonham AC, Joad JP: Neurones in commissural nucleus tractus solitarii required for full expression of the pulmonary C fibre reflex in rat. J Physiol 1991;441:95–112.
73 Kubin L, Kimura H, Davies RO: The medullary projections of afferent bronchopulmonary C fibres in the cat as shown by antidromic mapping. J Physiol 1991;435:207–228.
74 Torrealba F, Calderon F: Central projections of coarse and fine vagal axons of the cat. Brain Res 1990;510:351–354.
75 Bennett JA, Goodchild CS, Kidd C, McWilliam PN: Neurones in the brain stem of the cat excited by vagal afferent fibres from the heart and lungs. J Physiol 1985;369:1–15.
76 Donoghue S, Garcia M, Jordan D, Spyer KM: The brain-stem projections of pulmonary stretch afferent neurones in cats and rabbits. J Physiol 1982;322: 353–363.
77 Berger AJ, Averill DB: Projection of single pulmonary stretch receptors to solitary tract region. J Neurophysiol 1983;49:819–830.
78 Davies RO, Kubin L, Pack AI: Pulmonary stretch receptor relay neurones of the cat: location and contralateral medullary projections. J Physiol 1987;383: 571–585.
79 Keller JT, Beduk A, Saunders MC: Central brainstem projections of the superior vagal ganglion of the cat. Neurosci Lett 1987;75:265–270.
80 Kalia M, Welles RV: Brain-stem projections of the aortic nerve in the cat – a study using tetramethyl benzidine as the substrate for horseradish-peroxidase. Brain Research 1980;188:23–32.
81 Hellner K, von Baumgarten L: On a terminal area of afferent, cardiovascular fibers of the vagus nerve in he rhombencephalon of the cat. Pflügers Arch Gesamte Physiol Menschen Tiere 1961;273:223–234.
82 Kubin L, Davies RO: Sites of termination and relay of pulmonary rapidly adapting receptors as studied by spike-triggered averaging. Brain Res 1988;443: 215–221.
83 Lipski J, Ezure K, Wong She RB: Identification of neurons receiving input from pulmonary rapidly adapting receptors in the cat. J Physiol 1991;443: 55–77.
84 Coleridge HM, Coleridge JCG: Reflexes evoked from traheobronchial tree and lungs; in Cherniack NS, Widdicombe JG (eds): Handbook of Physiology. Section 3, The Respiratory System, Vol. II. Control of Breathing. Washington, American Psychological Society, 1986, pp 395–429.
85 Widdicombe JG: Pulmonary and respiratory tract receptors. J Exp Biol 1982;100:41–57.
86 Goehler LE, Relton JK, Dripps D, et al: Vagal paraganglia bind biotinylated interleukin-1 receptor antagonist: a possible mechanism for immune-to-brain communication. Brain Res Bull 1997;43:357–364.
87 Goehler LE, Gaykema FJH, Tilders SF, Maier SF, Watkins LR: Localization of immune and inflammatory markers in the rat vagus nerve and liver hilus. Soc Neurosci Abstr 1996;22:88.
88 Böck P: The paraganglia; in Oksche A, Vollrath L (eds): Handbuch der mikroskopischen Anatomie des Menschen. New York, Springer, 1982, pp 1–315.
89 Hollinshead WH: The innervation of the supracardiac bodies in the cat. J Comp Neurol 1940;73: 37–47.
90 Knoche H, Schmitt G: Über die Chemo- und Pressorezeptorenfelder am Coronarkreislauf. Z Zellforsch Mikrosk Anat 1963;61:524–560.
91 Dolezel S, Kovalcik V, Kriska M: Monoamines in the glomus pulmonale. Experientia 1968;24:442–443.

92 Becker AE, Drukker J, Meijer AE: Histochemical characteristics of chemoreceptor organs (glomera). Histochemie 1967;11:195–204.

93 Watzka M, Scharf JH: Paraganglia at and near the ganglion nodosum vagi in the adult. Z Zellforsch Mikrosk Anat 1951;36:141–150.

94 McLean JR, Burnstock G: Innervation of the lungs of the sleepy lizard (*Trachysaurus rugosus*). I. Fluorescent histochemistry of catecholamines. Comp Biochem Physiol 1967;22:809–813.

95 McLean JR, Burnstock G: Innervation of the lungs of the toad (*Bufo marinus*). II. Fluorescent histochemistry of catecholamines. Comp Biochem Physiol 1967;22:767–773.

96 Blumcke S: Experimental and morphological studies on the efferent bronchial innervation. I. The peribronchial plexus. Beitr Pathol Anat 1968;137: 239–286.

97 Bock P: The fine structure of the guinea pig peribronchial micro-paraganglia. Z Zellforsch Mikrosk Anat 1970;110:243–257.

98 Mann SP: The innervation of mammalian bronchial smooth muscle: the localization of catecholamines and cholinesterases. Histochem J 1971;3:319–331.

99 Jacobowitz D, Kent KM, Fleisch JH, Cooper T: Histofluorescent study of catecholamine-containing elements in cholinergic ganglia from the calf and dog lung. Proc Soc Exp Biol Med 1973;144:464–466.

100 Knight DS: A light and electron microscopic study of feline intrapulmonary ganglia. J Anat 1980;131: 413–428.

101 Scheuermann DW, Groodt-Lasseel MH, Stilman C, Meisters ML: A correlative light-, fluorescence- and electron-microscopic study of neuroepithelial bodies in the lung of the red-eared turtle, *Pseudemys scripta elegans*. Cell Tissue Res 1983;234:249–269.

102 Scheuermann DW, Groodt-Lasseel MH, Stilman C: A light and fluorescence cytochemical and electron microscopic study of granule-containing cells in the intrapulmonary ganglia of *Pseudemys scripta elegans*. Am J Anat 1984;171:377–399.

103 Heym C, Williams TH: Evidence for autonomic paraneurons in sympathetic ganglia of a shrew (*Tupaia glis*). J Anat 1979;129(Pt 1):151–164.

104 Abe H, Watanabe H, Yamamoto TY: Relationship between granule-containing cells and blood vessels in the rat autonomic ganglia. Anat Rec 1983;205:65–72.

105 Balaguer L, Romano J, Ruiz-Pesini P: Serotonin immunoreactivity in the autonomic intrapulmonary ganglia of the fetal sheep. Neurosci Lett 1991; 133:151–153.

106 Lauweryns JM, Peuskens JC: Neuro-epithelial bodies (neuroreceptor or secretory organs?) in human infant bronchial and bronchiolar epithelium. Anat Rec 1972;172:471–481.

107 Pack RJ, Widdicombe JG: Amine-containing cells of the lung. Eur J Respir Dis 1984;65:559–578.

108 Scheuermann DW: Morphology and cytochemistry of the endocrine epithelial system in the lung. Int Rev Cytol 1987;106:35–88.

109 Lauweryns JM, Cokelaere M: Hypoxia-sensitive neuro-epithelial bodies. Intrapulmonary secretory neuroreceptors, modulated by the CNS. Z Zellforsch Mikrosk Anat 1973;145:521–540.

110 Lauweryns JM, Cokelaere M, Theunynck P, Deleersnyder M: Neuroepithelial bodies in mammalian respiratory mucosa: light optical, histochemical an ultrastructural studies. Chest 1974;65(suppl): 22S–29S.

111 Lauweryns JM, Liebens M: Microspectrography of formaldehyde and fluorescamine-induced fluorescence in rabbit pulmonary neuroepithelial bodies: demonstration of a new, probably polypeptide intracytoplasmic substance. Experientia 1977;33: 1510–1511.

112 Eaton JA Jr, Fedde MR: Identification of two populations of biogenic amine-containg cells in the mouse lung. Cell Tissue Res 1977;176:243–249.

113 Lauweryns JM, de Bock, V, Verhofstad AA, Steinbusch HW: Immunohistochemical localization of serotonin in intrapulmonary neuro-epithelial bodies. Cell Tissue Res 1982;226:215–223.

114 Sonstegard KS, Mailman RB, Cheek JM, Tomlin TE, DiAugustine RP: Morphological and cytochemical characterization of neuroepithelial bodies in fetal rabbit lung. I. Studies of isolated neuroepithelial bodies. Exp Lung Res 1982;3:349–377.

115 Lauweryns JM, Cokelaere M, Theunynck P: Neuroepithelial bodies in the respiratory mucosa of various mammals: a light optical, histochemical and ultrastructural investigation. Z Zellforsch Mikrosk Anat 1972;135:569–592.

116 Lauweryns JM, Van Lommel AT, Dom RJ: Innervation of rabbit intrapulmonary neuroepithelial bodies. Quantitative and qualitative ultrastructural study after vagotomy. J Neurol Sci 1985;67: 81–92.

117 Lauweryns JM, de B, V, Guelinckx P, Decramer M: Effects of unilateral hypoxia on neuroepithelial bodies in rabbit lungs. J Appl Physiol 1983;55: 1665–1668.

118 Lauweryns JM, Van Lommel A: The intrapulmonary neuroepithelial bodies after vagotomy: demonstration of their sensory neuroreceptor-like innervation. Experientia 1983;39:1123–1124.

119 Van Lommel A, Lauweryns JM, De Leyn P, Wouters P, Schreinemakers H, Lerut T: Pulmonary neuroepithelial bodies in neonatal and adult dogs: histochemistry, ultrastructure, and effects of unilateral hilar lung denervation. Lung 1995;173:13–23.

120 Van Lommel A, Lauweryns JM: Neuroepithelial bodies in the Fawn Hooded rat lung: morphological and neuroanatomical evidence for a sensory innervation. J Anat 1993;183:553–566.
121 Hung KS, Hertweck MS, Hardy JD, Loosli CG: Ultrastructure of nerves and associated cells in bronchiolar epithelium of the mouse lung. J Ultrastruct Res 1973;43:426–437.
122 Glorieux R: Les cellules argentaffines du poumon et leurs connexions avec le système nerveux. Arch Biol 1963;74:377–390.
123 Lauweryns JM, Cokelaere M, Deleersynder M, Liebens M: Intrapulmonary neuro-epithelial bodies in newborn rabbits. Influence of hypoxia, hyperoxia, hypercapnia, nicotine, reserpine, L-DOPA and 5-HTP. Cell Tissue Res 1977;182:425–440.
124 Taylor W: Pulmonary argyrophil cells at high altitude. J Pathol 1977;122:137–144.
125 Gould VE, Linnoila RI, Memoli VA, Warren WH: Neuroendocrine components of the bronchopulmonary tract: hyperplasias, dysplasias, and neoplasms. Lab Invest 1983;49:519–537.
126 Johnson NF, Wagner JC, Wills HA: Endocrine cell proliferation in the rat lung following asbestos inhalation. Lung 1980;158:221–228.
127 Sheppard MN, Johnson NF, Cole GA, Bloom SR, Marangos PJ, Polak JM: Neuron specific enolase (NSE) immunostaining detection of endocrine cell hyperplasia in adult rats exposed to asbestos. Histochemistry 1982;74:505–513.
128 Day R, Lemaire I, Masse S, Lemaire S: Pulmonary bombesin in experimentally induced asbestosis in rats. Exp Lung Res 1985;8:1–13.
129 Tabassian AR, Nylen ES, Linnoila RI, Snider RH, Cassidy MM, Becker KL: Stimulation of hamster pulmonary neuroendocrine cells and associated peptides by repeated exposure to cigarette smoke. Am Rev Respir Dis 1989;140:436–440.
130 Wang NS, Chen MF, Schraufnagel DE, Yao YT: The cumulative scanning electron microscopic changes in baby mouse lungs following prenatal and postnatal exposures to nicotine. J Pathol 1984;144:89–100.
131 Kleinerman J, Marchevsky AM, Thornton J: Quantitative studies of APUD cells in airways of rats. The effects of diethylnitrosamine and NO_2. Am Rev Respir Dis 1981;124:458–462.
132 Reznik-Schuller H: Ultrastructural alterations of APUD cells during nitrosamine-induced lung carcinogenesis. J Pathol 1977;121:79–82.
133 Cutz E, Chan W, Sonstegard KS: Identification of neuro-epithelial bodies in rabbit fetal lungs by scanning electron microscopy: a correlative light, transmission and scanning electron microscopic study. Anat Rec 1978;192:459–466.
134 Avadhanam KP, Plopper CG, Pinkerton KE: Mapping the distribution of neuroepithelial bodies of the rat lung. A whole-mount immunohistochemical approach. Am J Pathol 1997;150:851–859.
135 Hung KS: Innervation of rabbit fetal lungs. Am J Anat 1980;159:73–83.
136 Hoyt RF Jr, Sorokin SP, Feldman H: Small-granule (neuro)endocrine cells in the infracardiac lobe of a hamster lung. Number, subtypes, and distribution. Exp Lung Res 1982;3:273–298.
137 Sorokin SP, Hoyt RF Jr, Grant MM: Development of neuroepithelial bodies in fetal rabbit lungs. I. Appearance and functional maturation as demonstrated by high-resolution light microscopy and formaldehyde-induced fluorescence. Exp Lung Res 1982;3:237–259.
138 Cho T, Chan W, Cutz E: Distribution and frequency of neuro-epithelial bodies in post-natal rabbit lung: quantitative study with monoclonal antibody against serotonin. Cell Tissue Res 1989;255:353–362.
139 Larsell O, Dow RS: The innervation of the human lung. Am J Anat 1933;52:125–146.
140 Elftman AG: The afferent and parasympathetic innervation of the lungs and trachea of the dog. Am J Anat 1943;72:1–27.
141 Honjin R: On the nerve supply of the lung of the mouse, with special reference to the structure of the peripheral vegetative nervous system. J Comp Neurol 1956;105:587–625.
142 Spencer H, Leof D: The innervation of the human lung. J Anat 1964;98:599–609.
143 Fröhlich F: Die 'Helle Zelle' der Brochialschleimhaut und ihre Beziehungen zum Problem der Chemoreceptoren. Frankf Z Pathol 1949;60:517–559.
144 Shul'ga MI: Islet receptors of the lungs. Fed Proc Transl Suppl 1965;24:605–607.
145 Cook RD, King AS: A neurite-receptor complex in the avian lung: electron microscopical observations. Experientia 1969;25:1162–1164.
146 Jeffery P, Reid L: Intra-epithelial nerves in normal rat airways: a quantitative electron microscopic study. J Anat 1973;114:35–45.
147 Jeffery PK, Reid L: New observations of rat airway epithelium: a quantitative and electron microscopic study. J Anat 1975;120:295–320.
148 Hung KS, Loosli CG: Bronchiolar neuro-epithelial bodies in the neonatal mouse lungs. Am J Anat 1974;140:191–199.
149 Lauweryns JM, Goddeeris P: Neuroepithelial bodies in the human child and adult lung. Am Rev Respir Dis 1975;111:469–476.
150 Hung KS: Fine structure of tracheo-bronchial epithelial nerves of the cat. Anat Rec 1976;185:85–91.

151 Wasano K: Neuro-epithelial bodies in the lung of the rat and the mouse. Arch Histol Jpn 1977; 40(suppl):207–219.
152 Taira K, Shibasaki S: A fine structure study of the non-ciliated cells in the mouse tracheal epithelium with special reference to the relation of 'brush cells' and 'endocrine cells'. Arch Histol Jpn 1978;41: 351–366.
153 Edmondson NA, Lewis DJ: Distribution and ultrastructural characteristics of Feyrter cells in the rat and hamster airway epithelium. Thorax 1980;35: 371–374.
154 Goniakowska-Witalinska L: Endocrine-like cells in the lungs of the newt, *Triturus alpestris* Laur. Cell Tissue Res 1980;210:521–524.
155 Goniakowska-Witalinska L: Neuroepithelial bodies in the lung of the tree frog, *Hyla arborea* L. A scanning and transmission electron microscopic study. Cell Tissue Res 1981;217:435–441.
156 Al-Ugaily LH, Pack RJ, Widdicombe JG: The innervation of the murine airway. J Physiol 1983;340: 54P.
157 DiAugustine RP, Jahnke GD, Talley F: Endocrine cells of the guinea pig upper airways. Morphology, distribution, and deposition after xenotransplantation in the nude mouse; in Becker KL, Gazder AF (eds): The Endocrine Lung in Health and Disease. Philadelphia, Saunders, 1984, pp 232–248.
158 Stahlman MT, Gray ME: Ontogeny of neuroendocrine cells in human fetal lung. I. An electron microscopic study. Lab Invest 1984;51:449–463.
159 Bensch KG, Gordon GB, Miller LR: Studies on the bronchial counterpart of the Kultschitzky (argentaffin) cell and innervation of bronchial glands. J Ultrastruct Res 1965;12:668–686.
160 Rietveld S, Everaerd W, Creer TL: Stress-induced asthma: a review of research and potential mechanisms. Clin Exp Allergy 2000;30:1058–1066.
161 Pisi G, Olivieri D, Chetta A: The airway neurogenic inflammation: clinical and pharmacological implications. Inflamm Allergy Drug Targets 2009;8: 176–181.
162 McDonald DM, Mitchell RA, Gabella G, Haskell A: Neurogenic inflammation in the rat trachea. II. Identity and distribution of nerves mediating the increase in vascular permeability. J Neurocytol 1988;17:605–628.
163 McDonald DM: Respiratory tract infections increase susceptibility to neurogenic inflammation in the rat trachea. Am Rev Respir Dis 1988;137:1432–1440.
164 McDonald DM: Neurogenic inflammation in the rat trachea. I. Changes in venules, leucocytes and epithelial cells. J Neurocytol 1988;17:583–603.
165 Dey RD, Shannon WA Jr, Hagler HK, Said SI: Histochemical and ultrastructural characterization of serotonin-containing cells in rabbit tracheal epithelium. J Histochem Cytochem 1983;31:501–508.
166 Kirkeby S, Romert P: Argyrophilic cells in the larynx of the guinea-pig demonstrated by the method of Grimelius. J Anat 1977;123:87–92.
167 Ericson LE, Hakanson R, Larson B, Owman C, Sundler F: Fluorescence and electron microscopy of amine-storing enterochromaffin-like cells in tracheal epithelium of mouse. Z Zellforsch Mikrosk Anat 1972;124:532–545.
168 Cutz E, Chan W, Wong V, Conen PE: Ultrastructure and fluorescence histochemistry of endocrine (APUD-type) cells in tracheal mucosa of human and various animal species. Cell Tissue Res 1975; 158:425–437.
169 Dey RD, Echt R, Dinerstein RJ: Morphology, histochemistry, and distribution of serotonin-containing cells in tracheal epithelium of adult rabbit. Anat Rec 1981;199:23–31.
170 Terzakis JA, Sommers SC, Andersson B: Neurosecretory appearing cells of human segmental bronchi. Lab Invest 1972;26:127–132.
171 Moosavi H, Smith P, Heath D: The Feyrter cell in hypoxia. Thorax 1973;28:729–741.
172 Hernandez-Vasquez A, Will JA, Quay WB. Quantitative characteristics of the Feyrter (APUD) cells of the neonatal rabbit lung in normoxia and chronic hypoxia. Thorax 1977;32:449–456.
173 Stahlman MT, Kasselberg AG, Orth DN, Gray ME: Ontogeny of neuroendocrine cells in human fetal lung. II. An immunohistochemical study. Lab Invest 1985;52:52–60.
174 Selye H: The Stress of Life. New York, McGraw-Hill, 1976.
175 Stansfeld CE, Wallis DI: Properties of visceral primary afferent neurons in the nodose ganglion of the rabbit. J Neurophysiol 1985;54:245–260.
176 Undem BJ, Weinreich D: Electrophysiological properties and chemosensitivity of guinea pig nodose ganglion neurons in vitro. J Auton Nerv Syst. 1993; 44:17–33.
177 Franklin KBJ, Paxinos G: The Mouse Brain in Stereotaxic Coordinates, ed 3. New York, Academic Press, 2007.

Dr. Christopher A. Lowry
Department of Integrative Physiology and Center for Neuroscience, University of Colorado Boulder
1725 Pleasant St
Boulder, CO 80309–0354 (USA)
Tel. +1 303 492 6029, E-Mail christopher.lowry@colorado.edu

Bienenstock J (ed): Allergy and the Nervous System.
Chem Immunol Allergy. Basel, Karger, 2012, vol 98, pp 142–162

Allergen-Induced Neuromodulation in the Respiratory Tract

Letitia A. Weigand · Bradley J. Undem

Asthma and Allergy Center, Johns Hopkins University, Baltimore, Md., USA

Abstract

Many of the symptoms of allergic airway disease such as sneezing, coughing, excessive secretions, reflex bronchoconstriction, and dyspnea occur secondary to changes in the activity of the airway nervous system. In addition, many subjects with allergic airway disease have a heightened sensitivity to non-immunologic irritants in the environment. The symptoms and heightened sensitivities may be explained largely as a consequence of allergen-induced neuromodulation. Mediators associated with allergic inflammation can modulate primary afferent nerves, their connecting neurons in the central nervous system, as well as efferent autonomic neurons innervating the airways. This modulation can take the form of acute electrophysiological changes, or more persistent phenotypic changes at the level of gene transcription, i.e. neuroplasticity. Some of the known mechanisms that underlie this modulation are reviewed here.

When an allergen interacts with cell-bound (predominately mast cell- and basophil-bound) IgE, it sets in motion a cascading sequence of inflammatory events that ultimately lead to the symptoms of allergic disease [1]. The nature of the symptoms depends on the tissue in which the cells are activated. Most commonly, allergic individuals suffer from cutaneous, gastrointestinal, and/or respiratory symptoms. In each case it is the nervous system that is largely responsible for transducing the local allergic inflammatory reaction to the symptoms of the disease observed, i.e. the intense itching and flare responses in cutaneous allergy, the discomfort and changes in motility in GI allergy, and the sneezing, itching, coughing, increase in mucus secretion, and bronchonconstriction of respiratory allergic reactions.

This chapter focuses on the respiratory tract and will emphasize the allergic response in the lower airways and lungs (beginning with the trachea). Although the sensory fibers in the skin are derived from neurons situated in the dorsal root ganglion and the upper airways and lower airways are innervated by trigeminal and vagal fibers, respectively, the mechanisms by which these sensory nerves are modulated by local inflammatory events are often quite similar [2]. Therefore, the general principles to be discussed are directly relevant to the upper (nasal) airways as well as other organs, with the main distinction being in the nature of the neural pathways involved.

We first provide a very brief overview of the innervation of the respiratory tract. This is then followed by a discussion of specific mechanisms by which these nerves are modulated during an allergic reaction.

Neurobiology of the Respiratory Tract

The peripheral nerves in the respiratory tract function to maintain homeostasis and to defend the lungs against hazardous stimuli. Most of the innervation to the respiratory tract is provided by the right and left vagus nerves. The vagi carry both sensory afferent nerves that transmit information about conditions within the airways and lungs into the CNS, and parasympathetic efferent nerves that conduct action potentials from the brainstem back to the lungs and airways.

Sensory Afferent Innervation of the Respiratory Tract

The vagal sensory afferent innervation to the lungs arises from cell bodies that are situated within two distinct vagal sensory ganglia, namely the nodose ganglion and the jugular ganglion [3]. These ganglia are located along the cervical vagus immediately outside the CNS, and contain cell bodies that project axons peripherally via the vagus nerves to terminals that detect local stimuli in the lungs and airways. The central projections of the neurons terminate largely within the nucleus tractus solitarious (nTS) in the brainstem [4].

There are three basic types of vagal sensory afferent nerves within the respiratory tract that can be distinguished physiologically on the basis of conduction velocity [4]. One group of fibers are fast myelinated fibers (Aβ-fibers) derived from the larger diameter neurons with the nodose ganglion. These nerves conduct action potentials at velocities around 10–50 m/s (depending on the species). Another group of fibers innervating the airways are nodose-derived neurons that conduct action potentials around 2–8 (m/s), and are referred to as Aδ-fibers. The third groups of fibers are small unmyelinated fibers that conduct action potentials around 1 m/s [4]. These are derived from both nodose and jugular ganglia and are referred to as C-fibers.

The vagal afferent nerves can also be subdivided based on their stimulus profile. Many of the fast myelinated fibers are low-threshold mechanosensors that are selectively activated by tissue distention [5]. These are often referred to as stretch receptors ('receptor' in this case being the term sensory biologist often use for a sensory nerve). The stretch receptors are further subdivided into rapidly adapting and slowly adapting receptors (RARs and SARs) [6].

The slower Aδ-fibers have been described in detail in the guinea pig where they are located exclusively in the extrapulmonary airways (trachea/main bronchi) [7]. They do not to respond efficiently to tissue stretch, but are exquisitely sensitive to punctate mechanical stimuli (light touch) applied to the mucosal surface [7, 8].

The vagal C-fibers are much less sensitive to mechanical stimuli, but can be activated by noxious stimuli, and by events commonly associated with tissue inflammation [9]. These fibers therefore fit the general definition of Sherrington's 'nociceptors' [10]. The vagal C-fibers can be further distinguished based on the location of the terminals (bronchial and pulmonary C-fibers) [9], or on the location of their cell bodies and embryonic origin (placodally derived nodose ganglia or neural crest-derived jugular ganglia) [11, 12]. In summary, at the most general level there are at least 5 subtypes of vagal afferent nerves (SARs, RARs, touch-sensitive extrapulmonary Aδ-fibers, nodose C-fibers, and jugular C-fibers). The consequences of activation of vagal sensory nerves will depend strictly on the nature of the nerve activated.

It should be kept in mind that the mammalian respiratory tract is also innervated by spinal sensory afferent nerves with cell bodies situated in dorsal root ganglia. These nerves typically get brief mention in discussions about respiratory afferent nerves. This absence of attention is not due to studies showing their lack of involvement in respiratory physiology and sensations, rather it is due to the embarrassing lack of information about these nerves in general. The majority of spinal sensory neurons innervating the airways and lungs are qualitatively similar to jugular vagal neurons in that they are relatively small in diameter and express neuropeptides [3, 13]. Based on these features it is likely that many, but not all, have a nociceptive C-fiber phenotype.

Vagal sensory afferents that innervate the respiratory tract terminate within the central nervous system in distinct subnuclei in the middle and caudal regions of the nucleus tractus solitarius (nTS) [14, 15]. Input from primary vagal afferent nerve fibers leads to modulation of higher order neurons in various regions of the CNS, including respiratory centers within the medulla and the dorsal motor nucleus that influences breathing pattern and parasympathetic outflow [14].

Autonomic Efferent Innervation of the Respiratory Tract

Parasympathetic

Extrinsic efferent nerves innervating the lower respiratory tract in humans are predominately parasympathetic. Preganglionic nerve fibers arise from cell bodies located in the region of the nucleus ambiguous and the dorsal motor nucleus of the brainstem [16–18]. The axon terminals of these neurons synapse onto parasympathetic postganglionic neurons whose cell bodies are located in small ganglia within the walls of the trachea and bronchi [19, 20]. The cell bodies in the ganglia project axons that terminate at effector cells including smooth muscle, glands, and vasculature, beginning in the conducting airways and extending out to the bronchioles [21]. Parasympathetic stimulation of these effectors leads to airway smooth muscle contraction, increased mucous secretion, and vasodilation within both the bronchial and pulmonary vasculature [22].

The neurons within the ganglia may be cholinergic or non-cholinergic/non-adrenergic (NANC) in nature [23]. The so-called NANC neurons typically use NO and/or vasoactive intestinal peptide (VIP) as neurotransmitters that function to relax airway smooth muscle [23]. In many species including humans, the parasympathetic nervous system provides the only contractile (cholinergic) and relaxant (NO/VIP) innervation to airway smooth muscle.

Sympathetic
In most species including humans, there is little sympathetic innervation to bronchial smooth muscle (although the bronchial smooth muscle relaxation can be mediated humorally via epinephrine-dependent activation of stimulation of β_2-adrenergic receptors). The sympathetic nervous system is primarily involved in control of the bronchial and pulmonary vasculature [22]. Stimulation of sympathetic nerves has largely a contractile effect on vascular smooth muscle via α-adrenergic receptors [22], and can also exert non-adrenergic control over the bronchial and pulmonary vascular systems via neuropeptide Y [24].

Axon Reflexes and Peripheral Reflexes
The central reflexes mediated by respiratory afferent nerves involve effects on the pattern of respiration, and on autonomic (mainly parasympathetic) output to effector cells in the airways. Activation of afferent nerves may also lead to local reflex regulation independently of CNS involvement. Neuropeptides that are stored in the terminals of sensory afferent nerves (mainly neural crest-derived C-fibers) [25, 26] can be released locally secondary to the initiation of an action potential that occurs within the nerve terminal membrane [27]. The transmitters released as a result of this 'axon reflex' can then act on neighboring effector cells leading to vasodilation, increases in vascular permeability, and leukocyte infiltration producing the characteristic neurogenic inflammatory reaction [28].

Neuropeptide-laden C-fiber terminals are often found surrounding the principle neurons of bronchial parasympathetic ganglia [25, 29–31]. The release of neuropeptides caused by activation of these afferent nerves causes increases in electrical excitability of the parasympathetic neurons and an increase in synaptic transmission [31–33]. This local afferent-efferent response is often referred to as a 'peripheral reflex'.

Allergen-Induced Neuromodulation

Mast cells are consistently found in close proximity to nerves [34–37]. Because of this intimate anatomical relationship, mast cell mediators released downstream of allergen exposure inevitably interact directly with receptors expressed on nerves. Allergen-induced neuromodulation can be acute or long-lasting. The acute modulation occurs

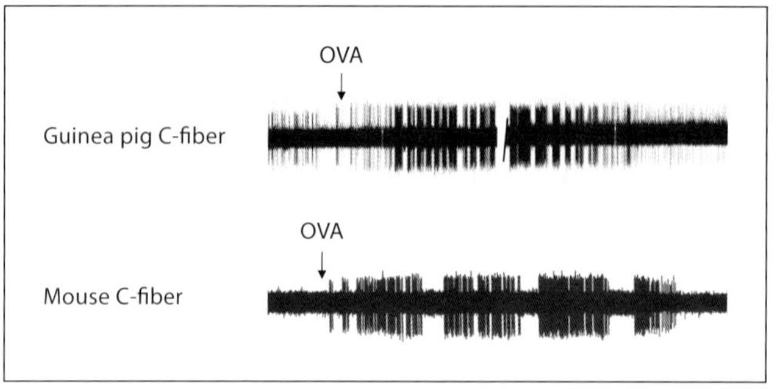

Fig. 1. Allergen-induced activation of bronchopulmonary C-fibers from guinea pig and mouse lungs. Recordings of action potential discharge in response to ovalbumin (OVA) in a single C-fiber in lungs isolated from sensitized guinea pig and mouse [Weigand and Undem, unpubl. data].

in the form of the electrophysiological changes in the nerve membrane. Long-lasting neuromodulation involves changes in gene transcription at the level of the neuronal cell bodies. This may result in qualitative phenotypic changes in the neuron-a process often referred to as neuroplasticity.

Allergen-Induced Afferent Neuromodulation

Acute Activation of Afferent Nerves

The most obvious modulatory effect of allergen challenge on airway afferent nerve activity is seen in the overt activation of vagal C-fibers. Examples of allergen-induced action potential discharge in vagal airway C-fibers in the mouse and guinea pig are illustrated in figure 1.

The induction of action potentials presupposes the initiation of a generator potential. That is to say, allergen challenge by some mechanism leads to the depolarization of the C-fiber terminal membrane and this depolarization is sufficient to reach action potential threshold. The initiating generator potential is most likely due to the effect of autacoids acting on receptors in the nerve membrane. The simplest mechanism to envisage is where the chemical mediator or autacoid interacts with ligand-gated cation channels. Some of the ligand-gated ion channels expressed by airway vagal C-fibers that are relevant to allergen induced afferent nerve activation include P2X purinergic receptors, 5-HT3 receptors, and certain transient receptor potential (TRP) channels, namely TRP-vanniloid-1 (TRPV1) and TRP-ankyrin-repeat-1 (TRPA1) (table 1).

Purinergic P2X Receptor. ATP strongly activates vagal C-fibers, most notably those that arise from the nodose ganglion [12, 38]. ATP can also activate the low-threshold stretch-sensitive afferent nerves in the airways [7]. ATP is a ubiquitous intracellular chemical, but is also known to be released from cells [39], and is present extracellularly in inflammatory reactions where it is available to interact with P2X receptors [40]. There are at least 7 ionotropic P2X receptors (P2X1–7) [41]. The ATP-gated ion channel most that is likely involved in the strong membrane depolarization and action potential discharge in nodose airway afferent nerves is the heteromeric P2X2/3 receptor [42].

Table 1. Influence of mediators associated with allergic inflammation on vagal bronchopulmonary C-fibers

Mediator	Mechanism (receptor)
Activating mediators	
ATP	P2X2/3
Adenosine	A1, A2a
5-HT	5-HT3
H^+	TRPV1, ASICs
Bradykinin	B2
Histamine	H1
Sensitizing mediators	
PGD2	?
PGE2	EP2, EP3
Major basic protein	?
Tryptase	PAR2

Examples of endogenous mediators known to acutely activate (cause action potential discharge) or sensitize (increase excitability) of bronchopulmonary C-fibers. Mechanisms for activation are listed if known. See text for references.

5-HT3 Receptors. Among the large family of 5-HT receptors, the only ligand-gated ion channel is 5-HT3 [43]. 5-HT is a strong activator of vagal airway C-fibers [9], especially nodose C-fibers, and this activation is abolished by 5-HT3 receptor antagonists [44]. The major biogenic amine stored in rodent mast cells is 5-HT, whereas in humans, and other laboratory animals, histamine is the predominant amine [45]. It is not surprising that in rodent allergy, 5-HT likely plays a major role in evoking various respiratory neuronal responses [46–48]. Although, not the predominant amine, 5-HT is also found in human mast cell granules, so it may also play some role in evoking symptoms in human allergy [49].

Transient Receptor Potential-Vanilloid-1 (TRPV1). TRPV1 is the receptor for the vanilloid capaicin (the active ingredient in hot peppers) [50]. Virtually all vagal C-fibers innervating the airways express TRPV1 [12]. TRPV1 can be gated by the low pH that may be associated with airway inflammation [50–53]. Studies with TRPV1 knockout mice, or TRPV1 antagonists indicate that more than 50% of the acid-induced action potential discharge in airway C-fibers is mediated via TRPV1; the remaining activity is likely due to activation of certain acid-sensing ion channels [54–56]. TRPV1 can also be gated by certain eicosanoids, especially 12 and 15 lipoxygenase products of arachidonic acid [57], and by signal transduction mechanisms that are induced by activation of certain G-protein-coupled receptors (GPCRs) [58–60]. As discussed below, this may be relevant to vagal airway C-fiber activation via histamine, bradykinin and adenosine.

TRP-Ankyrin Repeat-1 (TRPA1). Like TRPV1, TRPA1 is largely restricted to a subset of nociceptive sensory nerves, including vagal sensory nerves [61–63]. Single cell RT-PCR analysis of airway-specific vagal sensory neurons demonstrates the selective expression of TRPA1 in those neurons that also express TRPV1 (a marker for nociceptive function) [64]. TRPA1 is a polymodal sensor that can be activated by a large variety of structurally disparate chemicals [65]. The acute allergic reaction is associated with large increases in PGD2, the major prostanoid formed by tissue mast cells [66]. PGD2 itself does not activate TRPA1, but its major metabolite deoxy $D^{12,14}$ prostaglandin J_2 causes action potential discharge in airway C-fibers that is entirely dependent on TRPA1 [67]. Likewise a metabolite of PGE2, another prostanoid elevated at sites of allergic inflammation, strongly activates TRPA1 [67]. Several molecules associated with the oxidative stress of airway inflammation are also strong activators of airway C-fibers strictly via TRPA1-dependent mechanisms [68, 69].

In humans and experimental animals, inhalation of allergen often leads to both an immediate acute bronchoconstriction and also a so-called 'late-phase' bronchoconstrictive response. In guinea pigs, the late-phase response can be inhibited by blocking either muscarinic cholinergic receptors or by blocking TRPA1. This is consistent with the conclusion that the late-phase response involves a parasympathetic cholinergic reflex initiated by the production of TRPA1 agonists and the consequent activation of vagal nociceptors [70]. Interestingly, in TRPA1–/– mice the allergen-induced inflammatory response per se is inhibited, raising the possibility that some of the cellular inflammation in this model is neurogenic in nature [71].

GPCR Agonists. In general, GPCR agonists are relatively ineffective in overtly evoking action potential discharge in airway afferent nerves. When a GPCR agonist leads to action potential generation, it is often a secondary effect, e.g. as a mechanical consequence of bronchial smooth muscle contraction or edema formation in the lungs [72]. Bradykinin, however, a mediator associated with allergic inflammation, strongly and directly evokes action potential discharge in airway vagal C-fibers [12, 73]. The question arises, how does GPCR activation lead to the membrane depolarization of a generator potential? The evidence supports several potential mechanisms. There are multiple signaling pathways by which activation of the G_q-linked receptors leads to the opening of TRPV1 [57]. The action potential discharge induced by bradykinin in vagal airway C-fibers is inhibited, but not abolished by TRPV1 inhibitors or in TRPV1–/– mice [54, 60]. There is also evidence that G_q-coupled receptors can lead to the opening of TRPA1 in the membrane [74], and this too could contribute to the overall generator potential. Finally, data show that the elevation in intracellular calcium can lead to the opening of calcium-activated chloride channels in airway C-fiber neurons, causing chloride to leave the neurons which leads to membrane depolarization [75, 76]. Blocking chloride channels in airway vagal C-fibers results in ~50% reduction in bradykinin-induced action potential discharge [75].

Histamine also leads to action potential generation is some airway C-fibers [9]. Inasmuch as H1 receptors are often G_q coupled receptors, similar activating mechanisms as those described for bradykinin are likely involved. Indeed, both TRPV1 and *pirt*, and endogenous modulator of TRPV1, has been found to be essential for histamine-induced itch in mice [77].

Adenosine, another mediator released upon mast cell activation [78], effectively activates vagal respiratory C-fibers, in particular those C-fibers arising from the nodose ganglion [79, 80]. In guinea pigs, activation of either A1 or A2a adenosine receptors can lead to action potential discharge [79]. The signaling events and ion channels responsible for adenosine-induced activation have not been worked out.

Acute Increases in Electrical Excitability of Afferent Airway Nerves

Mediators associated with allergic inflammation can acutely modulate afferent nerve activity without overtly causing a generator potential and subsequent action potential discharge (table 1). Autacoids can interact with GPCR receptors that lead to phosphorylation of certain ion channels that alone does not depolarize the membrane, but lowers the action potential threshold, or changes the pattern and frequency of action potential discharge.

An example of allergen-induced change in excitability can be seen in the extrapulmonary punctate-sensitive Aδ-fibers in the guinea pig trachea. Challenging the airway with allergen leads to mast cell activation and mediator release in the tissues, but does not cause action potentials in these so-called 'cough receptors' [81]. However, following allergen challenge the amount of mechanical force required to activate these nerves is substantially reduced [81] (fig. 2). Likewise, allergen challenge is associated with an acute increase in the excitability of bronchopulmonary C-fibers, such that the same degree of lung inflation or concentration of a chemical stimulus such as 5-HT, adenosine, or capsaicin, leads to a much stronger action potential discharge [80, 82] (fig. 2).

Prostanoids. Allergic inflammation is associated with elevation of most prostanoids in the airway tissues [83–85]. Virtually all the prostanoids have been associated with increases in afferent nerve activity in the airways [86]. PGD2 is the primary prostanoid synthesized by tissue mast cells, and can increase the excitability of nodose C-fiber neurons through inhibition of a potassium channel responsible for the slow after-spike membrane hyperpolarization current [87]. A similar mechanism of increased excitability is seen with prostacyclin and accounts for some of the increased nodose C-fiber excitability by bradykinin [88]. PGE2 increases the excitability of airway C-fibers through EP2 receptor stimulation and consequent modulation of certain sodium channels in the C-fiber membrane [89]. PGE2 may also increase excitability via EP3 receptor activation, leading to increases in cough sensitivity [90].

Major Basic Protein. Major basic protein is associated with the allergic reaction as a consequence of eosinophil activation. When studied in vivo major basic protein can lead to striking increases in the excitability of vagal airway C-fibers [91]. MBP appears to increase the neuronal excitability by blocking certain potassium channels [92].

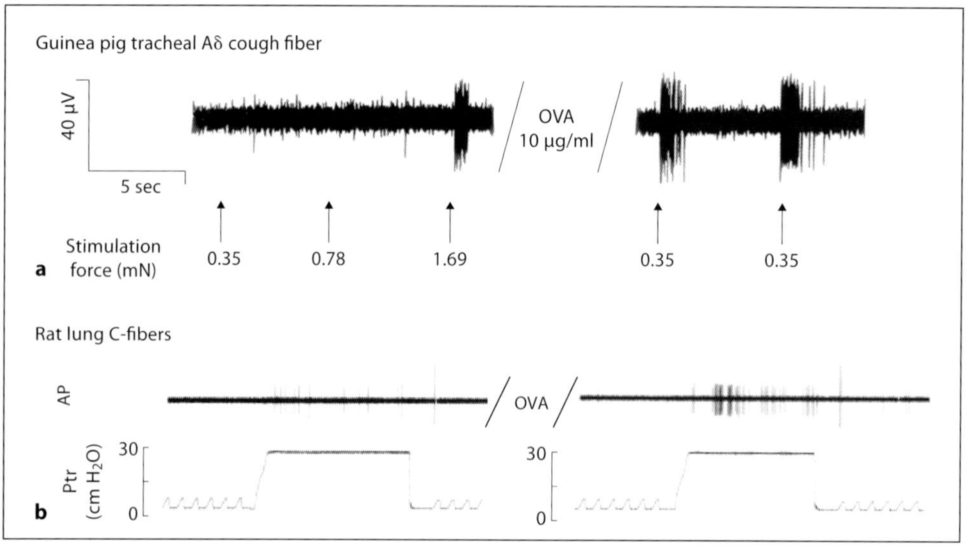

Fig. 2. Allergen-induced increases in afferent neural excitability. **a** Recording of the mechanical threshold from a single nodose Aδ-fiber (cough receptor) in trachea isolated from an OVA-sensitized guinea pig. Allergen challenge did not overtly activate the nerve; however, it reduced the threshold for mechanical activation from 1.69 mN of applied force before, to 0.35 mN after OVA exposure (see Riccio et al. [81] for details). **b** An in vivo recording of mechanical (inflation: Ptr = tracheal pressure)-induced action potential (AP) discharge of a pulmonary C-fiber in a rat before and after allergen (OVA) challenge. OVA challenge did not overtly activate the C-fiber, but increased the fiber's response to mechanical activation. Adapted from Zhang et al. [82].

Leukotriene D4. Cysteinyl-leukotrines are produced in large quantities upon mast cell activation [93]. Activation of the Cys-LT1 receptors with LTD_4 potently augments the action potential-driven tachykinin release from airway C-fibers [94]. Activation of cys-LT1 receptors leads to an increase in airway vagal C-fiber membrane resistance, presumably by inhibiting certain potassium channels [95]. Activation of cys-LT1 receptors also increases excitability of C-fibers innervating the upper airways, leading to a substantial increase in histamine-induced action potential discharge frequency [96].

Mast Cell Tryptase. Antigenic stimulation of mast cells leads to the release of granule associate mast cell tryptase [93]. Mast cell tryptase selectively and effectively activates PAR2 [97]. Activation of PAR2 on airway specific vagal sensory C-fiber neurons increases their excitability and responsiveness to subsequent stimulation [98].

Allergen-Induced Sensory Neuroplasticity

Either by overt activation or by increasing excitability, mediators associated with the allergic reaction in the airways will lead to increases in the number and frequency of action potentials arising in the CNS from nerve terminals in the respiratory tract. This quantitative increase likely explains many of the acute symptoms of the allergic response (sneezing, coughing, reflex bronchoconstriction and secretion). The allergic reaction can also lead to changes in gene expression in the afferent neurons. This neuroplasticity can qualitatively change the communication between the airways and brainstem, an effect that may outlast the acute inflammatory response.

Neurotrophic Factors. The cell bodies that contain the nuclei of vagal afferent neurons are situated in the nodose and jugular ganglia, far removed from the site of inflammation at the airway wall; however, the effects of inflammation at the nerve terminal can induce changes in gene expression at the cell body via the actions of neurotrophic factors. Neurotrophic factors interact with high affinity receptors at the nerve terminal, after which the factor-receptor complex is internalized, and via retrograde transport mechanisms, travels to the cell body where it can modify gene transcription [99]. In the adult guinea pig, all afferent nerve phenotypes innervating the airways express multiple neurotrophic factor receptor subtypes [100]. Based on the receptor expression, the neurotrophic factors likely to be relevant to the function of airway primary afferent nerves include the neurotrophins, namely NGF, brain-derived neurotrophic factor (BDNF), NT-3 and NT-4; and the glial-derived neurotrophic factor- (GDNF) related ligands (GFLs), namely GDNF, nurturin, artemin, and persephin. Mast cell activation and allergic airway inflammation is commonly associated with the production of neurotrophins [101]. Allergen challenge is also associated with increases in GDNF production in the airway mucosa of actively sensitized guinea pigs [102].

Neuroplasticity and Neuropeptides. Several studies in humans and laboratory animals have revealed that allergic airway inflammation is associated with elevations in sensory neuropeptides [103, 104]. When released from the peripheral terminals of nociceptors, neuropeptides such as substance P and calcitonin gene-related peptide (CGRP) can have strong influences on the microvasculature that contribute to the overall inflammatory reaction [28]. Neuropeptides are also released from the central terminals of afferent nerves where they exert modulatory influences on synaptic transmission between the primary and secondary neurons [105, 106]. In healthy airways, the afferent neurons that express substance P and CGRP are largely confined to neural crest derived C-fibers [3, 26]. However, following allergic inflammation or exogenously applied NGF, these peptides are expressed in the low threshold Aβ stretch receptors (RAR/SAR) [44] as well as the extrapulmonary Aδ cough fibers [107, 108]. In contrast to nociceptive C-fibers, stretch receptors are activated during eupneic breathing. Therefore, rather than being released (peripherally and centrally) from C-fibers only after inflammatory and noxious input to C-fibers, that allergic response may lead to release of these potent bioactive peptides with each breath.

TRP Receptors. Allergic inflammation may also lead to expression of genes that define the nerve activation profile. Allergic airway inflammation in rats increases

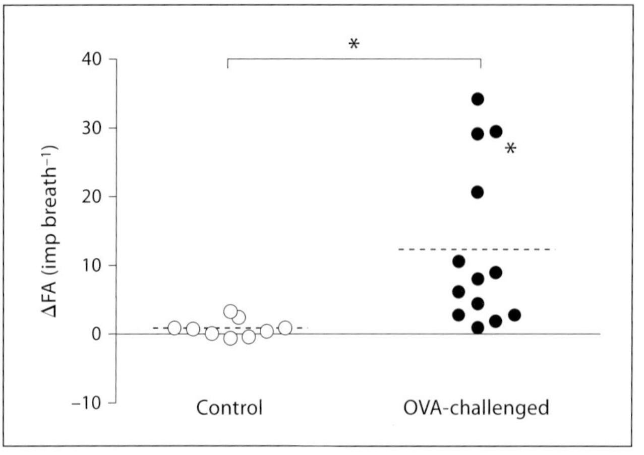

Fig. 3. Allergen-induced sensory neuroplasticity in rat vagal RAR fibers. The response of RAR fibers to capsaicin in control rats and in rats that were challenged with OVA. Note that in control rats RARs do not respond to capsaicin (this nerve phenotype typically does not express the capsaicin receptor TRPV1). After repetitive OVA challenge (3 days/week for 3 weeks) the RAR changed its phenotype such that it expressed TRPV1 and responded to capsaicin. From Zhang et al. [108].

the expression of TRPV1 in airway nodose neurons [109]. In healthy airways, this ion channel is limited to nociceptive-type nerves, mainly C-fibers [12, 109]. A few days after allergen inhalation, TRPV1 was found to be expressed on low-threshold mechanosensitive SAR and RAR fibers [109] (fig. 3). In guinea pigs, both TRPV1 and TRPA1 genes are induced in the extrapulmonary Aδ cough fiber neurons upon allergic inflammation or treatment with neurotrophic factors [102, 110]. Under normal conditions, these cough-causing nerves do not express TRPA1 or TRPV1 and are not activated by irritants produced or inhaled into the extrapulmonary airways [111]. In susceptible individuals in which this type of phenotypic change in TRP channel expression occurs, one can envision stimuli leading to urge to cough sensations, and parasympathetic reflex drive that in healthy subjects would go unnoticed.

Allergic Neuromodulation in the CNS

The synapse between the vagal afferent nerve and the second order neurons in the brain occurs in the nucleus tractus solitarious (nTS) [14, 15]. Although there are mast cells resident within the CNS [112], it is unlikely that they would interact directly with inhaled allergen. Nonetheless, allergic inflammation in the airways can lead to neuromodulation within the CNS. The sensitization of central neural processing by peripheral inflammation is referred to as central sensitization, and has been studied extensively as it pertains to pain in the somatosensory system [113]; however, it is less well characterized in the vagal-visceral system. The idea that allergic airway inflammation can lead to changes in the excitability of

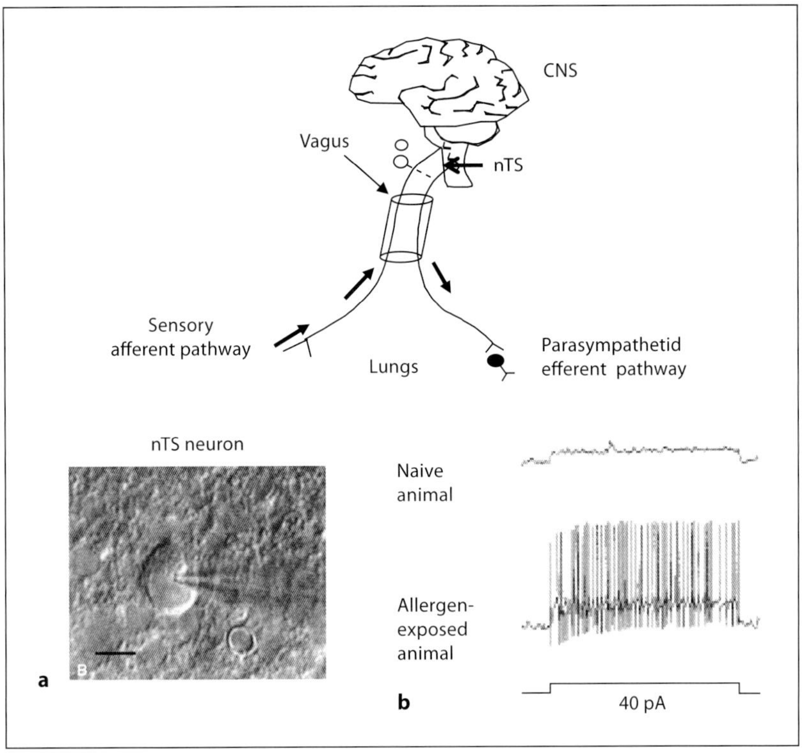

Fig. 4. Allergen-induced increases in electrical excitability in CNS neurons. Allergic sensitization and subsequent allergen challenge increases excitability in neurons within the CNS. Top: Diagram showing the general brainstem location of the nTS. Bottom: **a** Photomicrograph of a patch-clamped neuron in a brain slice from the caudomedial nTS where vagal sensory afferents terminate. **b** Whole cell patch clamp recordings of depolarizing current pulses applied to individual nTS neurons from naïve or allergen-sensitized and challenged rhesus monkeys. Monkeys were sensitized and repeatedly challenged with house dust mite allergen prior to the experiments. Note that a subthreshold (40 pA) depolarizing current step is suprathreshold for action potential discharge in the allergen challenged animals. From Chen et al. [114].

neurons in the brainstem (nTS) has directly been observed in monkeys. The electrical excitability of nTS neurons (in the region where the airway afferent nerve endings terminate) isolated from monkeys sensitized and repeatedly exposed to house dust mite, was enhanced compared to the neurons isolated from healthy monkeys [114] (fig. 4).

One mechanism by which peripheral inflammation can lead to central sensitization is by nociceptor activation. This leads to the release of transmitters and neuropeptides from their central terminals that by multiple mechanisms may sensitize the central synapses. After vagal C-fiber activation, central sensitization leads to a situation where the magnitude of the stimulus to nodose tracheal Aδ-fibers required to reach cough threshold is substantially reduced [115]. Vagal C-fiber activation can also centrally sensitize parasympathetic reflexes. For example, stimulation of laryngeal C-fibers strongly augmented the parasympathetic reflexes evoke by activation of intrapulmonary mechanosensitive RAR A-fibers [116].

Allergic Neuromodulation of Efferent (Autonomic) Nerves

Acute Activation and Increases in Parasympathetic Nerve Excitability

By increasing the activity in afferent nerves, allergic inflammation in the airways will lead to a reflex increase in parasympathetic preganglionic nerve activity [117–119]. Mast cell activation in the airways can also directly modulate parasympathetic nerve activity. The first point of modulation occurs at the synapse within the bronchial parasympathetic ganglia. Mast cells can be found surrounding bronchial parasympathetic ganglia [120], and antigenic activation of these mast cells leads to membrane depolarization and increases in electrical activity of the principal parasympathetic neurons therein [48, 120, 121]. Action potentials arise rhythmically along preganglionic axons at relatively high frequency (~50 Hz) [122]. Under normal conditions, much of the preganglionic activity is filtered out at the ganglia as the excitatory post synaptic potentials fail to reach the firing threshold of the postganglionic neurons [122]. By increasing the excitability of these neurons, allergen exposure can increase synaptic efficacy and decrease the filtering function of the ganglia resulting in increases in parasympathetic drive [120, 123] (fig. 5). Classic mast cell mediators such as histamine and PGD2 appear to play a role in regulating parasympathetic nerve excitability [120, 123]. There is also evidence that the autonomic neurons themselves express high affinity IgE receptors, in which case the allergen may directly interact with neurons independently of mast cell activation [124].

The second point of modulation occurs at the postganglionic parasympathetic nerve-effector junction. Allergic inflammation can modulate acetylcholine release at the nerve terminal leading to a larger end-organ response (e.g. smooth muscle contraction) per action potential [125]. One mechanism through which this occurs is by the inhibition of muscarinic M2 receptors function on the nerve endings [126, 127]. Activation of the M2 receptor by locally released acetylcholine during high frequency stimulation leads to feedback inhibition of subsequent transmitter secretion [126]. By inhibiting M2 receptor activity, allergic inflammation in the airways inhibits the negative feedback system thereby amplifying the cholinergic parasympathetic response [128, 129]. This is discussed in more detail elsewhere in this volume.

Allergen-Induced Neuroplasticity in the Parasympathetic Nerves

Allergen challenge has been also associated with phenotypic changes in airway parasympathetic neurons. Following allergic airway inflammation in the guinea pig, there is a phenotypic switch in the NANC (VIP/NO) parasympathetic neurons such that they begin to express choline acetyltransferase [130]. Such change could lead to an overall increase in the cholinergic contractile vs. NANC relaxant innervation to the smooth muscle.

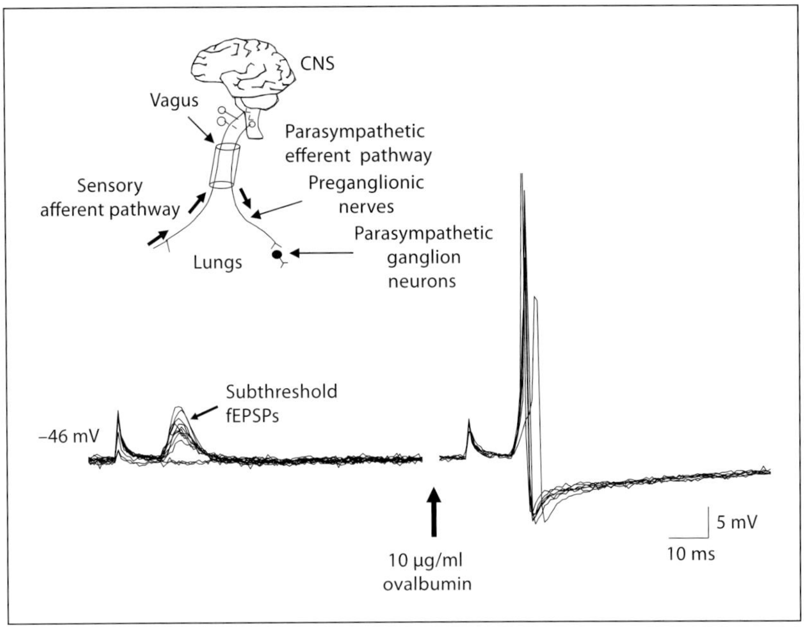

Fig. 5. Allergen increases the synaptic efficacy in bronchial parasympathetic cholinergic ganglion neurons. Top: diagram showing location of parasympathetic ganglion neurons. Bottom: intracellular electrophysiological recording of vagus nerve-stimulated fast excitatory post-synaptic potentials (fEPSPs) in a single bronchial parasympathetic cholinergic ganglionic neuron from an OVA-sensitized guinea pig before and after allergen challenge. The fEPSPs are due to stimulation of nicotinic receptors by acetylcholine released from the preganglionic terminals. The fEPSPs before OVA are often subthreshold for action potential discharge (filter out the activity), but become suprathreshold for action potential generation after allergen challenge. See Myers and coworkers [121, 123] for details.

Clinical Allergy and the Neural Hypersensitive State

The above sections make clear that the allergic reaction in the respiratory tract is associated with overt activation, increases in electrical excitability, as well as phenotypic changes in sensory, central, and autonomic neurons. Much of the literature reviewed in the above sections is based on studies with experimental animals and isolated neurons. It is more difficult to characterize allergic neuronal hypersensitivity in human subjects. Although much of the activation of sensory nerves in the lower airways is not associated with corresponding conscious sensations, studies of human sensations are instructive when addressing hypotheses relating to allergy and neural hypersensitivity.

Patients with allergic rhinitis commonly complain of exaggerated nasal symptoms induced by various perfumes and other strong odors, smoke, as well as by changes in atmospheric conditions. In a questionnaire delivered as part of a screening protocol in 350 individuals with allergic rhinitis, 60% listed smoke as one of the triggers

Fig. 6. Evidence for increases in neuronal responses in human allergy. Human subjects were challenged intranasally with the C-fiber stimulant capsaicin and secretions (largely reflex parasympathetic in nature) were measured. Individuals with allergic rhinitis exhibited remarkable hypersensitivity to the capsaicin challenge compared to their nonallergic counterparts. From Sanico et al. [141].

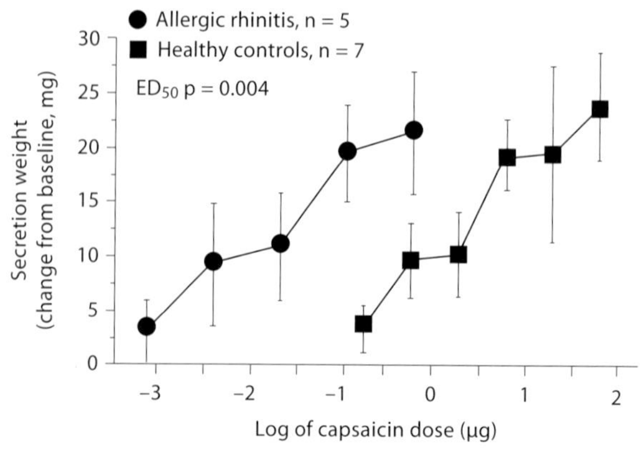

of their nasal symptoms, 58% other irritants and 47% cold air [131]. These percentages were even higher in the volunteers with perennial versus seasonal allergic rhinitis. Objective demonstration of this clinical observation has been produced by Shusterman et al. [132] who found that nasal exposure to low levels of chlorine gas leads to stronger responses in individuals with seasonal allergic rhinitis compared to healthy controls. Likewise, the same concentration of an inflammatory mediator capable of activating sensory C-fibers leads to much stronger sensations and effects (sneezing and parasympathetic reflex secretions) when studied in the context of allergic inflammation. This can be observed whether the sensory nerve stimulus is capsaicin, histamine, bradykinin or endothelin [133–136] (fig. 6).

In the lower respiratory tract, where conscious sensations are not as acute as in the nose, the same principle is observed. With a questionnaire aimed at determining triggers of an asthmatic attack, it is clear that triggers associated directly or indirectly with sensory nerve stimulation are among the most prominent culprits [137]. Analogous to observations in the upper airways, inhalation of an innocuous concentration of sulfur dioxide into the lower airways produces little effect in healthy airways, but leads to strong reflex bronchoconstriction in those suffering from asthma [138]. It has been argued that the classical airways hyperreactivity that typifies asthma may in fact be a 'hyperreflexivity' in many subjects [111]. In this light, it should be kept in mind that methacholine, often thought to act only as a direct bronchial smooth muscle agonist, can also act as an initiator of parasympathetic cholinergic reflex contractions [139]. It should not be surprising that virtually all of the increase in airway resistance in moderate to severe asthma that can be reversed with a beta-adrenoceptor agonist is cholinergic in nature; i.e. an antimuscarinic drug such as tiopropium is as effective as a beta agonist in reducing airway resistance in these subjects [140].

Conclusions

Allergic airway disease is characterized as an inflammatory disorder. Yet the most troubling symptoms can only be understood within the context of the nervous system. The reflex arc that innervates the lungs can be impacted by the allergic reaction at all levels; from the sensory afferent nerve terminals, to the synaptic communication in CNS, to the autonomic transmission within the airway walls. Many of the symptoms of allergic airway disease have analogies in inflammatory diseases in tissues innervated by the somatosensory system. In such tissues, acute pain is experienced, as well as painful sensations to normally innocuous stimuli such as light touch (allodynia). In the case of allergic airway disease, rather than pain there is cough, sneeze, dyspnea, excessive secretions, and, arguably, airway hyperreactivity. There are also inappropriate sensations such as the itchy urge to cough despite nothing in the airway (allotussive sensations) or strong dyspneic sensations with very modest compromises in airflow (allodyspnea). Although these symptoms are linked to changes in neural control of respiratory function, there are as yet few therapies available that specifically target the airway nervous system. A better understanding of the mechanisms controlling airway afferent nerves, their connections in the CNS, and the autonomic process at the neuro-effector junction will likely present novel targets for future therapies aimed at limiting the suffering of those with allergic airway disease.

References

1 Bochner BS, Undem BJ, Lichtenstein LM: Immunological aspects of allergic asthma. Annu Rev Immunol 1994;12:295.
2 Christianson JA, Davis BM: The role of visceral afferents in disease; in Kruger L, Light AR (eds): Translational Pain Research: From Mouse to Man. Boca Raton, CRC Press, 2010.
3 Kummer W, Fischer A, Kurkowski R, Heym C: The sensory and sympathetic innervation of guinea-pig lung and trachea as studied by retrograde neuronal tracing and double-labeling immunohistochemistry. Neuroscience 1992;49:715.
4 Carr MJ, Undem BJ: Bronchopulmonary afferent nerves. Respirology 2003;8:291.
5 Adrian EO: Afferent impulses in the vagus and their effect on respiration. J Physiol 1933;79:332.
6 Knowlton GC, Larrabee MG: Unitary analysis of pulmonary volume receptors. Am J Physiol 1946; 147:100.
7 Canning BJ, Mazzone SB, Meeker SN, Mori N, Reynolds SM, Undem BJ: Identification of the tracheal and laryngeal afferent neurones mediating cough in anaesthetized guinea-pigs. J Physiol 2004; 557:543.
8 McAlexander MA, Myers AC, Undem BJ: Adaptation of guinea pig vagal airway afferent neurones to mechanical stimulation. J Physiol 1999;521: 239.
9 Coleridge JCG, Coleridge HM: Afferent vagal C-fiber innervation of the lungs and airways and its functional significance. Rev Physiol Biochem Pharmacol 1984;99:1–110.
10 Sherrington CS: In Schafer EA (ed.): Textbook of Physiology. Edinburgh, Pentland, 1900, pp 1–698.
11 Baker CV, Schlosser G: The evolutionary origin of neural crest and placodes. J Exp Zool B 2005;304: 269.
12 Undem BJ, Chuaychoo B, Lee MG, Weinreich D, Myers AC, Kollarik M: Subtypes of vagal afferent C-fibres in guinea-pig lungs. J Physiol 2004;556: 905.
13 Oh EJ, Mazzone SB, Canning BJ, Weinreich D: Reflex regulation of airway sympathetic nerves in guinea-pigs. J Physiol 2006;573:549.
14 Kubin L, Alheid GF, Zuperku EJ, McCrimmon DR: Central pathways of pulmonary and lower airway vagal afferents. J Appl Physiol 2006;101:618.

15 Kalia M, Mesulam MM: Brain stem projections of sensory and motor components of the vagus complex in the cat. I. The cervical vagus and nodose ganglion. J Comp Neurol 1980;193:435.
16 Hadziefendic S, Haxhiu MA: CNS innervation of vagal preganglionic neurons controlling peripheral airways: a transneuronal labeling study using pseudorabies virus. J Auton Nerv Syst 1999;76:135.
17 Haxhiu MA, Jansen AS, Cherniack NS, Loewy AD: CNS innervation of airway-related parasympathetic preganglionic neurons: a transneuronal labeling study using pseudorabies virus. Brain Res 1993;618: 115.
18 Perez Fontan JJ, Velloff CR: Labeling of vagal motoneurons and central afferents after injection of cholera toxin B into the airway lumen. Am J Physiol Lung Cell Mol Physiol 2001;280:L152.
19 Dey RD: Airways ganglia; in Raeburn D, Giembycz MA (eds): Airways Smooth Muscle: Structure, Innervation, and Neurotransmission. Basel, Birkhauser, 1995.
20 Myers AC: Transmission in autonomi ganglia. Respir Physiol 2001;125:99.
21 Canning BJ, Fischer A: Neural regulation of airway smooth muscle tone. Respir Physiol 2001;125:113.
22 Widdicombe JG: Neural control of airway vasculature and edema. Am Rev Respir Dis 1991;143:S18.
23 Canning BJ, Undem BJ: Evidence that distinct neural pathways mediate parasympathetic contractions and relaxations of guinea-pig trachealis. J Physiol 1993;471:25.
24 Franco-Cereceda A, Matran R, Alving K, Lundberg JM: Sympathetic vascular control of the laryngeotracheal, bronchial, and pulmonary circulation in the pig: evidence for non-adrenergic mechanisms involving neuropeptide Y. Acta Physiol Scand 1995; 155:193.
25 Kummer W: Ultrastructure of calcitonin gene-related peptide-immunoreactive nerve fibers in guinea-pig peribronchial ganglia. Regul Pept 1992; 37:135.
26 Riccio MM, Kummer W, Biglari B, Myers AC, Undem BJ: Interganglionic segregation of distinct vagal afferent fibre phenotypes in guinea-pig airways. J Physiol 1996;496:521.
27 Chahl LA: Antidromic vasodilation and neurogenic inflammation. Pharmacol Ther 1988;37:217–224.
28 Baluk P, Nadel JA, McDonald DM: Calcitonin gene-related peptide in secretory granlues of serous cells in the rat tracheal epithelium. Am J Respir Cell Mol Biol 1992;8:446.
29 Martling CR, Saria A, Fischer JA, Hokfelt T, Lundberg JM: Calcitonin gene-related peptide and the lung: neuronal coexistence with substance P, release by capsaicin and vasodilatory effect. Regul Pept 1988;20:125.
30 Lundberg JM, Hokfelt T, Martling CR, Saria A, Cuello C: Substance P-immunoreactive sensory nerves in the lower respiratory tract of various mammals including man. Cell Tissue Res 1984;235: 251.
31 Myers AC, Undem BJ: Electrophysiological effects of tachykinins and capsaicin on guinea-pig bronchial parasympathetic ganglion neurons. J Physiol 1993;470.
32 Myers AC, Undem BJ, Kummer W: Anatomical and electrophysiological comparison of the sensory innervation of bronchial and tracheal parasympathetic ganglion neurons. J Auton Nerv Syst 1996;61: 162.
33 Canning BJ, Reynolds SM, Anukwu LU, Kajekar R, Myers AC: Endogenous neurokinins facilitate synaptic transmission in guinea pig airway parasympathetic ganglia. Am J Regul Integr Comp Physiol 2002;283:R320.
34 Stead RH, Dixon MF, Bramwell NH, Riddell RH, Bienenstock J: Mast cells are closely apposed to nerves in the human gastrointestinal mucosa. Gastroentereology 1989;98:575.
35 Bienenstock J, Perdue M, Blennerhassett M, Stead R, Kakuta N, Sestini P, Bancheri C, Marshall J: Inflammatory cells in the epithelium. Mast cell/ nerve interactions in the lung in vitro and in vivo. Am Rev Respir Dis 1988;138:S31.
36 Heine H, Forster FJ: Histophysiology of mast cells in skin and other organs. Arch Dermatol Res 1975;253:225.
37 Alving K, Sundstrom C, Matran R, Panula P, Hokfelt T, Lundberg JM: Association between histamine-containing mast cells and sensory nerves in the skin and airways of controls and capsaicin-treated pigs. Cell Tissue Res 1991;264:529.
38 Pelleg A, Hurt CM: Mechanism of action of ATP on canine pulmonary vagal C fibre nerve terminals. J Physiol 1996;490:265.
39 Burnstock G: Purinergic nerves. Pharmacol Rev 1972;24:509.
40 Bours MJ, Dagnelie PC, Giuliani AL, Wesselius A, Di Virgilio F: P2 receptors and extracellular ATP: a novel homeostatic pathway in inflammation. Front Biosci 2011;3:1443–1456.
41 Burnstock G: Purine and pyrimidine receptors. Cell Mol Life Sci 2007;64:1471.
42 Cockayne DA, Dunn PM, Zhong Y, Rong W, Hamilton SG, Knight GE, Ruan HZ, Ma B, Yip P, Nunn P, McMahon SB, Burnstock G, Ford AP: P2X2 knockout mice and P2X2/P2X3 double knockout mice reveal a role for the P2X2 receptor subunit in mediating multiple sensory effects of ATP. J Physiol 2005;567:621.

43 Pytliak M, Vargova V, Mechirova V, Felsoci M: Serotonin receptors – from molecular biology to clinical applications. Physiol Res 2011;60:15.

44 Chuaychoo B, Lee MG, Kollarik M, Undem BJ: Effect of 5-hydroxytryptamine on vagal C-fiber subtypes in guinea pig lungs. Pulm Pharmacol Ther 2005;18:355.

45 Kitamura Y: Heterogeneity of mast cells and phenotypic change between subpopulations. Annu Rev Immunol 1989;7:59.

46 Eum SY, Norel X, Lefort J, Labat C, Vargaftig BB, Brink C: Anaphylactic bronchoconstriction in BP2 mice: interactions between serotonin and acetylcholine. Br J Pharmacol 1999;126:312.

47 Cyphert JM, Kovarova M, Allen IC, Hartney JM, Murphy DL, Wess J, Koller BH: Cooperation between mast cells and neurons is essential for antigen-mediated bronchoconstriction. J Immunol 2009;182:7430.

48 Weigand LA, Myers AC, Meeker S, Undem BJ: Mast cell-cholinergic nerve interaction in mouse airways. J Physiol 2009;587:3355.

49 Kushner-Sukhov NM, Brown JM, Wu Y, Kirshenbaum A, Metcalfe DD: Human mast cells are capable of serotonin synthesis and release. J Allergy Clin Immunol 2007;119:498.

50 Caterina MJ, Julius D: The vanilloid receptor: a molecular gateway to the pain pathway. Annu Rev Neurosci 2001;24:487.

51 Ugawa S, Ueda T, Ishida Y, Nishigaki M, Shibata Y, Shimada S: Amiloride-blockable acid-sensing ion channels are leading acid sensors expressed in human nociceptors. J Clin Invest 2002;110:1185.

52 Gu Q, Lee LY: Characterizations of acid-signaling in rat vagal pulmonary sensory neurons. Am J Physiol Lung Cell Mol Physiol 2006;291:L58.

53 Jacobus WE, Taylor GJ 4th, Hollis DP, Nunnally RL: Phosphorus nuclear magnetic resonance of perfused working rat hearts. Nature 1977;265:756.

54 Kollarik M, Undem BJ: Activation of bronchopulmonary vagal afferent nerves with bradykinin, acid and vanilloid receptor agonists in wild-type and TRPV1-/- mice. J Physiol 2004;555:115.

55 Fox AJ, Urban L, Barnes PJ, Dray A: Effects of capsazepine against capsaicin-and proton-evoked excitation of single airway C-fibres and vagus nerve from guinea-pig. Neuroscience 1995;67:741–752.

56 Kollarik M, Undem BJ: Mechanisms of acid-induced activation of airway afferent nerve fibres in guinea-pig. J Physiol 2002;543:591.

57 Hwang SW, Cho H, Kwak J, Lee SY, Kang CJ, Jung J, Cho S, Min KH, Suh YG, Kim D, Oh U: Direct activation of capsaicin receptors by products of lipoxygenases: endogenous capsaicin-like substances. Proc Natl Acad Sci USA 2000;97:6155.

58 Chuang HH, Prescott ED, Kong H, Shields S, Jordt SE, Basbaum AI, Chao MV, Julius D: Bradykinin and nerve growth factor release the capsaicin receptor from Ptdlns (4,5), P2-mediated inhibition. Nature 2001;411:957–962.

59 Shin J, Cho H, Hwang SW, Jung J, Shin CY, Lee SY, Kim SH, Lee MG, Choi YH, Kim J, Haber NA, Reichling DB, Khaser S, Levine JD, Oh U: Bradykinin-12-lipoxygenase-VR1 signaling pathway for inflammatory hyperalgesia. Proc Natl Acad Sci USA 2002;99:10150.

60 Carr MJ, Kollarik M, Meeker SN, Undem BJ: A role for TRPV1 in bradykinin-induced excitation of vagal airway afferent nerve terminals. J Pharmacol Exp Ther 2003;304:1275.

61 Story GM, Peier AM, Reeve AJ, Eid SR, Mosbacher J, Hricik TR, Earley TJ, Hergarden AC, Andersson, DA, Hwang SW, McIntire P, Jegla T, Bevan S, Patapoutian A: ANKTM1, a TRP-like channel expressed in nociceptive neurons, is activated by cold temperatures. Cell 2003;112:819.

62 Bandell M, Story GM, Hwang SW, Viswanath V, Eid SR, Petrus MJ, Early TJ, Patapoutian A: Noxious cold ion channel TRPA1 is activated by pungent compounds and bradykinin. Neuron 2004;41:849.

63 Jordt SE, Bautista DM, Chuang HH, McKemy DD, Zygmunt PM, Hogestatt ED, Meng ID, Julius D: Mustard oils and cannabinoids excite sensory nerve fibres through the TRP channel ANKTM1. Nature 2004;427:260.

64 Nassenstein C, Kwong K, Taylor-Clark T, Kollarik M, Macglashan DM, Braun A, Undem BJ: Expression and function of the ion channel TRPA1 in vagal afferent nerves innervating mouse lungs. J Physiol 2008;586:1595.

65 Bessac BF, Jordt SE: Breathtaking TRP channels: TRPA1 and TRPV1 in airway chemosensation and reflex control. Physiology 2008;23:360.

66 Lewis RA, Soter NA, Diamond PT, Austen KF, Oates JA, Roberts LJ 2nd: Prostaglandin D2 generation after activation of rat and human mast cells with anti-IgE. J Immunol 1982;129:1627.

67 Taylor-Clark TE, Undem BJ, MacGlashan DW Jr, Ghatta S, Carr MJ, McAlexander MA: Prostaglandin-induced activation of nociceptive neurons via direct interaction with transient recpetor potential A1 (TRPA1). Mol Pharmacol 2008;2008:274.

68 Taylor-Clarke TE, McAlexander MA, Nassenstein C, Sheardown SA, Wilson S, Thornton J, Carr MJ, Undem BJ: Relative contributions of TRPA1 and TRPV1 channels in the activation of vagal bronchopulmonary C-fibres by the endogenous autacoid 4-oxononenal. J Physiol 2008;586:3447.

69 Taylor-Clark TE, Ghatta S, Bettner W, Undem BJ: Nitrooleic acid, an endogenous product of nitrative stress, activates nociceptive sensory nerves via the direct activation of TRPA1. Mol Pharmacol 2009;75:820.

70 Raemdonck K, de Alba J, Birrell MA, Grace M, Maher SA, Irvin CG, Fozard JR, O'Byrne PM, Belvisi MG: A role for sensory nerves in the late asthmatic response. Thorax 2012;67:19–25.

71 Caceres AI, Brackmann M, Elia MD, Bessac BF, del Camino D, D'Amours M, Witek JS, Fanger CM, Chong JA, Hayward NJ, Homer RJ, Cohn L, Huang X, Moran MM, Jordt SE: A sensory neuronal ion channel essential for airway inflammation and hyperreactivity in asthma. Proc Natl Acad Sci USA 2009;106:9099.

72 Lee MG, Kollarik M, Chuaychoo B, Undem BJ: Ionotropic and metabotropic receptor mediated airway sensory nerve activation. Pulm Pharmacol Ther 2004;17:355.

73 Fox AJ, Barnes PJ, Urban L, Dray A: An in vitro study of the properties of single vagal afferents innervating guinea-pig airways. J Physiol 1993;469: 21.

74 Bautista DM, Jordt SE, Nikai T, Tsuruda PR, Read AJ, Poblete J, Yamoah EN, Basbaum AI, Julius D: TRPA1 mediates the inflammatory actions of environmental irritants and proalgesis agents. Cell 2006;124:1269.

75 Lee MG, MacGlashan DW Jr, Undem BJ: Role of chloride channels in bradykinin-induced guinea pig airway vagal C-fibre activation. J Physiol 2005;566: 205.

76 Oh EJ, Weinreich D: Bradykinin decreases K(+) and increases CL(–) conductances in vagal afferent neurones of the guinea pig. J Physiol 2004;558:513.

77 Patel KN, Liu Q, Meeker S, Undem BJ, Dong X: Pirt, a TRPV1 modulator, is required for histamin-dependent and -independent itch. PLoS One 2011;6: e20559.

78 Marquardt DL, Gruber HE, Wasserman SI: Adenosine release from stimulated mast cells. Proc Natl Acad Sci USA 1984;81:6192.

79 Chuaychoo B, Lee MG, Kollarik A, Pullmann R Jr, Undem BJ: Evidence for both adenosine A1 and A2A receptors activating single vagal sensory C-fibres in guinea pig lungs. J Physiol 2006;575: 481.

80 Kuo YL, Lai CJ: Ovalbumin sensitizes vagal pulmonary C-fiber afferents in Brown Norway rats. J Appl Physiol 2008;105:611.

81 Riccio MM, Myers AC, Undem BJ: Immunomodulation of afferent neurons in guinea-pig isolated airway. J Physiol 1996;491:499.

82 Zhang G, Lin RL, Wiggers M, Lee LY: Sensitizing effects of chronic exposure and acute inhalation of ovalbumin aerosol on pulmonary C fibers in rats. J Appl Physiol 2008;105:128.

83 Undem BJ, Raible DC, Adkinson NF, Adams GK: Effect of removal of epithelium on antigen-induced smooth muscle contraction and mediator release from guinea pig isolated trachea. J Pharmacol Exp Ther 1988;244:659.

84 Schulman ES, Adkinson NF Jr, Newball HH: Cyclooxygenase metabolites in human lung anaphylaxis: airway vs. parenchyma. J Appl Physiol 1982;53:589.

85 Liu MC, Hubbard WC, Proud D, Stealey BA, Galli SJ, Kagey-Sobotka A, Bleeker ER, Lichtenstein LM: Immediate and late inflammatory responses to ragweed antigen challenge of the peripheral airways in allergic asthmatics. Cellular, mediator, and permeablility changes. Am Rev Respir Dis 1991;144:51.

86 Coleridge HM, Coleridge JC, Ginzel KH, Baker DG, Banzett RB, Morrison MA: Stimulation of 'irritant' receptors and afferent C-fibres in the lungs by prostaglandins. Nature 1976;264:451.

87 Weinreich D, Wonderlin WF: Inhibition of calcium-dependent spike after-hyperpolarization increases excitability of rabbit visceral sensory neurones. J Physiol 1987;394:415.

88 Weinreich D, Koschorke GM, Undem BJ, Taylor GE: Prevention of the excitatory actions of bradykinin by inhibition of PGI2 formation in nodose neurons of the guinea-pig. J Physiol 1995;483:735.

89 Kwong K, Lee LY: PGE2 sensitizes cultured pulmonary vagal sensory neurons to chemical and electrical stimuli. J Appl Physiol 2002;93:1419.

90 Maher SA, Birrell MA, Belvisi MG: Prostaglandin E2 mediates cough via the EP3 receptor: implications for future disease therapy. Am J Respir Crit Care Med 2009;180:923.

91 Lee LY, Gu Q, Gleich GJ: Effect of human eosinophil granule-derived cationic proteins on C-fiber afferents in the rat lung. J Appl Physiol 2001;91:1318.

92 Gu Q, Wiggers ME, Gleich GJ, Lee LY: Sensitization of isolated rat vagal pulmonary sensory neurons by eosinophil-derived cationic proteins. Am J Physiol Lung Cell Mol Physiol 2008;294.

93 Metcalfe DD, Baram D, Mekori YA: Mast Cells. Physiol Rev 1997;77:1033.

94 Ellis JL, Undem BJ: Role of peptidoleukotrienes in capsaicin-sensitive sensory fibre-mediated responses in guinea-pig airways. J Physiol 1991;436:469.

95 McAlexander MA, Myers AC, Undem BJ: Inhibition of 5-lipoxygenase diminishes neurally evoked tachykinergic contraction of guinea pig isolated airway. J Pharmacol Exp Ther 1998;285:602.

96 Taylor-Clarke TE, Nassenstein C, Undem BJ: Leukotriene D4 increases the excitability of capsaicin-sensitive nasal sensory nerves to electrical and chemical stimuli. Br J Pharmacol 2008;154:1359.

97 Macfarlane SR, Seatter MJ, Kanke T, Hunter GD, Plevin R: Proteinase-activated receptors. Pharmacol Rev 2001;53:245.

98 Gu Q, Lee LY: Hypersensitivity of pulmonary chemosensitive neurons induced by activation of protease-activated receptor-2 in rats. J Physiol 2006;574:867.

99 Zweifel LS, Kuruvilla R, Ginty DD: Functions and mechanisms of retrograde neurotrophin signalling. Nat Rev Neurosci 2005;22:146.

100 Lieu T, Kollarik M, Myers AC, Undem BJ: Neurotrophin and GDNF family ligand receptor expression in vagal sensory nerve subtypes innervating the adult guinea pig respiratory tract. Am J Physiol Lung Cell Mol Physiol 2011;300:L790.

101 Nockher WA, Renz H: Neurotrophins in allergic diseases: from neuronal growth factors to intercellular signaling molecules. J Allergy Clin Immunol 2006;117:583.

102 Lieu T, Myers AC, Meeker S, Undem BJ: TRPV1 induction in low-threshold mechanosensory neurons by allergen challenge and neurotrophic factors. Am J Physiol Lung Cell Mol Physiol 2012 Feb 17; Epub ahead of print.

103 Gronenberg DA, Quarcoo D, Forssard N, Fischer A: Neurogenic mechanisms in bronchial inflammatory diseases. Allergy 2004;59:1139.

104 Fischer A, Hoffmann B: Nitric oxide synthase in neurons and nerve fibers of lower airways and in vagal sensory ganglia of man. Am J Respir Crit Care Med 1996;154:209.

105 Mazzone SB, Geraghty DP: Respiratory actions of tachykinins in the nucleus of the solitary tract: characterization of receptors using selective agonists and antagonists. Br J Pharmacol 2000;129:1121.

106 Bolser DC, DeGennaro FC, O'Reilly S, McLeod RL, Hey JA: Central antitussive activity of the NK1 and NK2 tachykinin receptor antagonists, CP-99,994, and SR 48968, in the guinea-pig and cat. Br J Pharmacol 1997;121:165.

107 Myers AC, Kajekar R, Undem BJ: Allergic inflammation-induced neuropeptide production in rapidly adapting afferent nerves in guinea pig airways. Am J Physiol Lung Cell Mol Physiol 2002;282:L775.

108 Hunter DD, Myers AC, Undem BJ: Nerve growth factor-induced phenotypic switch in guinea pig airway sensory neurons. Am J Respir Crit Care Med 2000;161:1985.

109 Zhang G, Lin RL, Wiggers M, Snow DM, Lee LY: Altered expression of TRPV1 and sensitivity to capsaicin in pulmonary myelinated afferents following chronic airway inflammation in the rat. J Physiol 2008;586:5771.

110 Lieu T, Undem BJ: Neuroplasticity in vagal afferent neurons involved in cough. Pulm Pharmacol Ther 2011;24:276.

111 Undem BJ, Carr MJ: The role of nerves in asthma. Curr Allergy Asthma Rep 2002;2:159.

112 Silver R, Silverman AJ, Vitkovic L, Lederhendler II: Mast cells in the brain: evidence and functional significance. Trends Neurosci 1996;19:25.

113 Woolf CJ: Central sensitization: implications for the diagnosis and treatment of pain. Pain 2011;152:S2.

114 Chen CY, Bonham AC, Schelegle ES, Gershwin LJ, Plopper CG, Joad JP: Extended allergen exposure in asthmatic monkeys induces neuroplasticity in nucleus tractus solitarius. J Allergy Clin Immunol 2001;108:557.

115 Mazzone SB, Mori N, Canning BJ: Synergistic interactions between airway afferent nerve subtypes regulating the cough reflex in guinea-pigs. J Physiol 2005;569:559.

116 Mazzone SB, Canning BJ: Synergistic interactions between airway afferent nerve subtypes mediating reflex bronchospasm in guinea pigs. Am J Physiol Regul Integr Comp Physiol 2002;283:R86.

117 Coleridge HM, Coleridge JCG, Baker DG, Ginzel KH, Morrison MA: Comparison of the effects of histamine and prostaglandin on afferent C-fiber endings and irritant receptors in the intrapulmonary airways. Adv Exp Med Biol 1978;99:291.

118 Mills JE, Widdicombe JG: Role of the vagus nerves in anaphylaxis and histamine-induced bronchoconstriction in guinea-pigs. Br J Pharmacol 1970;39:724.

119 Coleridge HM, Coleridge JC, Schultz HD: Afferent pathways involved in reflex regulation of airway smooth muscle. Pharmacol Ther 1989;42:1.

120 Myers AC, Undem BJ, Weinreich D: Influence of antigen on membrane properties of guinea pig bronchial ganglion neurons. J Appl Physiol 1991;71:970.

121 Myers AC, Undem BJ: Antigen depolarizes guinea pig bronchial parasympathetic ganglion neurons by activation of histamine H1 receptors. Am J Physiol 1995;268:L879.

122 Mitchell RA, Herbert DA, Baker DG, Basbaum CB: In vivo activity of tracheal parasympathetic ganglion cells innervating tracheal smooth muscle. Brain Res 1987;437:157.

123 Kajekar R, Undem BJ, Myers AC: Role of cyclooxygenase activation and prostaglandins in antigen-induced excitability changes of bronchial parasympathetic ganglia neurons. Am J Physiol Lung Cell Mol Physiol 2003;284:L581.
124 van der Kleij H, Charles N, Karimi K, Mao YK, Foster J, Janssen L, Chang Yang P, Kunze W, Rivera J, Bienenstock J: Evidence for neuronal expression of functional Fc (epsilon and gamma) receptors. J Allergy Clin Immunol 2010;125:757.
125 Fryer AD, Jacoby DB: Muscarinic receptors and control of airway smooth muscle. Am J Respir Crit Care Med 1998;158:5154.
126 Fryer AD, Maclagan J: Muscarinic inhibitory receptors in pulmonary parasympathetic nerves in the guinea-pig. Br J Pharmacol 1984;83:973.
127 Kilbinger H, Schneider R, Siefken H, Wolf D, D'Agostino G: Characterization of prejunctional muscarinic autoreceptors in guinea-pig trachea. Br J Pharmacol 1991;103:1757.
128 Larsen GL, Fame TM, Renz H, Loader JE, Graves J, Hill M, Gelfand EW: Increased acetylcholine release in tracheas from allergen-exposed IgE-immune mice. Am J Physiol 1994;266:L263.
129 Fryer AD, Wills-Karp M: Dysfunction of M2 muscarinic receptors in pulmonary parasympathetic nerves after antigen challenge in guinea-pigs. J Appl Physiol 1991;71:2255.
130 Pan J, Rhode HK, Undem BJ, Myers AC: Neurotransmitters in airway parasympathetic neurons altered by neurotrophin-3 and repeated allergen challenge. Am J Respir Crit Care Med 2009;43: 452.
131 Revicki DA, Leidy NK, Brennan-Diemer F, Thompson C, Togias A: Development and preliminary validation of the mulitattribute Rhinitis Symptom Utility Index. Qual Life Res 1998;7:693.
132 Shusterman DJ, Murphy MA, Balmes JR: Subjects with seasonal allergic rhinitis and nonrhinitic subjects react differentially to nasal provocation with chlorine gas. J Allergy Clin Immunol 1998;101:732.
133 Riccio MM, Proud D: Evidence that enhanced nasal reactivity to bradykinin in patients with symptomatic allergy is mediated by neural reflexes. J Allergy Clin Immunol 1996;97:1252.
134 Riccio MM, Reynolds CJ, Hay DW, Proud D: Effects of intranasal administration of endothelin-1 to allergic and nonallergic individuals. Am J Respir Crit Care Med 1995;152:1757.
135 Majchel AM, Proud D, Freidhoff L, Creticos PS, Norman PS, Naclerio RM: The nasal response to histamine challenge: effect of pollen season and immunotherapy. J Allergy Clin Immunol 1992;90: 85.
136 Philip G, Baroody FM, Proud D, Naclerio RM, Togias AG: The human nasal response to capsaicin. J Allergy Clin Immunol 1994;94:1035.
137 Ritz T, Steptoe A, Bobb C, Harris AH, Edwards M: The asthma trigger inventory: validation of a questionnaire for perceived triggers of asthma. Psychosom Med 2006;68:956.
138 Sheppard D, Wong WS, Uehara CF, Nadel JA, Boushey HA: Lower threshold and greater bronchomotor responsiveness of asthmatic subjects to sulfur dioxide. Am Rev Respir Dis 1980;122:873.
139 Wagner EM, Jacoby DB: Methacholine causese reflex bronchoconstriction. J Appl Physiol 1999;88: 294.
140 Peters SP, Kunselman SJ, Icitovic N, et al: Tiotropium bromide step-up therapy for adults with uncontrolled asthma. N Engl J Med 2010;363:1715.
141 Sanico AM, Philip G, Proud D, Naclerio RM, Togias A: Comparison of nasal mucosal responsiveness to neuronal stimulation in non-allergic and allergic rhinitis: effects of capsaicin nasal challenge. Clin Exp Allergy 1998;28:92.

Dr. Bradley J. Undem
Asthma and Allergy Center, Johns Hopkins University
5501 Hopkins Bayview Circle
Baltimore, MD 21224 (USA)
Tel. +1 410 550 2160, E-Mail bundem1@jhmi.edu

Bienenstock J (ed): Allergy and the Nervous System.
Chem Immunol Allergy. Basel, Karger, 2012, vol 98, pp 163–175

Role of Microbiome in Regulating the HPA Axis and Its Relevance to Allergy

Nobuyuki Sudo

Department of Psychosomatic Medicine, Graduate School of Medical Sciences, Kyushu University, Fukuoka, Japan

Abstract

There has been an increasing and intense interest in the role that gut bacteria play in maintaining the health of the host. Gut microbiota have an estimated mass of 1–2 kg, number 100 trillion and together possess 100 times the number of genes in the human genome. In addition to their well-established role in the postnatal maturation of the mammalian immune system, they are also responsible for an enormous array of metabolic activities that include effects on the digestion of food and the production of a host of biologically active substances. Moreover, it is also rapidly becoming apparent that the gut microbiome plays a major role in the development and regulation of neuroendocrine systems such as the hypothalamic-pituitary-adrenal axis, a central integrative system crucial for the successful physiological adaptation of the organism to stress. In fact, our previous study on gnotobiotic mice demonstrated that exposure to gut microbes is a postnatal environmental determinant that regulates the development of the hypothalamic-pituitary-adrenal axis stress response and also the set point for this axis.

This article focuses on the ability of commensal microbiota to regulate the hypothalamic-pituitary-adrenal (HPA) axis response, which plays a critical role in regulating allergic reactions.

The human gut is sterile at birth. Immediately after birth, it becomes colonized by numerous types of microorganisms. During the first weeks of life, tremendous temporal and interindividual variations are evident in the infant's microbial populations (microbiome). By 1 year of age, while babies retain their unique bacterial profiles, these converge toward a profile characteristic of the adult individual gastrointestinal tract [1]. Gut microbiota have now been estimated to consist of at least 1,800 genera and up to 40,000 species of bacteria based on the analysis of 16S ribosomal RNA. They have an estimated mass of 1–2 kg, number 100 trillion [2] and together possess 100 times the number of genes present in the human genome [3]. These bacteria not only play a principal role in the postnatal maturation of the mammalian immune system, but also aid in the digestion and absorption of macromolecules and act as a barrier to gut pathogens by blocking attachment to gut binding sites, which is the first step of bacterial pathogenicity [4]. Moreover, it is also rapidly becoming apparent that the gut microbiome plays a major role in the development and regulation of neuroendocrine systems such as the HPA axis [5–7].

A large number of papers have already described a possible causal link between gut microbiota and an increased risk of developing allergic diseases in the context of the 'hygiene hypothesis' [8–10]. However, this chapter will focus on the ability of commensal microbiota to set the HPA axis response, which is critically important for regulating allergic reactions.

HPA Axis Sensitivity to Stress Is Determined by Early-Life Environmental Factors

The HPA axis is considered to be a central integrative system crucial for the successful physiological adaptation of the organism to stress. During stress corticotropin-releasing hormone (CRH) and arginine vasopressin, the principal hypothalamic regulators of the HPA axis are released. CRH stimulates the secretion of adrenocorticotropin hormone (ACTH) from the anterior pituitary into the hypophyseal portal system via collateral fibers in the systemic circulation. ACTH leads to the secretion of glucocorticoids (GCs; cortisol in humans and corticosterone in rodents) from the adrenal cortex, the main target of ACTH. GCs are the final effectors of the HPA axis. GCs regulate multiple bodily functions and prepare the individual to cope with the demand of metabolic, physical and psychological stressors [11, 12].

Importantly, the HPA axis is subjected to programming by early life events. For example, as adults, neonatally handled animals exhibit dampened HPA responses to stress compared with nonhandled animals [13]. In contrast, adult animals exposed to repeated periods of prolonged maternal deprivation as neonates display increased HPA response to stress [14]. These effects persist into adulthood and the resulting hyperactivity of HPA responses are associated with the incidence of age-related neuropathology [13], such as memory impairment in animals [15, 16] and humans [17].

Normal Functioning of the HPA Axis is Necessary for Diminishing Ongoing Allergic Reactions

It is well known that the HPA activity is involved in the regulation of allergic reaction. For example, in an animal model evaluating the extent of itching on the basis of the number of compound 48/80-induced scratching behaviors, inhibition of an endogenous glucocorticoid activity by RU-486 significantly increased the degree of scratching behavior after the injection of compound 48/80 (fig. 1) [18]. Moreover, surgical removal of the adrenal glands also significantly increased the compound

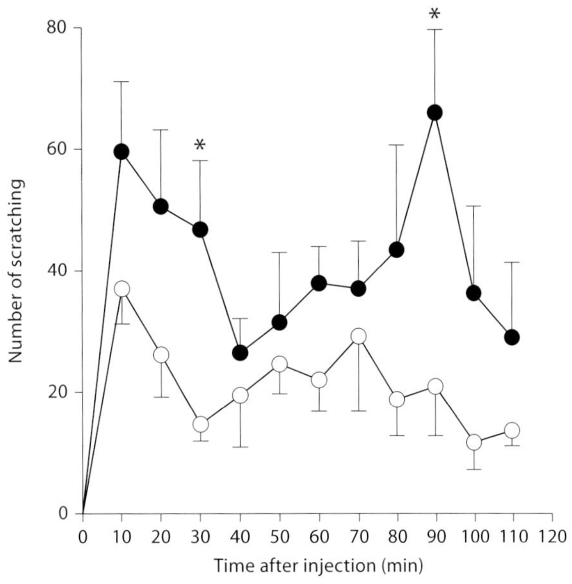

Fig. 1. Effects of RU-486 on the compound 48/80-induced scratching behavior. The mice were administered RU-486 (closed circle) or a corresponding vehicle (open circle) 1 h prior to the injection of compound 48/80. All data are expressed as the mean ± SE. A significant group difference between the RU-486- and vehicle-treated animals was found by an ANOVA. * $p < 0.05$ was considered to indicate a significant difference from the corresponding values in the vehicle group.

48/80-induced scratching behavior without affecting the locomotor activity, indicating that endogenous glucocorticoids exert their anti-pruritogenic effects independently of changes in behavior. We also confirmed the importance of the HPA axis function in an alternative animal model of bronchial asthma [19]. As shown in figure 2, adult mice that were subjected to either foot-shock stress (physical stress) or communication-box stress (psychological stress) during their 4th week of life, exhibited increases in the number of eosinophils and total mononuclear cells in their bronchoalveolar lavage (BAL) and a significant attenuation of the increase in the serum corticosterone levels following OVA challenge in comparison with the control group. The enhanced airway allergy in the communication stress group was at least partially attributed to HPA dysfunction, since the inhibition of transient corticosterone elevation following communication stress by RU-486 pretreatment resulted in the normalization of such OVA-induced eosinophil increases in the BAL in adults.

Since all these results were obtained during animal experiments, they are not directly applicable to the human clinical situation. However, several clinical reports suggested that reduced HPA axis activity may be involved in the maintenance and exacerbation of atopy [20–22]. In fact, the pathogenic significance of a dysfunctional HPA axis in skin atopy is clearly indicated by an incidental observation by Laue et al. [23]. They reported that after treatment with the glucocorticoid receptor antagonist RU-486, healthy volunteers showed atopy-like symptoms such as erythema and eczematous skin. None of the subjects had a prior history of atopy. More importantly,

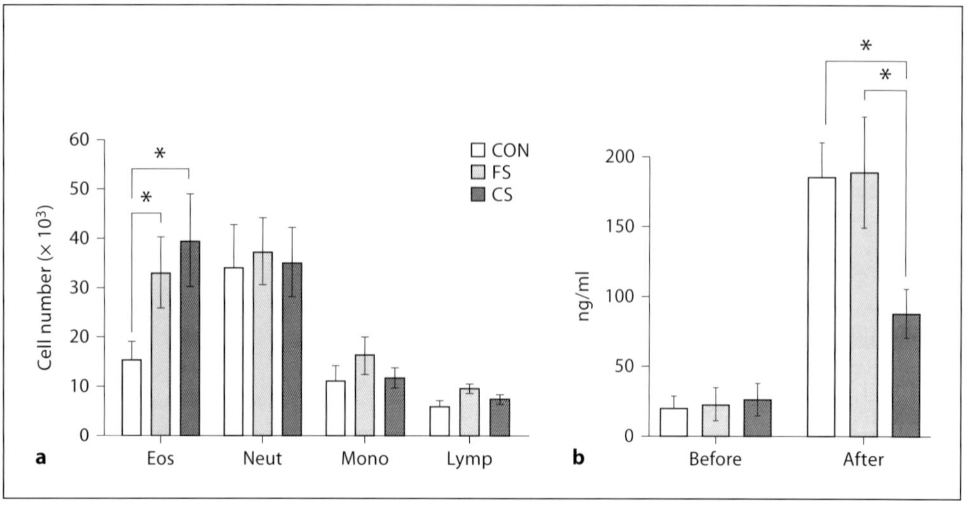

Fig. 2. Number of BAL cells after antigen challenge in actively sensitized mice. CON, FS, and CS indicate the groups exposed to the control conditions, physical stress by electric foot-shock, and psychological stress by the communication box, respectively. The subpopulation cell number (EOS = eosinophils; NEUT = neutrophils; MONO = monocytes; LYMP = lymphocytes) was assessed 24 h after OVA airway challenge. All values are expressed as the means ± SE. * $p < 0.05$ was considered to be significantly different from the corresponding value of the CON group.

based on a series of excellent studies, Buske-Kirschbaum and colleagues [24, 25] suggested that a hyporesponsive HPA axis may not be a characteristic feature limited to skin atopy, but may actually be a phenomenon generally linked to allergic inflammation, regardless of the organ affected. This idea has been confirmed by others showing lower cortisol responses to a stressful laboratory procedure, i.e. blood sampling in adolescents with different forms of allergy, such as atopic dermatitis [26].

Regardless of the mechanism responsible for why patients with allergies have a hyporesponsive HPA axis, it is clear that the normal functioning of the HPA axis is critically important for adequately controlling allergic inflammation.

Gut Microbiota Play a Critical Role in Determining the Setpoint of the HPA Axis

As described earlier, the HPA axis is susceptible to environmental influences especially early in life. Therefore, we speculated that indigenous microbiota, a major environmental force affecting the host physiology, might alter the development of the HPA response.

To test this hypothesis, we investigated the HPA response to stress by comparing genetically identical mice that had no exposure to microorganisms (germfree: GF), mice raised with a normal functional microbiota but not with specific pathogens (specific pathogen free: SPF), and mice raised with a selected group of organisms

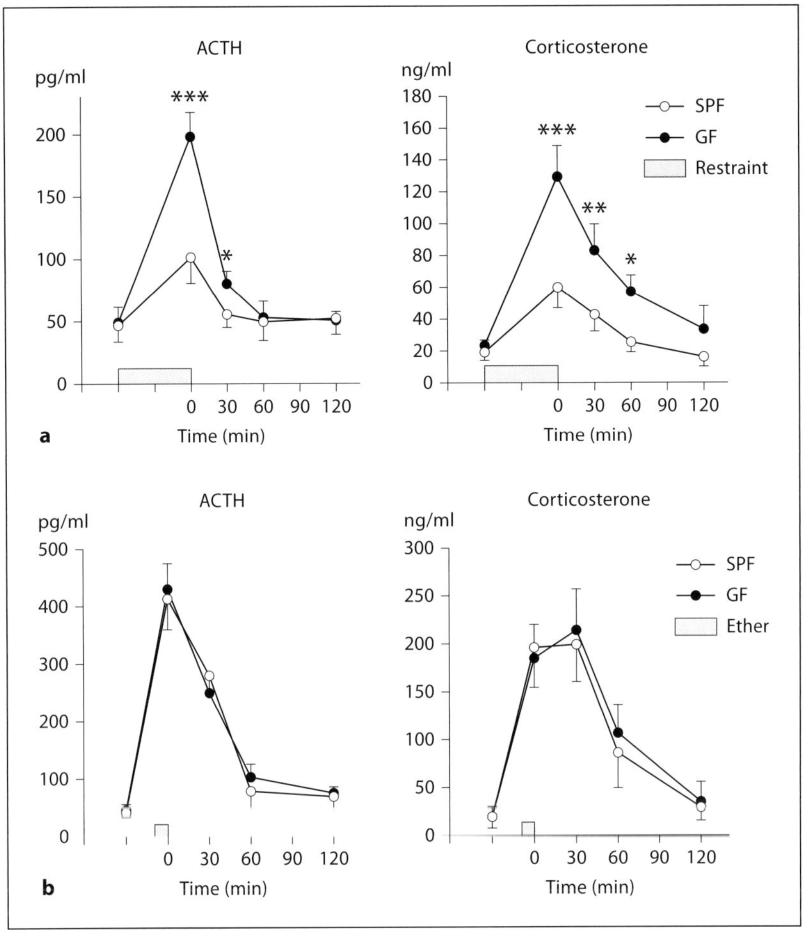

Fig. 3. Plasma ACTH and corticosterone levels increased after restraint stress, but not ether exposure, in GF mice. **a** The mice were subjected to a 1-hour period of restraint stress. The baseline data were obtained by cardiac puncture from mice that were killed by cervical dislocation before stress exposure. *** $p < 0.001$, ** $p < 0.01$, * $p < 0.05$ in a posthoc Dunnett's test between the GF and SPF groups. **b** GF and SPF mice failed to show any difference in the HPA response to ether exposure.

(gnotobiotic) [5]. As shown in figure 3a, the plasma ACTH and corticosterone elevation in response to 1 h restraint stress was substantially higher in GF mice than in SPF mice. When the mice were exposed to ether stimulus, no significant difference in the plasma ACTH or corticosterone responses were found between these two groups of animals (fig. 3b).

To further elucidate the involvement of gut microbiota in the HPA stress response, gnotobiotic mice whose flora were composed of a single strain of bacterium at the neonatal stage were tested for their susceptibility to restraint stress as adults. Monoassociation with *Bifidobacterium infantis*, which is a representative inhabitant of the neonate gut, dampened the HPA stress response to the level observed in the

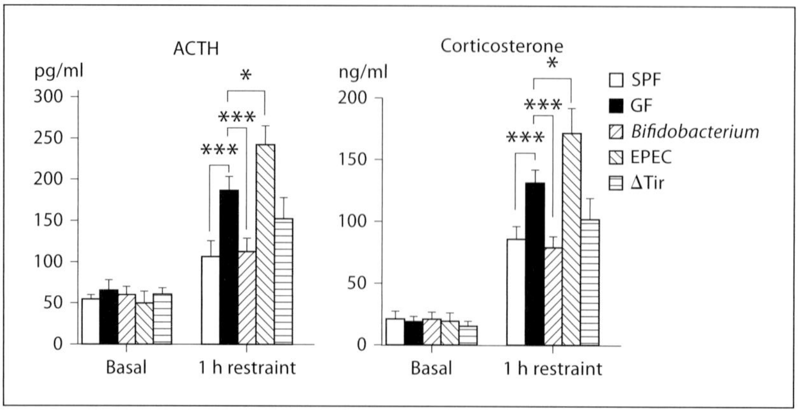

Fig. 4. Effects of restraint stress on plasma ACTH and corticosterone levels in gnotobiotic mice. The plasma ACTH and corticosterone levels were measured before or immediately after 1 h restraint in GF, SPF and monoassociated mice at 9 weeks of age. *** $p < 0.001$, * $p < 0.05$ by Dunnett's test.

SPF mice (fig. 4). In accord with a previous report indicating that neonatal endotoxin treatment increases the HPA stress response later in life [27, 28], the hormonal stress response in rabbit-derived EPEC-monoassociated mice was substantially higher than that in GF mice, although no such exaggerated response was found in the mice reconstituted with an EPEC mutant strain, ΔTir [29], which is not internalized due to defects in the translocated intimin receptor.

Next, the effects of a complete SPF flora on the hormonal response to stress were examined. The enhanced HPA stress response of GF mice was partially corrected at 3 weeks after reconstitution with SPF feces at an early stage of development (fig. 5a), while such a correction was not found when reconstitution was performed later in life (fig. 5b). Therefore, the microbe-induced reversal of the HPA axis set-point extended into adulthood, but only if bacterial colonization occurred before the animals reached 6 weeks of age. Colonization as adults was ineffective, thus suggesting that there is a critical window of susceptibility to these effects with regard to the bacteria-host interaction.

Recently, Gareau et al. [30] have reported that probiotic treatment consisting of *Lactobacillus rhamnosus* and *Lactobacillus helveticus* can ameliorate the enhanced HPA axis activity induced by maternal separation stress in rats, suggesting that probiotics normalize the activity of the HPA axis. Although the precise mechanism is unclear, they speculate that the expression of IL10 and its receptor in pituitary and hypothalamic tissues may be an important endogenous regulator of HPA axis activity. Taken together, these findings suggest that intervention with probiotics may protect infants from developing allergy later in life not only via modulating the immunological function, e.g. inducing Th1 and Treg cells, but also via the normalization of the HPA activity.

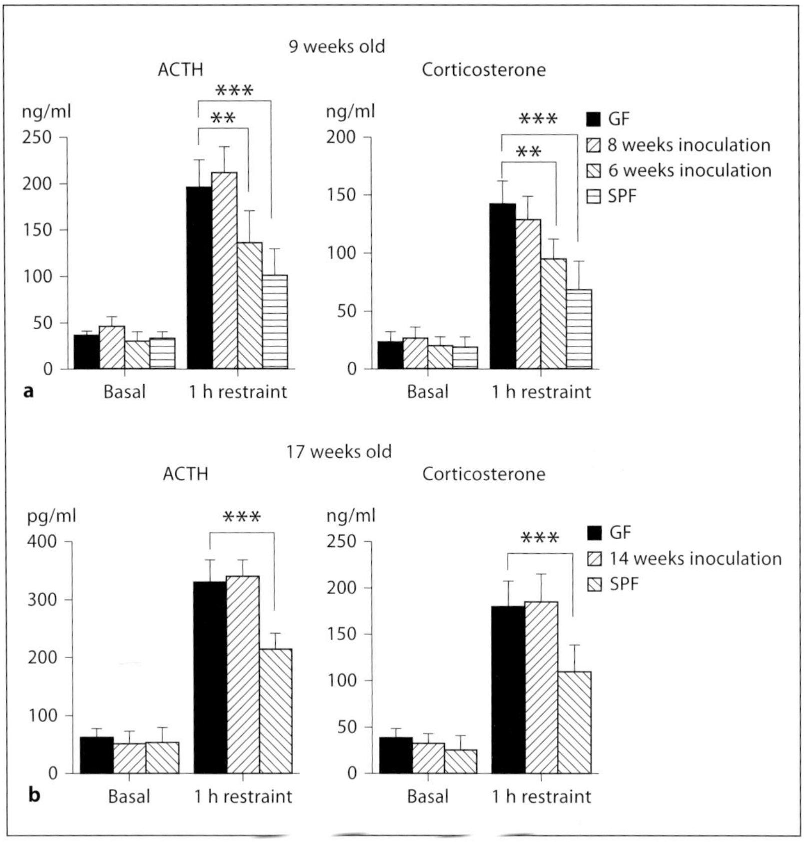

Fig. 5. Effects of restraint stress on the plasma ACTH and corticosterone levels in the mice reconstituted with SPF feces. SPF flora-reconstituted mice were established by orally introducing fresh SPF mouse feces into the GF mice at either 1 or 3 weeks before they were subjected to the stress protocol. Restraint stress was applied to the reconstituted mice at 9 (**a**) and 17 weeks of age (**b**). *** $p < 0.001$, ** $p < 0.01$ by Dunnett's test.

Brain Network Recognizes Signaling of Microbial Colonization in Gut and Elicits Transient Increases in Plasma Corticosterone Levels

The above studies suggest that the brain may recognize the colonization of bacteria inside the gut. However, precisely how this occurs and what pathways are involved in this process still remains unclear. As shown in figure 6a, the administration of *B. infantis* to GF mice triggered a small but significant increase in plasma IL-6 levels at 12 h after inoculation without elevating the plasma IL-1β levels. Interestingly, an increase in the c-Fos mRNA level in the hypothalamus was already noted at 6 h after inoculation (fig. 6b). Such a c-Fos response was accompanied by a concomitant increase in the plasma corticosterone level following exposure to microbes (basal 20 ± 11 ng/ml, 6 h 142 ± 36 ng/ml ($p < 0.001$ vs. basal value), 12 h 35

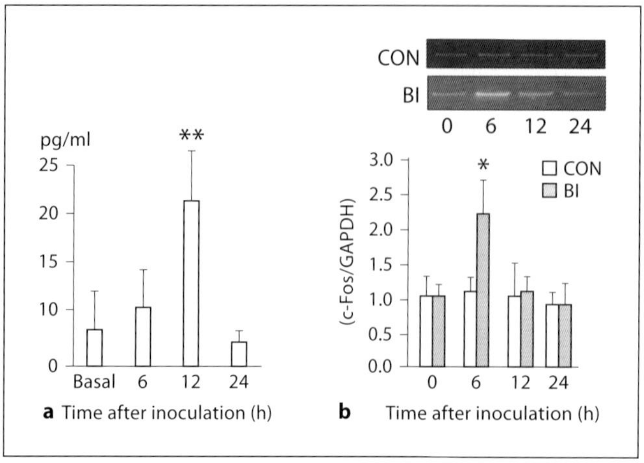

Fig. 6. The kinetics of the change in IL-6 levels in the plasma and the c-Fos gene expression in the hypothalamus upon exposure to *B. infantis*. GF mice at 5 weeks of age received a gavage of either 0.5 ml skim milk containing 1×10^9 CFU *B. infantis* (BI) or skim milk alone (CON), and plasma and brain samples were collected before (0), and 6, 12 or 24 h after *Bifidobacterium* inoculation. **a** Plasma IL-6 levels were analyzed by the B9 cell bioassay. **b** A typical RT-PCR product with c-Fos specific primers revealed PCR products with the predicted 247-bp length of c-Fos mRNA (upper panel). The bar graphs show the relative band intensities on the densitometric analysis as the ratios of c-Fos to GAPDH mRNA after 30 cycles of amplification (lower panel). ** $p < 0.01$ and * $p < 0.05$ were considered significantly different from the corresponding basal values.

± 26 ng/ml, 24 h 30 ± 19 ng/ml: n = 5–7 per time-point). Moreover, pretreatment with an anti-IL-6 antibody failed to affect the elevated c-Fos response in the hypothalamus or the corticosterone response in the plasma following exposure to *B. infantis*. In contrast, neonatal treatment with capsaicin partially suppressed the *Bifidobacterium*-induced c-fos elevation in the hypothalamus (fig. 7). Taken together, these results indicate that the brain can recognize the signals following bacterial colonization and subsequently activate the HPA axis via transient corticosterone elevation, which is mediated at least partly through a capsaicin-sensitive nerve.

Possible Gut Microbe-Derived Neurotransmitters and Gases Involved in Microbiome-Brain Signaling

The exact mechanisms by which gut bacteria-induced local changes in the gut epithelium and the enteric nervous system communicate with the brain and possibly alter its function and activity remain to be elucidated. As described above, capsaicin-sensitive nerves play an important role in the signaling from the gut microbes to the central nervous system; however, the underlying pathways are highly complex, and

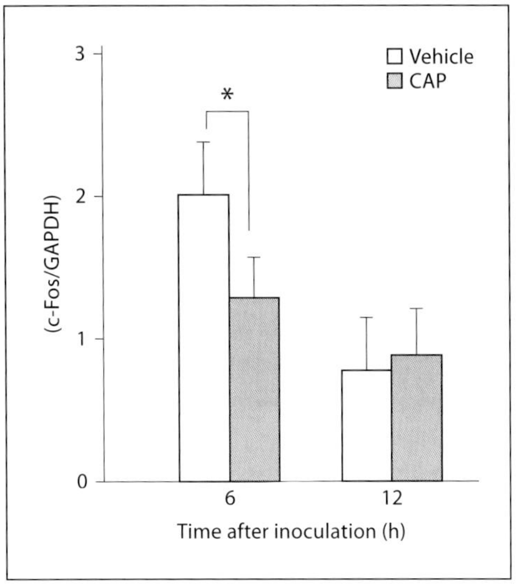

Fig. 7. Effects of neonatal capsaicin treatment on the PVN c-Fos response upon exposure to *Bifidobacterium*. GF mice were treated with either capsaicin (CAP) or the corresponding vehicle 2 days after birth. At 5 weeks of age, these two groups of mice were given *B. infantis* and their hypothalamus c-Fos responses were examined as described above. * $p < 0.05$ was considered to indicate a significant difference from the corresponding values in the VEH group.

it is unlikely that only one pathway or series of molecules is involved [6]. However, some possible pathways we feel may be involved are reviewed below.

It is not widely appreciated that commensal organisms produce neuroactive molecules such as serotonin, melatonin, gamma-aminobutyric acid (GABA) catecholamines, histamine and acetylcholine [31]. However, GABA is produced by many bacteria, especially Lactobacilli, and this property may serve to protect the organism from the acid environment encountered in the stomach, since its synthesis involves proton exchange for the uptake of glutamate [32]. A recent publication by Wikoff et al. [33] involving a metabolomic assessment of the plasma has shown that conventionalization of the microbiome of GF mice resulted in the appearance of a 2.8-fold increase in serotonin and other neuroactive metabolites. This clearly indicates the significance of the direct or indirect effects of microbes on the development and function of the neuroendocrine system. In addition, certain organisms, including *Lactobacilli* are able to convert nitrate to NO, a potent regulator of both the immune and nervous systems while hydrogen sulfide (H_2S), which is produced by some gut microbiota, has been shown to modulate gut motility through actions at the vanilloid receptor TRPV1 in capsaicin-sensitive nerve fibers [34]. *Lactobacilli* have also been shown to increase the activity of indoleamine 2,3-dioxygenase (IDO), an enzyme involved in the catabolism of tryptophan and the formation of the neuroactive compounds kynurenic and quinolinic acid [35].

Iyer et al. [31] have proposed the interesting theory that the evolutionary history of prokaryotic genes encoding many of the enzymes involved in the synthetic and metabolic pathways of catecholamines, histamine, acetylcholine and GABA is best described by scenarios that include late horizontal gene transfer from bacteria. This concept is substantiated by a growing body of evidence that bacteria produce small molecules which are formally involved in bacteria-bacteria communication and have now become involved in bacteria-host communication. The fact that some species of bacteria have a receptor-like molecule to take up GABA [36], and the fact that GABA and its receptor are found in the host gut epithelia [37], suggest that the GABA derived from gut microbiota may actually be involved in 'inter-kingdom signaling' [38], another aspect of which has previously been referred to with respect to stress-microbe interactions [39]. While we emphasize GABA in this context, it is but one of many examples of the bacterial synthesis of neuroactive molecules which remain to be explored.

Epigenetics May Be a Key Mechanism Explaining the Modification of the HPA Axis by the Microbiome

Recent topics related to epigenetic regulation are reviewed below, because some critical molecules involved in the HPA stress response, such as GR and CRF, are now known to be susceptible to epigenetic modifications [40].

Epigenetic modulation of gene transcription, a recently proposed mechanism for regulating the gene expression changes underlying neural plasticity, might likewise be affected by early-life adversity. Epigenetic modifications are most commonly regulated by either direct methylation of DNA or by posttranslational modifications of histones, both of which can either promote or repress gene transcription [41, 42]. In the central nervous system, DNA methylation has historically been viewed as a static process after neural development and cell differentiation; however, recent data continue to highlight the dynamic role of DNA methylation in gene regulation [43–45]. Furthermore, there is growing evidence for the role of epigenetic modifications in support of adult cognition and emotional health. For example, a landmark study by Meaney and colleagues [46] reported that increased pup licking and grooming (LG) and arched-back nursing (ABN) by rat mothers altered the offspring epigenome at a GR gene promoter in the hippocampus. The offspring of mothers that showed high levels of LG and ABN were found to have differences in DNA methylation, as compared to offspring of 'low-LG-ABN' mothers. These differences emerged over the first week of life, were reversed with cross-fostering, persisted into adulthood and were associated with altered histone acetylation and transcription factor (NGFI-A) binding to the GR promoter. Central infusion of a histone deacetylase inhibitor removed the group differences in histone acetylation, DNA methylation, NGFI-A binding, GR expression and HPA responses to stress, suggesting a causal relationship among the epigenomic states, GR expression and the maternal effect on stress responses in the offspring. These findings are further emphasized by the fact that a mouse model of depression demonstrated the changes in BDNF gene expression after chronic adult stress to be attributable to the epigenetic modification of the BDNF gene in the hippocampus [47].

The molecules involved in the epigenetic regulation associated with the microbiota-induced changes in the set-point of the HPA axis and how they achieve their effects are still unclear. However, while the available evidence is still scant, some possible candidates have been suggested. These include short-chain fatty acids (SCFAs), which are the end products of anaerobic bacterial fermentation in the gastrointestinal tract. Under physiological conditions, their production is entirely dependent on commensal microbes, and there are only negligible amounts of SCFAs detectable in GF mice [48]. Butyric acid is produced by obligate anaerobic bacteria, such as the Clostridium species, and is also a prototype member of an emerging class of drugs, the histone deacetylase inhibitors [49]. Recent findings have implicated epigenetic modifications in the etiology of mood disorders via chromatin remodeling and changes in histone acetylation [47]. In addition, Schroeder et al. [50] showed that systemic injection of butyrate induced histone hyperacetylation in the hippocampus and frontal cortex, and exerted antidepressant-like effects in mice that were associated with increased BDNF transcripts in the frontal cortex. Whether or not physiological levels of butyric can have the same effects on the brain is so far unknown. However, it is interesting to imagine that the butyric acid produced in the gut could affect the physiological function of the brain, because the brain BDNF levels in the cortex of GF mice (which have no butyric acid) were substantially lower than those of SPF mice that have considerably high levels of butyric acid [5].

Conclusion and Perspectives

Gut microbiota in the neonatal period can have long-lasting and profound effects on the adult HPA axis, which plays an important role in diminishing ongoing allergic reactions. However, several important questions still remain to be elucidated. For example, it is currently unclear what mechanisms are responsible for the microbiota-induced modulation of the HPA axis activity. If epigenetic modifications are involved, the molecules and/or target genes modified by this regulation still need to be identified. Another important question is whether or not our findings, which were based on animal experiments, are also applicable to humans. Namely, can indigenous microbiota affect the HPA stress response in human infants? This may be answered by longitudinal birth cohort studies with precise clinical data, including fecal microbial data and the salivary cortisol response to stressors (e.g. vaccination).

Clearly, further studies are still required to elucidate the actual role of GI commensal microbes in the regulation of the HPA set-point, but such studies would allow for the design of new therapeutic approaches to allergic and other diseases in terms of alleviating dysfunctional HPA axis activity.

References

1 Palmer C, Bik EM, DiGiulio DB, Relman DA, Brown PO: Development of the human infant intestinal microbiota. PLoS Biol 2007;5:e177.

2 Frank DN, Pace NR: Gastrointestinal microbiology enters the metagenomics era. Curr Opin Gastroenterol 2008;24:4–10.

3 Kurokawa K, Itoh T, Kuwahara T, Oshima K, Toh H, Toyoda A, Takami H, Morita H, Sharma VK, Srivastava TP, Taylor TD, Noguchi H, Mori H, Ogura Y, Ehrlich DS, Itoh K, Takagi T, Sakaki Y, Hayashi T, Hattori M: Comparative metagenomics revealed commonly enriched gene sets in human gut microbiomes. DNA Res 2007;14:169–181.

4 Finlay BB: Cell adhesion and invasion mechanisms in microbial pathogenesis. Curr Opin Cell Biol 1990;2:815–820.

5 Sudo N, Chida Y, Aiba Y, Sonoda J, Oyama N, Yu XN, Kubo C, Koga Y: Postnatal microbial colonization programs the hypothalamic-pituitary-adrenal system for stress response in mice. J Physiol Lond 2004;558:263–275.

6 Forsythe P, Sudo N, Dinan T, Taylor VH, Bienenstock J: Mood and gut feelings. Brain Behav Immun 2010;24:9–16.

7 Collins SM, Bercik P: The relationship between intestinal microbiota and the central nervous system in normal gastrointestinal function and disease. Gastroenterology 2009;136:2003–2014.

8 Guarner F, Bourdet-Sicard R, Brandtzaeg P, Gill HS, McGuirk P, van Eden W, Versalovic J, Weinstock JV, Rook GAW: Mechanisms of disease: the hygiene hypothesis revisited. Nat Clin Pract Gastroenterol Hepatol 2006;3:275–284.

9 Noverr M, Huffnagel G: Does the microbiota regulate immune responses outside the gut? Trends Microbiol 2004;12:562–568.

10 Rautava S, Kalliomaki M and Isolauri E: New therapeutic strategy for combating the increasing burden of allergic disease: Probiotics – a nutrition, allergy, mucosal immunology and intestinal microbiota (NAMI) research group report. J Allergy Clin Immunol 2005;116:31–37.

11 Chrousos G, Gold P: The concepts of stress and stress system disorders – overview of physical and behavioral homeostasis. JAMA 1992;267:1244–1252.

12 Turnbull AV, Rivier CL: Regulation of the hypothalamic-pituitary-adrenal axis by cytokines: actions and mechanisms of action. Physiol Rev 1999;79:1–71.

13 Meaney MJ, Aitken DH, van Berkel C, Bhatnagar S, Sapolsky RM: Effect of neonatal handling on age-related impairments associated with the hippocampus. Science 1988;239:766–768.

14 Schmidt M, Oitzl MS, Levine S, De Kloet ER: The HPA system during the postnatal development of CD1 mice and the effects of maternal deprivation. Dev Brain Res 2002;139:39–49.

15 Landfield PW, Waymire JC, Lynch G: Hippocampal aging and adrenocorticoids: quantitative correlations. Science 1978;202:1098–1102.

16 Landfield PW, Baskin RK, Pitler TA: Brain aging correlates: retardation by hormonal-pharmacological treatments. Science 1981;214:581–584.

17 Lupien SJ, de Leon M, de Santi S, Convit A, Tarshish C, Nair NP, Thakur M, McEwen BS, Hauger RL, Meaney MJ: Cortisol levels during human aging predict hippocampal atrophy and memory deficits. Nat Neurosci 1998;1:69–73.

18 Hirayama K, Sudo N, Sueyasu M, Sonoda J, Chida Y, Oishi R, Kubo C: Endogenous glucocorticoids inhibit scratching behavior induced by the administration of compound 48/80 in mice. Eur J Pharmacol 2003;481:59–65.

19 Chida Y, Sudo N, Sonoda J, Hiramoto T, Kubo C: Early-life psychological stress exacerbates adult mouse asthma via the hypothalamus-pituitary-adrenal axis. Am J Resp Crit Care Med 2007;175:316–322.

20 Buske-Kirschbaum A, Jobst S, Wustmans A, Kirschbaum C, Rauh W, Hellhammer D: Attenuated free cortisol response to psychosocial stress in children with atopic dermatitis. Psychosom Med 1997;59:419–426.

21 Buske-Kirschbaum A, Geiben A, Höllig H, Morschhäuser E, Hellhammer D: Altered responsiveness of the hypothalamus-pituitary-adrenal axis and the sympathetic adrenomedullary system to stress in patients with atopic dermatitis. J Clin Endocrinol Metab 2002;87:4245–4251.

22 Rupprecht M: Cortisol, corticotropin, and β-endorphin responses to corticotropin-releasing hormone in patients with atopic eczema. Psychoneuroendocrinology 1995;20:543–551.

23 Laue L, Lotze MT, Chrousos GP, Barnes K, Loriaux DL, Fleisher TA: Effect of chronic treatment with the glucocorticoid antagonist RU 486 in man: toxicity, immunological, and hormonal aspects. J Clin Endocrinol Metab 1990;71:1474–1480.

24 Buske-Kirschbaum A: Cortisol responses to stress in allergic children: interaction with the immune response. Neuroimmunomodulation 2009;16:325–332.

25 Buske-Kirschbaum A, Ebrecht M, Hellhammer DH: Blunted HPA axis responsiveness to stress in atopic patients is associated with the acuity and severeness of allergic inflammation. Brain Behav Immun 2010;24:1347–1353.

26 Wamboldt MZ, Laudenslager M, Wamboldt FS, Kelsay K, Hewitt J: Adolescents with atopic disorders have an attenuated cortisol response to laboratory stress. J Allergy Clin Immunol 2003;111:509–514.
27 Shanks N, Larocque S, Meaney MJ: Neonatal endotoxin exposure alters the development of the hypothalamic-pituitary-adrenal axis. Early illness and later responsivity to stress. J Neurosci 1995;15:376–384.
28 Shanks N, Windle RJ, Perks PA, Harbuz MS, Jessop DS, Ingram CD, Lightman SL: Early-life exposure to endotoxin alters hypothalamic-pituitary-adrenal function and predisposition to inflammation. Proc Natl Acad Sci USA 2000;97:5645–5650.
29 Kenny B, DeVinney R, Stein M, Reinscheid DJ, Frey EA, Finlay BB: Enteropathogenic *E. coli* (EPEC) transfers its receptor for intimate adherence into mammalian cells. Cell 1997;91:511–520.
30 Barreau F, Ferrier L, Fioramonti J, Bueno L: Neonatal maternal deprivation triggers long term alterations in colonic epithelial barrier and mucosal immunity in rats. Gut 2004;53:501–506.
31 Iyer LM, Aravind L, Coon SL, Klein DC, Koonin EV: Evolution of cell-cell signaling in animals: did late horizontal gene transfer from bacteria have a role? Trends Genet 2004;20:292–299.
32 Higuchi T, Hayashi H, Abe K: Exchange of glutamate and gamma-aminobutyrate in a *Lactobacillus* strain. J Bacteriol 1997;179:3362–3364.
33 Wikoff WR, Anfora AT, Liu J, Schultz PG, Lesley SA, Peters EC, Siuzdak G: Metabolomics analysis reveals large effects of gut microflora on mammalian blood metabolites. Proc Natl Acad Sci USA 2009;106:3698–3703.
34 Schicho R, Krueger D, Zeller F, Von Weyhern CW, Frieling T, Kimura H, Ishii I, De Giorgio R, Campi B, Schemann M: Hydrogen sulfide is a novel prosecretory neuromodulator in the guinea-pig and human colon. Gastroenterology 2006;131:1542–1552.
35 Forsythe P, Inman MD, Bienenstock J: Oral treatment with live *Lactobacillus reuteri* inhibits the allergic airway response in mice. Am J Respir Crit Care Med 2007;175:561–569.
36 Guthrie GD, Nicholson-Guthrie CS: Gamma-aminobutyric acid uptake by a bacterial system with neurotransmitter binding characteristics. Proc Natl Acad Sci USA 1989;86:7378–7381.
37 Nakajima K, Tooyama I, Kuriyama K, Kimura H: Immunohistochemical demonstration of GABAB receptors in the rat gastrointestinal tract. Neurochem Res 1996;21:211–215.
38 Hughes DT, Sperandio V: Inter-kingdom signalling: communication between bacteria and their hosts. Nat Rev Microbiol 2008;6:111–120.
39 Freestone PP, Sandrini SM, Haigh RD, Lyte M: Microbial endocrinology: how stress influences susceptibility to infection. Trends Microbiol 2008;16: 55–64.
40 Roth TL, Lubin FD, Funk AJ, Sweatt JD: Lasting epigenetic influence of early-life adversity on the BDNF gene. Biol Psychiatry 2009;65:760–769.
41 Chahrour M, Jung SY, Shaw C, Zhou X, Wong ST, Qin J, Zoghbi HY: MeCP2, a key contributor to neurological disease, activates and represses transcription. Science 2008;320:1224–1229.
42 Suzuki MM, Bird A: DNA methylation landscapes: provocative insights from epigenomics. Nat Rev Genet 2008;9:465–476.
43 Siegmund KD, Connor CM, Campan M, Long TI, Weisenberger DJ, Biniszkiewicz D, Jaenisch R, Laird PW, Akbarian S: DNA methylation in the human cerebral cortex is dynamically regulated throughout the life span and involves differentiated neurons. PLoS One 2007;2:e895.
44 Brown SE, Weaver IC, Meaney MJ, Szyf M: Regional-specific global cytosine methylation and DNA methyltransferase expression in the adult rat hippocampus. Neurosci Lett 2008;440:49–53.
45 Kangaspeska S, Stride B, Metivier R, Polycarpou-Schwarz M, Ibberson D, Carmouche RP, Benes V, Gannon F, Reid G: Transient cyclical methylation of promoter DNA. Nature 2008;452:112–115.
46 Weaver ICG, Cervoni N, Champagne FA, D'Alessio AC, Sharma S, Seckl JR, Dymov S, Szyf M, Meaney MJ: Epigenetic programming by maternal behavior. Nat Neurosci 2004;7:847–854.
47 Tsankova NM, Berton O, Renthal W, Kumar A, Neve RL, Nestler EJ: Sustained hippocampal chromatin regulation in a mouse model of depression and antidepressant action. Nat Neurosci 2006;9: 519–525.
48 Hoverstad T, Midtvedt T: Short-chain fatty acids in germfree mice and rats. J Nutr 1986;116:1772–1776.
49 Tsankova N, Renthal W, Kumar A, Nestler EJ: Epigenetic regulation in psychiatric disorders. Nat Rev Neurosci 2007;8:355–367.
50 Schroeder FA, Lin CL, Crusio WE, Akbarian S: Antidepressant-like effects of the histone deacetylase inhibitor, sodium butyrate, in the mouse. Biol Psychiatry 2007;62:55–64.

Dr. Nobuyuki Sudo
Department of Psychosomatic Medicine, Graduate School of Medical Sciences, Kyushu University
3–1–1 Maidashi, Higashi-ku
Fukuoka 812–8582 (Japan)
Tel. +81 92 642 5316, E-Mail nobuyuki@med.kyushu-u.ac.jp

Bienenstock J (ed): Allergy and the Nervous System.
Chem Immunol Allergy. Basel, Karger, 2012, vol 98, pp 176–195

Autonomic Regulation of Anti-Inflammatory Activities from Salivary Glands

Ronald D. Mathison[a] · Joseph S. Davison[a] · Chris D. St. Laurent[b] · A. Dean Befus[b]

[a]Faculty of Medicine, University of Calgary, Calgary, Alta., and [b]550A Heritage Medical Research Centre, Faculty of Medicine and Dentistry, University of Alberta, Edmonton, Alta., Canada

Abstract

The cervical sympathetic nerves which innervate the medial basal hypothalamus-hypophyseal complex, primary and secondary lymph organs, and numerous glands, such as the pineal, thyroid, parathyroid and salivary glands form a relevant neuroimmunoendocrine structure that is involved in the regulation of systemic homeostasis. The superior cervical ganglia and the submandibular glands form a 'neuroendocrine axis' called the cervical sympathetic trunk submandibular gland (CST-SMG) axis. The identification of this axis usurps the traditional view of salivary glands as accessory digestive structures and reinforces the view that they are important sources of systemically active immunoregulatory and anti-inflammatory factors whose release is intimately controlled by the autonomic nervous system, and in particular the sympathetic branch. An end component of the CST-SMG axis is the synthesis, processing and release of submandibular rat-1 protein (SMR1), a prohormone, that generates several different peptides, one from near its N-terminus called sialorphin and another from its C-terminus called – submandibular gland peptide-T (SGP-T). SGP-T formed the template for tripeptide fragment (FEG) and its metabolically stable D-isomeric peptide feG, which are potent inhibitors of allergy and asthma (IgE-mediated allergic reactions) and several non-IgE-mediated inflammations. The translation from rat genetics and proteomics to humans has yielded structural and functional correlates that hopefully will lead to the development of new medications and therapeutic approaches for difficult to treat disorders. Although the CST-SMG axis has barely been explored in humans recognition of the importance of this axis could facilitate an understanding and improved management of periodontal disease, and other diseases with a more systemic and nervous system basis such as asthma, autoimmunity, graft-versus-host disease and even Parkinson's disease.

The close anatomical relationship of salivary glands with the oral cavity and their elaboration of digestive enzymes (lingual lipase and amylase) give them a digestive tract association, although salivary secretions are critically important for defense of the teeth and the soft tissues of the oral cavity and upper alimentary tract. Depending upon species adaptations, salivary secretions also act as pheromones for sexual signaling or territorial and kinship marking, are used to spin webs, cocoons and nests, function in both aggressive (e.g. venoms) and passive (e.g. toxin neutralization) defense mechanisms, participate in maintaining the health of the integument (e.g. licking of wounds, and newborn and infant offspring) [1, 2], and contribute to the maintenance of systemic functions.

The recognition that salivary glands work in close relationship to many body functions, organs and glands came with the identification of participatory roles for the submandibular (submaxillary) glands in reproduction [3], the recognition of sexual dimorphism in gland structure and function [4] and the identification of their endocrine secretions [5, 6]. The discovery of kallikrein in salivary glands [7] facilitated the concept that salivary gland factors exhibit regulatory functions, and solidification came three decades later with the identification of nerve growth factor (NGF) and epidermal growth factor (EGF) in mouse submandibular glands [8, 9]. Numerous biologically active factors exhibiting a range of functions including digestion, growth and differentiation, enzymatic control, homeostatic regulation, and adaptation to stress [10–12] are found in salivary glands. These factors, for the most part polypeptides, are secreted from salivary glands both into the oral cavity (exocrine secretion) and the blood (endocrine secretion). Nonetheless, salivary glands are still generally regarded as exocrine glands that dispense their protein and fluid externally into a lumen or a duct, although this orthodox view was deemed erroneous more than 75 years ago when it was shown that the pancreas and the parotid, two classical exocrine glands, release amylase directly into the blood stream [5, 6, 13]. From these and other observations salivary glands are now considered 'duacrine' glands – capable of both exocrine and endocrine secretion [14].

The endocrine secretions from salivary glands participate in the maintenance of the integrity of esophageal and gastrointestinal mucosa [15], promote hepatic regeneration [16] and mammary gland tumor genesis [17], are essential for maintenance of the reproductive system [18], protect against induction of liver tumors in young mice, but promote tumor growth in old mice [19], and modulate the severity of systemic inflammatory responses [20].

Given the importance of submandibular gland factors in the regulation of many essential body functions, it would be anticipated that their synthesis and release are subject to intimate control not only by the hypothalamic-pituitary-adrenal and gonadal axes [12, 21], but also by the sympatho-adrenal [22] and the autonomic nervous systems [23, 24]. An important regulatory component for the salivary glands is the cervical sympathetic trunk-submandibular gland (CST-SMG) axis – a neuroendocrine-immune track that confers a high level of control over submandibular glands that has profound impact on the regulation of systemic homeostasis and inflammation [25]. Although the submandibular glands have been more intensely studied and appear to be richer in regulatory factors than the parotid glands, the parotid also contains NGF [26], EGF and IGF-1 [27] that are probably localized to small granules that develop in the striated ducts under the influences of androgen and thyroid hormone influences [28], much as large granules are affected by these hormones in the submandibular glands. Nonetheless, autonomic nerve regulation of these two glands may be differentially regulated as sympathetic nerves negatively regulate NGF levels in the submandibular glands, but not the parotid glands [29]. Thus, our understanding of autonomic regulation of salivary gland function is still in development, and the CST-SMG axis will probably eventually become a CST-salivary gland axis (CST-SG axis) that also involves coordinate regulation between the different salivary glands [30].

Cervical Sympathetic Trunk-Submandibular Gland Axis

Neuroimmunoendocrinology, which studies the complex interplay and mutual interactions between the nervous, endocrine and immune systems, had its genesis in 1946 with recognition that the hypothalamic-pituitary-adrenal (HPA) axis plays a critical role in regulating the stress response. A key ingredient of adrenal-mediated actions, cortisone, is a powerful immunodepressant that reduces inflammation and attendant pain and swelling. Over the last several decades neuroimmunoendocrinology studies revealed that the central and peripheral nervous systems both stimulate and inhibit innate and adaptive immune responses through hormonal and neuronal pathways, which are in turn influenced by immune mediators and cytokines. A functional interaction between these systems maintains a balance between health and disease.

The nervous system influences the immune system through two major pathways – neuroendocrine axes and the autonomic nervous system (sympathetic and parasympathetic nerves), and has been extensively reviewed (see [31] for references). An exciting example of such neuroimmunological interactions is the cholinergic anti-inflammatory pathway [32]. Aside from the HPA axis other neuroimmunoendocrine relevant structures located in the head and neck (cervical-cephalic) region are the cervical sympathetic nerves that innervate the medial basal hypothalamus-hypophyseal complex, primary and secondary lymph organs, and numerous glands, such as the pineal, thyroid, parathyroid and salivary glands [33]. This branch of the autonomic nervous system modulates exocrine, endocrine and paracrine relationships in secretory cells that extend their influence to regulation of systemic homeostasis.

One week after decentralization of the superior cervical ganglia (SCG; fig. 1), by a process involving the submandibular glands, reductions occur in late-phase pulmonary inflammation following induction of anaphylaxis in sensitized rats [34], chemotactic responses and functions of circulating neutrophils [35], as well as mast cell-mediated TNF-dependent cytotoxicity [36]. The protective effect of decentralization of the SCG was abolished with concurrent bilateral removal of the submandibular glands [37]. Since antigen challenge produces increases excitability of the neurons in the SCG that can last minutes to several hours [38–40], it is probable that the superior

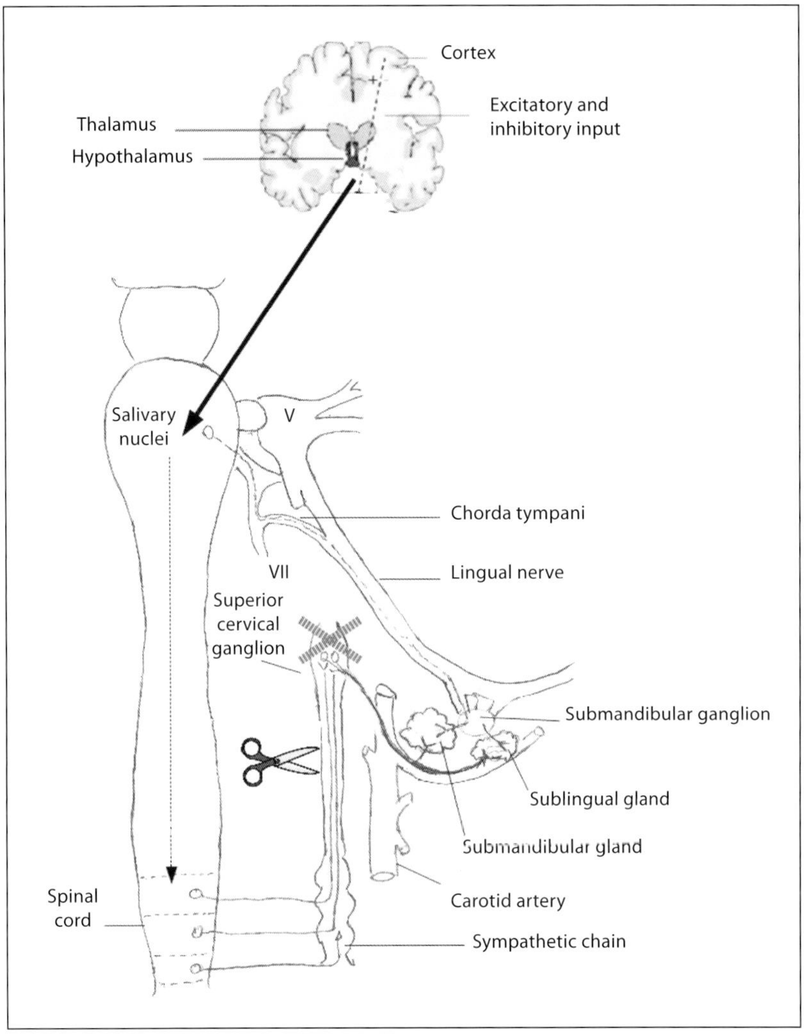

Fig. 1. The cervical sympathetic trunk submandibular gland axis – an important neuroimmunoendocrine structure found in the head and neck region. Afferent stimuli are integrated in the salivary nuclei of the medulla. The parasympathetic innervation of the submandibular (submaxillary) gland is carried in cranial nerve VII, and the sympathetic innervation originates in the SCG, which have their preganglionic nerves in thoracic segments T1-T4 of the spinal cord. The scissors indicate cutting of the cervical sympathetic nerve (decentralization) and the hatched cross indicates removal of the SCG (ganglionectomy). Adapted and modified from Knowledgerush. Parasympathetic. GNU Free Documentation License, 2011.

cervical innervation of the submandibular glands inhibits release of a 'factor' from these glands that down regulates the severity of allergic reactions [25] (fig. 2). A more generalized role for this axis in regulating systemic inflammation was later deduced in a model of endotoxin-induced acute hypotension, when either bilateral decentralization of the SCG or submandibular sialoadenectomy resulted in significantly larger

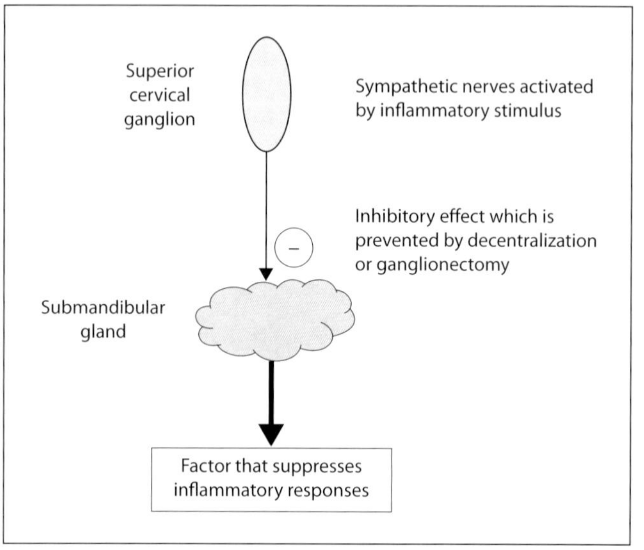

Fig. 2. Model for the CST-SMG axis and the regulation of inflammation.

drops in blood pressure compared to intact controls [41]. These observations support the suggestion that submandibular glands release a 'factor' that protects against not only acute hypotension induced by endotoxin but also allergic reactions. The release of this 'factor' is under the control of the cervical sympathetic nervous system, and led to our proposal of the 'cervical sympathetic trunk-submandibular (CST-SMG) axis' as an important neuroendocrine component that contributes to the modulation of systemic inflammatory responses [25, 37].

Innervation of the Submandibular Glands

Salivary gland secretion is a nerve-mediated reflex (fig. 1), with unstimulated flow of saliva providing a protective role for maintenance of oral health. The primary stimuli for release of saliva are smell, taste and mastication, although other factors such as noxious stimuli of physical and psychological origin, grooming and social behavior, alterations in light and darkness, oral hygiene, systemic diseases and medication use can impact release of saliva significantly. The two branches of the autonomic nervous system (parasympathetic and sympathetic) have considerable influence on the submandibular glands by controlling immediate secretion and exerting trophic effects so that volume and composition of the secretion is maintained and regulated according to functional requirements [24]. The parasympathetic nerves (cholinergic and NANC) arise in the salivary nuclei within the medulla oblongata and reach the glands through the facial nerve (cranial nerve VII). These nerves are primarily involved in fluid secretion as salivary flow essentially ceases if this innervation is interrupted. Approximately 90% of preganglionic sympathetic (adrenergic) innervation of the SCG originating in thoracic segments T1 to T3 [42] of the spinal cord, plays a negligible role in modulating salivary fluid flow, but acts primarily to regulate blood flow and protein secretion, thereby modulating saliva composition. In our studies the sympathetic component of this neuroimmunoendocrine structure was studied, primarily because of its role in regulating protein secretion, and the value of decentralization of SCG as an experimental model given that adrenergic nerves degenerate within 36–48 h of surgery, rendering neurotransmission nonfunctional (full postsynaptic paralysis) in the target organs [43, 44].

Submandibular Glands
The major salivary glands, parotid, submandibular and sublingual glands, are located in and around the mouth. The submandibular glands, located beneath the floor of the mouth, produce about 70% of the salivary volume under unstimulated conditions, whereas with stimulation (e.g. eating) the parotid produces the majority of saliva. The salivary glands have different secretory properties in that the parotid glands produce a serous watery secretion, whereas the submandibular glands produce a mixed serous and mucous secretion, and the sublingual glands secrete predominantly mucous saliva. These differences reflect the predominant presence of either serous cells (watery fluid) or mucous cells (mucous-rich secretions) in the glands. Saliva is a complex mixture of more than 2,000 products in its peptidome, of which only a quarter are derived from the salivary glands, indicating that other cells in the oral cavity (e.g. epithelial cells and leukocytes) make a significant quantitative contribution to saliva [45]. A proportion of the salivary gland secretions find their way into the blood.

Submandibular Rat-1 Protein, Its Derivatives and Human Homologues

Submandibular Gland Peptide T (SGP-T)
Since the reduction in allergy-induced pulmonary inflammation [34] and lipopolysaccaride (LPS)-induced hypotension [41] observed with cervical sympathetic denervation was dependent upon the presence of the submandibular glands, we proposed that an endocrine factor released from these glands was responsible for these effects. The heptapeptide SGP-T (submandibular gland peptide-T; TDIFEGG) was isolated from extracts of the gland and identified as the C-terminal amino acids (aa 138–144) of a 146 amino acid prohormone named SMR1 (submandibular rat-1 protein) [46] (fig. 3). The processing of the C-terminal of SMR1 (TDIFEGGGK) is not known, although the PeptideCutter [47] suggests that a probable product is DIFEGGG consequent to enzymatic actions of Asp-N endopeptidase and proteinase K. Further, enzymatic processing of the FEGGGK C-terminal sequence of SMR1 probably yields C-terminal amidated peptides upon removal of the basic residue (K) by a carboxypeptidase B-like enzyme, followed by generation of the alpha-amidated peptide by the multifunctional protein peptidylglycine alpha-amidating mono-oxygenase acting on glycine-extended peptides [48]. The salivary glands contain a carboxyl-terminal

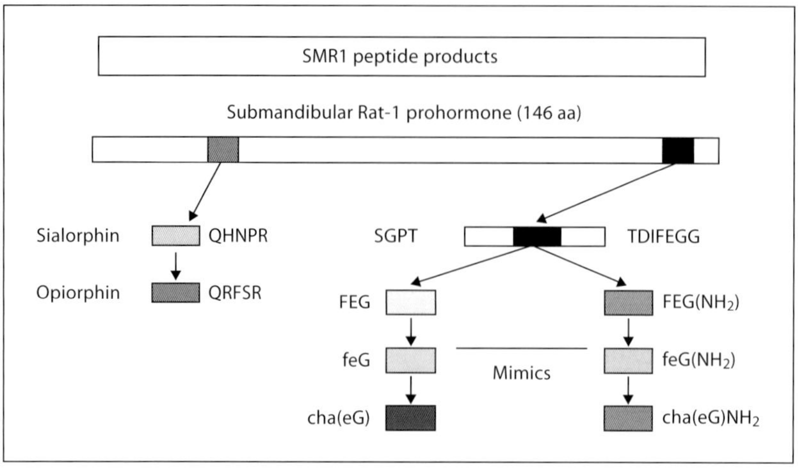

Fig. 3. Peptide derivatives of the SMR1 prohormone. Opiorphin is a human homologue of sialorphin.

peptide alpha-amidation enzymatic activity that effects post-translational processing of secretory polypeptides [49, 50]. Of potential relevance to the processing by peptidylglycine alpha-amidating mono-oxygenase-like enzymes and potential differential regulation of biologically active peptides by the various salivary glands is the observation that the enzyme occurs diffusely in both acinar and tubule cells of the sublingual gland, whereas it is confined to granular convoluted tubule cells in the submandibular glands [51].

Through structure-activity studies, the tripeptide FEG was identified as the minimal sequence of SGP-T required for inhibition of allergic reactions [52], and became the basis for the development of the metabolically stable D-isomeric peptides feG (D-phenylalanine-D-glutamate-glycine) and (cha)eG (D-cycloxylalanine-D-glutamate-Glycine) [53], and their amidated derivatives feG-NH_2 and (cha) eG-NH_2.

SMR1 prohormone was originally identified as a product of an androgen-regulated gene expressed in acinar cells of submandibular glands, prostate, urogenital tract and lungs of rats [54–56]. This gene, *Vcsa1* [57], the first described for the VCS (variable coding sequence) multigene family, encodes a precursor protein, submandibular rat1 protein (SMR1), which gives rise to several biologically active peptides, in addition to SGP-T. Of three structurally related peptides selectively matured by cleavage at dibasic amino acids near the N-terminal pentapeptide, QHNPR [58], has been most extensively investigated. The pentapeptide is known as sialorphin, because it is an endogenous salivary antinociceptive modulator consequent to inhibiting neutral endopeptidase [59]. Additional activities of sialorphin include modulation of systemic mineral ion homeostasis [60], regulation of intraspecific social behavior, such as an aggressive response to territorial challenge and/or sexual intercourse [61] and erectile function [59, 61–64], through relaxation of corporal smooth muscle tissue through a GPCR (G-protein coupled receptor) mechanism [62, 65].

A Human Homologue of Sialorphin – Opiorphin

Opiorphin (QRFSR) isolated from human saliva is the homologue of rat sialorphin. It blocks pain by inhibiting the enkephalin-inactivating ectopeptidases human neutral endopeptidase (hNEP) and human aminopeptidase-N (hAP-N) with consequent activation of endogenous opioid-dependent pathways [66]. Pain reduction by opiorphin does not show morphine-associated effects such as dependence and drug tolerance [67, 68], and by acting on delta-opioid receptor-dependent pathways, opiorphin has antidepressant-like effects [69, 70]. A role for opiorphin in erectile function is evident as the gene controlling its expression, *ProL1, is* downregulated in the corpora of men with erectile dysfunction [71], and overexpression is associated with experimental priapism, a persistent, often painful, penile erection that continues hours beyond, or is unrelated to, sexual stimulation [72, 73].

Human Homologues of SGP-T

Although a human homologue of SGP-T has not been identified, we sought to identify other proteins having peptide sequence similarity to TDIFEGG (SMR1). The focus was principally on peptide products that could be released into the bloodstream (endocrine hormones) or found on the extracellular membrane, and then either activate (agonist) or block (antagonist) a receptor site by mimicking an endogenous ligand found on another protein. Below are some findings of such proteins:

(1) Of particular interest due to close sequence homology to SGP-T (TDIFEGG) is calcium-binding and spermatid-specific protein 1 (CABS1) [74] with the TDIFELLK sequence located near its C-terminal. *CABS1* gene, responsible for synthesis of CABS1 protein, is located on human chromosome 5. *CABS1* greatest expression occurs in the testis (Geo Profile No. GDS3142), although some expression occurs in most tissues, including salivary glands and lungs. Further studies are required to identify potential processing and secretion products to verify CABS1 potential as a functional homologue of SGP-T in humans.

(2) A DIFELL sequence also is found in TBC1 domain family member 9B protein (TBC1–9B), which is located internally at amino acids 762 to 767 of a 1250 amino acid protein and has no obvious peptide cleavage sites. In contrast to CABS1 which is expressed almost exclusively in spermatids TBC1–9B (containing Tre-2, Bub2 and Cdc16) is expressed widely in most tissues, and has Rab GTPase activity involved in the control of cytokinesis [75]. Little is known about TBC1–9B, but the involvement of Rab proteins in integrin function [76], and protein kinase C (PKC) activity – two putative targets for SGP-T and analogue activity suggests some functional relationship (see section below – Cellular Mechanism of Action of SGP-T and feG).

(3) A DIFELL sequence is also found near the middle domain of vitronectin, a glycoprotein found in serum and the extracellular matrix. Vitronectin promotes cell

adhesion and spreading, and inhibits the membrane-damaging effect of the terminal cytolytic complement pathway [77]. The DIFELL sequence is not specifically known to participate in the functions of versican, and we found that the tripeptide derived from the heptapeptide SGP-T in SMR1, and with anti-inflammatory activity, feG (see below), does not modify the adhesion of circulating or peritoneal leukocytes to vitronectin (unpublished). Versican (chondroitin sulfate proteoglycan 2) contains a sequence TDIFEGSG (aa 2332–2340). This sequence is known as the short complement-like repeat (SCR) or the complement control protein (CCP) module. This domain is related to CD21 (the complement C3d receptor, CR2, Epstein Barr virus receptor or EBV-R) which is the receptor for EBV and for complement C3d, C3dg and iC3b, which activate immune cells, including B cells and neutrophils. The relation of versican to SGP-T actions requires further study.

(4) Modulation of potassium channels has potential use in asthma as blockers of some of these channels produce bronchodilation, reduce airways hyper-responsiveness, and reduce cough and mucus production [78]. Moreover, the transient receptor potential (TRP) cation channels have possible roles in asthma [79]. The TRP cation channel, subfamily M, member 7, isoform CRA_b (Genbank – EAW77406.1) has the IFEGG sequence (aa 289–293), although an association with the action of SGP-T/feG is improbable due to cytoplasmic localization of TRP [80]. On the other hand the potassium channel tetramerization domain containing 3 (*KCTD3*), identified as NY-REN-45 antigen (AAH94879) contains the sequence – KKGGFEGGGFLGRKK (aa 753–766) – and has enzymatic (trypsin and pepsin) cleavage sites that could generate FEG-like sequences, for example GGFEGGG. If the domain containing this sequence projects into the extracellular space it would be available for cleavage by plasma enzymes. Based on homology analysis *KCTD3* is probably involved in the voltage-gated potassium channel complex, and even though it is expressed in normal lung, testis, small intestine, breast, liver, and placenta [81], studies on this gene and its physiology are limited.

(5) Many protein kinase C (PKC) enzymes possess an FEG sequence near the C-terminal. All PKCs possess similar basic structures with an N-terminal regulatory domain and a C-terminal kinase domain, which is flanked C-terminally from the catalytic core by a segment of 50–70 amino acids and contains a highly conserved turn motif and a hydrophobic motif –FXXF. feG has sequence similarity to the hydrophobic motif of several protein kinases – PKCα,β (FEGF) and PKCδ (FAGF). Based on molecular modeling it is proposed that feG exerts its anti-inflammatory actions by binding to the hydrophobic pocket in the kinase domain that is normally occupied by the hydrophobic motif [82, 83]. PKC has a predominant intracellular location, but certain inflammation conditions induce its movement to the extracellular surface where it has possible roles in apoptosis [84, 85] and cell adhesion [86, 87].

This list of peptides that could mimic the actions of TDIFEGG (SGP-T) or its analogues may not be complete, but provides a starting point for identification of molecular targets for this potent anti-inflammatory peptide. Binding sites for SGP-T analogues, which probably exists for some isoforms of PKC [88], need to be verified.

Other Salivary Anti-inflammatory Peptides

The SMR1 found predominately in submandibular glands is only one of many anti-inflammatory proteins and peptides released from salivary glands. Consequent to almost continuous exposure of the oral cavity to bacteria and other infectious agents, saliva is replete with antimicrobial proteins and peptides, such as defensins, histatins, lactoferrin, peroxidase, lysozyme [89] and parotid secretory protein (PSP) [90]. PSP exhibits weak sequence similarity with LPS binding proteins, including bactericidal permeability-increasing protein and LPS-binding protein. PSP is proteolytically processed to release anti-inflammatory peptides that serve to control inflammation in the oral cavity [91], and possibly peripherally as endocrine secretion of this protein occurs with activation of the β-adrenergic receptors [92].

Biological Activities of FEG and Its Derivatives

The tripeptide FEG, which is present in the SGP-T sequence (fig. 3) and is the basis of the metabolically stable D-isomeric peptide feG, exerts anti-inflammatory activities in mice, rats, sheep, cats, dogs and on isolated human leukocytes [93–96], indicating that receptor sites for this peptide are present in all species studied to date. The biological actions of feG have been reviewed thoroughly [20] and only the main points are summarized here. feG is a potent inhibitor of IgE-mediated allergic reactions, in that it reduces:

- amplitude of intestinal smooth muscle contractions in rats [52, 94];
- airway smooth muscle contractions in rats [97];
- late-phase bronchoconstriction and airways hypersensitivity reactions in sheep; [98];
- pulmonary inflammation in rats [97] and mice;
- edema of the skin (wheal response) in rats and sheep.

In non-IgE-mediated inflammations, feG:

- reduces IgG-evoked increases in vascular permeability (Arthus reaction) in rats;
- reduces complement (C5a)-induced adhesion to and migration across human neutrophils to human umbilical vein endothelial cells [Issekutz A, unpubl.], and complement provoked migration of leukocytes into knee joints of rats;
- endotoxin-provoked alterations of intestinal motility [99] in rats;
- activation of leukocytes in intestinal smooth muscle in rats [99],
- severity of spinal cord injury in rats [100, 101],
- cerulein-induced pancreatitis and associated pulmonary inflammation in mice [96].

From this profile, which shows in vivo efficacy in a wide range of inflammatory models and species, an analogue of feG is the lead candidate for a new class of drugs that is being developed by AIM Therapeutics Inc. as a preventative anti-inflammatory drug candidate in moderate to severe asthma.

Carboxyamide Derivatives. Although feG has a broad spectrum of anti-inflammatory actions, enzymatic alteration of SGP-T to add an amide to the C-terminus generates peptides with a different profile of inhibitory activities. To mimic this enzymatic reaction feG(NH2) was prepared and found to have no effect on immediate hypersensitivity reactions [52], but reduces the severity of endotoxic hypotension, endotoxin-induced perturbation of intestinal motility [99], and adhesion of leukocytes to extravascular tissue [102].

Cellular Mechanism of Action of SGP-T and feG

Early results showed that SGP-T treatment inhibited neutrophil chemotaxis [103] and rolling on endothelial cells [102, 104]. feG also exerts anti-inflammatory actions through the inhibition of leukocyte adhesion [95, 102, 105] and reactive oxygen species production [82].

feG does not affect adhesion of unactivated human neutrophils, whereas if the cells are PAF-activated a significant inhibition of adhesion occurs [95]. A similar dependency on cell activation or priming of neutrophils/leukocytes for feG inhibition of adhesion is seen with rat peritoneal leukocytes [105]. feG significantly inhibits the binding of peritoneal leukocytes to fibrinogen and fibronectin, and may exert these anti-adhesive actions by interfering with cell adhesion molecules in that:

- binding of CD11b (αM integrin) and CD16b (FcγRIIIb: low-affinity IgG receptor IIIB) of human neutrophils and rat leukocytes [95] is reduced;
- expression of CD49d (α4 integrin) on peritoneal neutrophils and circulating leukocytes collected from ovalbumin sensitized rats 24 h after challenge [106] is downregulated; modulating PKC activity [82, 83]. PKC has been demonstrated to be externalized in several models of inflammation [84, 87], a position where it would be amendable to interaction with SGP-T and homologues for modulation of enzymatic activity and inflammatory processes.

Genomics of SMR1 and its Homologues

The *Vcsa1* gene which encodes rat SMR1 is a member of the VCS multigene family, whose members share a common gene structure but exhibit extensive sequence variation in the coding region of the genes [107, 108]. The origin of the VCS genes from a common ancestor is probably by tandem gene duplications, with insertions, deletions and mutations resulting in related but functionally distinct genes. The VCS genes, which are divided into two subgroups VCSA and VCSB, with respectively two *(Vcsa1* and *Vcsa2)* and one *(Vcs-beta1)* members, are found exclusively in mammals [109]. The VCSA family has evolved, exclusively in rodents, whereas VCSB family is found in all placental mammals [110]. Human members of the VCSB family include *ProL1*, *SMR3B* and *SMR3A* [108], and encode salivary and lacrimal secreted proline-rich proteins [111–113]. ProL1 and SMR3A serve as markers for erectile dysfunction in humans [71, 114].

The rat Vcsa1 protein has 32% sequence identity with SMR3A, suggestive of possible similar functional roles, although as a consequence of mutation or truncation the C-terminal TDIFEGG sequence is not present in any other product of the VCSA subfamily. As discussed above a genetically related protein to SMR1 in humans is CABS1 which possesses the TDIFELL sequence, although this sequence does not occur in the rat or mouse CABS1 protein. Possible functional relationships may nonetheless exist since *CABS1, PROL1, SMR3A* and *SMR3B* have similar locations on human chromosome 4q13.3, whereas in the in rats *Smr1* and *Cabs1* are clustered on chromosome 14, in the p21-p22 region with other members of the VCS family. The pentapeptides hypothetically derived from hSMR3A and hSMR3B differ by two amino acids from that of PROL1, QRGPR and QRFSR, respectively [71].

The SMR1 protein product of the rat *Vcsa1* gene is cleaved into at least two biologically active peptides, sialorphin (QHNPR) and SGP-T (TDIFEGG) (fig. 3). Whereas the N-terminal QHNPR sequence is conserved in all products of the rat VCSA family members, the C-terminal TDIFEGG sequence is absent due to mutation or truncation of the C-terminus [111]. With the absence of the VCSA subgroup of genes in non-rodent mammals, sialorphin and SGP-T may not be present, although homologues of these peptides are encoded by VCSB genes. The human VCSB gene *ProL1* encodes a protein that contains a QRFSR motif (opiorphin) that is functionally equivalent to rat sialorphin from the *Vcsa1* gene [66]. Vcsa1 expression is hormonally regulated by androgens [61, 115], and the expression of opiorphin family genes may be similarly regulated [71]. In the adult male rat, the main tissues where SMR1 transcript expression occurs significantly are in corporal smooth muscle, prostate, submandibular and parotid glands and lungs, suggestive of relatively specific tissue expression [54, 56, 63].

Autonomic Control of Salivary Gland Endocrine Secretion

The release of salivary gland peptides into saliva and blood is under the control of the autonomic nervous system as evidenced by increases in both exocrine and endocrine release of kallikrein after α-adrenergic stimulation [116, 117]. Stress is an important activator of endocrine release of salivary gland peptides as evidenced by increased circulating levels of glandular kallikrein under heat stress [118], NGF following aggressive behaviour [119, 120], brain-derived neurotrophic factor (BDNF) with acute immobilization stress [121], and sialorphin after acute (2 min) exposure to ether fumes [60]. A positive correlation between plasma sialorphin and adrenocorticotropin hormone (ACTH) levels was also seen [12]. Other salivary glands also receive their sympathetic innervation from the SCG, and also exhibit endocrine secretion by β-adrenergic pathways [92, 122]. The parotid and submandibular glands appear to be differentially regulated by the sympathetic and parasympathetic nerves as SCG ganglionectomy increased levels of NGF in the submandibular glands, but had no effect in the parotid gland [29]. Increased transcripts for NGF and EGF occur in submandibular glands following SCG ganglionectomy [41]. An interesting feature of endocrine secretion of amylase from the parotid gland is that primary regulation is via the parasympathetic nerves, and not the sympathetic nerves [123], but to date no studies have addressed this aspect in submandibular glands. SMR1 is secreted into saliva after the administration of β-adrenergic or cholinergic agonists, and bilateral removal of the cervical sympathetic ganglia increased its levels in salivary glands, whereas the protein was depleted after isoproterenol (β adrenergic agonist) injection, but not pilocarpine (a nonselective muscarinic receptor agonist) [56]. However, since SMR1 protein levels in blood 30 or 60 min after isoproterenol or pilocarpine treatment did not change, the intact prohormone is possibly not secreted into the bloodstream. In contrast, levels of circulating sialorphin, emanating from a processed SMR1 protein, increased approximately 10-fold (from 1 to 10 ng/ml) within 10–30 min after intraperitoneal injection of epinephrine (αβ-adrenergic agonist), or isoproterenol (β-adrenergic agonist) [58].

The expression of SMR1 in submandibular and parotid glands was increased 2- and 1.5-fold, respectively, after bilateral superior cervical ganglionectomy, although this increase was not due to increased transcription since SMR1 mRNA was not increased [56]. The increase in SMR1 in the glands probably results from decreased secretion of the protein and its products with loss of sympathetic stimulation.

Although removal of submandibular glands and their sympathetic denervation have profound immunological consequences on allergic- and septic-induced inflammatory responses, to date no studies have examined exocrine or endocrine release of relevant modulating peptides or hormones.

CST-SMG Axis in Humans

Does the CST-SMG axis exist in humans and have a similar role to that identified in rats – contributing to the maintenance of systemic health and regulation of inflammatory responses? Aside from a study showing that environmental lighting controls salivary gland flow from the submandibular glands [124], the evidence garnered to date does not strongly support this hypothesis. However, subtle features of CST-SMG axis regulation probably have evaded detection in humans, possibly partly due to the sparing of the SCG neurons in humans, which, unlike other sympathetic nerves, do not undergo marked pathological changes (neuroaxonal dystrophy) consequent to aging [125].

Xerostomia, the subjective complaint of dry mouth due to a lack of saliva induces various problems including dental caries, periodontitis, denture problems, mastication and swallowing problems, burning sensations, and distortion of the sense of taste (dysgeusia). Thus, proper salivary gland function is important for health, as periodontal disease is suggested to be a modest risk factor for adverse pregnancy outcomes and several systemic diseases such as myocardial infarction, diabetes mellitus, various lung diseases such as asthma, pneumonia and chronic obstructive pulmonary disease, Alzheimer's and rheumatoid arthritis [126, 127]. In addition, several other systemic diseases are associated with reduced salivary flow and among these are chronic inflammatory rheumatic disorders (rheumatoid arthritis, systemic lupus erythematosus, scleroderma), cytomegalovirus and other herpes viruses, hepatitis C, ectodermal dysplasia, chronic pancreatitis, celiac disease and others [128]. Although a role for the SCG in oral disease is not established, animal models clearly indicate that this innervation helps maintain health of the teeth since with SCG removal osteoclast-mediated bone resorption and inflammation increases [129–131], and healing after injury to the maxilla and mandible [132] is reduced.

Diseases of human salivary glands arise from a variety of causes such as obstruction (stone formation), infection, inflammation, tumors and autoimmunity (Sjögren's syndrome), which generally result in loss of function with decreased saliva production and an ensuing complaint of xerostomia. Several systemic diseases that affect the oral fluid's composition include cystic fibrosis, multiple sclerosis, graft-versus-host disease, diabetes mellitus, alcoholic liver cirrhosis, acquired human immunodeficiency syndrome, epilepsy, burning mouth syndrome and kidney dysfunction [133]. Other causes of insufficient saliva production include anxiety, dehydration, chemo- and radiation therapy, and some medications such as antidepressants, amphetamines and antihistamines. This loss of salivary flow affects mastication and swallowing and if prolonged results in sialadenitis, dental caries, periodontal disease, persistent oral infections, generally results in a decline in the quality of life [134, 135], and may contribute, as with rodents [136] to maintaining mucosal integrity due to low levels of salivary EGF possibly contributing to Barrett's columnar lined oesophagus [137, 138]. The increases in salivary chromogranin A [139] and IgA [140] (antibacterial and antimicrobial properties), after upper thoracic massage may contribute to enhanced immune defense associated with these therapies in cancer and HIV patients. Future studies, aided by an approach involving genomics and proteomics, should address changes associated with salivary gland anti-inflammatory factors (including the VCS-related genes and peptides) and reveal their roles in modulating systemic health and their regulation by the autonomic nervous system.

Conclusions

In rats, the cervical sympathetic trunk-submandibular gland axis contributes to the regulation of systemic inflammatory responses. The identification of this axis led to development of new drugs for the treatment of allergic inflammation. The role that this axis has in other diseases or in the overall maintenance of systemic health has not been extensively explored, although the importance of these glands in ulcer formation, hepatic function, reproduction and tumor genesis, and the richness of factors released from the salivary glands leads to the speculation that other connections and relations will undoubtedly be established. It is probable that the CST-SMG gland axis has similar functions in humans, given the similarities to rats in expressed genes and peptides produced. Progress in recognition of its probable importance in human health is slow, mainly due to a lack of recognition of the role the axis plays in systemic homeostasis, and the entrenched association of salivary gland function uniquely with food processing and oral health.

References

1 Tandler B, Gresik EW, Nagato T, Phillips CJ: Secretion by striated ducts of mammalian major salivary glands: review from an ultrastructural, functional, and evolutionary perspective. Anat Rec 2001;264:121.

2 Tucker AS: Salivary gland adaptations: modification of the glands for novel uses. Front Oral Biol 2010;14:21.

3 Hardin A: Connection between the parotid glands and the generative organs. Lancet 1886;127:134.

4 Lacassagne A: Reactions de la glande sous-maxillaire a l'hormone male, chez la souris et le rat. Compt Rend Soc Biol 1940;133:539.

5 Ogata T: On the internal secretion of the salivary glands. Trans 9th Cong Far East Assoc Trop Med, 1935, p 709.

6 Ogata T: The internal secretion of salivary gland. Endocrinol Jpn 1955;2:247.

7 Werle E, Von Roden P: Über das Vorkommen des Kallikreins in den Speicheldrüsen und im Mundspeichel. Biochem Z 1936;286:213.

8 Cohen S: Isolation of a mouse submaxillary gland protein accelerating incisor eruption and eyelid opening in the new-born animal. J Biol Chem 1962; 237:1555.

9 Cohen S: Purification of a nerve-growth promoting protein from the mouse salivary gland and its neuro-cytotoxic antiserum. Proc Natl Acad Sci USA 1960;46:302.

10 Barka T: Biologically active polypeptides in submandibular glands. J Histochem Cytochem 1980;28: 836.

11 Mori M, Takai Y, Kunikata M: Review: biologically active peptides in the submandibular gland. Role of the granular convoluted tubule. Acta Histochem Cytochem 1992;25:325.

12 Rougeot C, Rosinski-Chupin I, Mathison R, Rougeon F: Rodent submandibular gland peptide hormones and other biologically active peptides. Peptides 2000;21:443.

13 Antopol W, Schifrin A, Tuchman L: Blood amylase response to acetylcholine and its modification by physostigmine and atropine. Proc Soc Exp Biol Med 1934;32:383.

14 Isenman L, Liebow C, Rothman S: The endocrine secretion of mammalian digestive enzymes by exocrine glands. Am J Physiol 1999;276:E223.

15 Li L, Yu Z, Piascik R, Hetzel DP, Rourk RM, Namiot Z, Sarosiek J, McClallum RW: Effect of esophageal intraluminal mechanical and chemical stressors on salivary epidermal growth factor in humans. Am J Gastroenterol 1993;88:1749.

16 Noguchi S, Ohba Y, Oka T: Influence of epidermal growth factor on liver regeneration after partial hepatectomy in mice. J Endocrinol 1991;128:425.

17 Kurachi H, Okamoto S, Oka T: Evidence for the involvement of the submandibular gland epidermal growth factor in mouse mammary tumorigenesis. Proc Natl Acad Sci USA 1985;82:5940.

18 Tsutsumi O, Oka T: Epidermal growth factor deficiency during pregnancy causes abortion in mice. Am J Obstet Gynecol 1987;156:241.
19 Ramirez I, Soley M: Submandibular salivary glands: influence on growth rate and life span in mice. J Physiol Biochem 2011;67:225.
20 Mathison RD, Davison JS, Befus AD, Gingerich DA: Salivary gland derived peptides as a new class of anti-inflammatory agents: review of preclinical pharmacology of C-terminal peptides of SMR1 protein. J Inflamm 2010;7:49.
21 Arancibia S, Assenmacher I: Submaxillary glands in an endocrine context. J Biol Buccale 1985;13:185.
22 Bellavia S, Gallara R: Effect of photic stimuli on rat salivary glands. Role of sympathetic nervous system. Acta Odontol Latinoam 2000;13:3.
23 Garrett JR: The proper role of nerves in salivary secretion: a review. J Dent Res 1987;66:387.
24 Proctor GB, Carpenter GH: Regulation of salivary gland function by autonomic nerves. Auton Neurosci 2007;133:3.
25 Mathison R, Davison JS, Befus AD: Neuroendocrine regulation of inflammation and tissue repair by submandibular gland factors. Immunol Today 1994;15: 527.
26 Hazen-Martin DJ, Landreth G, Simson JA: Immunocytochemical localization of nerve growth factor in mouse salivary glands. Histochem J 1987; 19:210.
27 Hansson HA, Tunhall S: Epidermal growth factor and insulin-like growth factor I are localized in different compartments of salivary gland duct cells. Immunohistochemical evidence. Acta Physiol Scand 1988;134:383.
28 Kurabuchi S, Hosoi K: Immunocytochemical study of granular duct cells with a hormonally enhanced granular cell phenotype in the mouse parotid gland. Odontology 2009;97:57.
29 Ekstrom J, Reinhold AC: Increases in nerve growth factor immunoreactivity in the submandibular gland, but not in the parotid gland, of the rat following sympathetic denervation. Arch Oral Biol 2004; 49:3.
30 Schneyer CA, Humphreys-Beher M, Hall HD: Nerve growth factor effects on inhibition by submandibular gland ablation or autonomic denervation of activity-induced parotid growth. J Auton Nerv Syst 1992;37:137.
31 Borghetti P, Saleri R, Mocchegiani E, et al: Infection, immunity and the neuroendocrine response. Vet Immunol Immunopathol 2009;130:141–162.
32 Rosas-Ballina M, Tracey KJ: The neurology of the immune system: neural reflexes regulate immunity. Neuron 2009;64:28.
33 Cardinali DP, Esquiflno AI: Neuroimmunoendocrinology and autonomic nervous system. Biomed Rev 1998;9:47.
34 Ramaswamy K, Mathison R, Carter L, Kirk D, Green F, Davision JS, Befus AD: Marked anti-inflammatory effects of decentralization of the superior cervical ganglia. J Exp Med 1990;172:1819.
35 Carter L, Ferrari JK, Davison JS, Befus D: Inhibition of neutrophil chemotaxis and activation following decentralization of the superior cervical ganglia. J Leukocyte Biol 1992;51:597.
36 Bissonnette EY, Mathison R, Carter L, Davison, JS, Befus AD: Decentralization of the superior cervical ganglia inhibits mast cell mediated TNF-alpha-dependent cytotoxicity. 1. Potential role of salivary glands. Brain Behav Immun 1993;7:293.
37 Mathison R, Hogan A, Helmer D, et al: Role for the submandibular gland in modulating pulmonary inflammation following induction of systemic anaphylaxis. Brain Behav Immun 1992;6:117.
38 Cavalcante de Albuquerque AA, Leal-Cardoso JH, Weinreich D: Antigen-induced synaptic plasticity in sympathetic ganglia from actively and passively sensitized guinea-pigs. J Auton Nerv Syst 1996;61: 139.
39 Christian EP, Undem BJ, Weinreich D: Endogenous histamine excites neurones in the guinea-pig superior cervical ganglion in vitro. J Physiol 1989;409: 297.
40 Weinreich D, Undem BJ, Taylor G, Barry MF: Antigen-induced long-term potentiation of nicotinic synaptic transmission in the superior cervical ganglion of the guinea pig. J Neurophysiol 1995;73: 2004.
41 Mathison R, Befus D, Davison JS: Removal of the submandibular glands increases the acute hypotensive response to endotoxin. Circ Shock 1993;39:52.
42 Rando TA, Bowers CW, Zigmond RE: Localization of neurons in the rat spinal cord which project to the superior cervical ganglion. J Comp Neurol 1981; 196:73.
43 Cardinali DP, Stern JE: Peripheral neuroendocrinology of the cervical autonomic nervous system. Braz J Med Biol Res 1994;27:573.
44 Savastano LE, Castro AE, Fitt MR, et al: A standardized surgical technique for rat superior cervical ganglionectomy. J Neurosci Methods 2010;192:22.
45 Amado F, Lobo MJ, Domingues P, et al: Salivary peptidomics. Expert Rev Proteomics 2010;7:709.
46 Mathison RD, Befus AD, Davison JS: A novel submandibular gland peptide protects against endotoxic and anaphylactic shock. Am J Physiol 1997; 273:R1017.

47 Gasteiger E, et al: Protein identification and analysis tools on the ExPASy server; in Walker JM (ed): The Proteomics Protocols Handbook. Urbana, Humana Press, 2005.
48 Merkler DJ: C-terminal amidated peptides: production by the in vitro enzymatic amidation of glycine-extended peptides and the importance of the amide to bioactivity. Enzyme Microb Technol 1994;16:450.
49 von Zastrow M, Tritton TR, Castle JD: Exocrine secretion granules contain peptide amidation activity. Proc Natl Acad Sci USA 1986;83:3297.
50 Eipper BA, Myers AC, Mains RE: Peptidyl-glycine alpha-amidation activity in tissues and serum of the adult rat. Endocrinology 1985;116:2497.
51 Braas KM, Harakall SA, Ouafik L Eipper BA, May V: Expression of peptidylglycine alpha-amidating monooxygenase: an in situ hybridization and immunocytochemical study. Endocrinology 1992;130:2778.
52 Metwally E, Pires JM, Moore GJ, Befus AD, Davison JS, Mathison R: Submandibular gland tripeptide FEG (Phe-Glu-Gly) and analogues: keys to structure determination. Peptides 2002;23:193.
53 Mathison R: Anti-inflammatory Peptides. Patent US. Salpep Biotechnology Inc., 2006.
54 Rosinski-Chupin I, Rougeot C, Courty Y, Rougeon F: Localization of mRNAs of two androgen-dependent proteins, SMR1 and SMR2, by in situ hybridization reveals sexual differences in acinar cells of rat submandibular gland. J Histochem Cytochem 1993;41:1645.
55 Rosinski-Chupin I, Tronik D, Rougeon F: High level of accumulation of a mRNA coding for a precursor-like protein in the submaxillary gland of male rats. Proc Natl Acad Sci USA 1988;85:8553.
56 Morris KE, St Laurent CD, Hoeve RS Forsythe P, Suresh MR, Mathison RD, Befus AD: Autonomic nervous system regulates secretion of anti-inflammatory prohormone SMR1 from rat salivary glands. Am J Physiol Cell Physiol 2009;296:C514.
57 Courty Y, Rosinski-Chupin I, Rougeon F: Various transcripts are generated from the VCSA1 gene by alternative splicing and poly(A) processing in the rat submandibular gland. Gene 1995;162:291.
58 Rougeot C, Rosinski-Chupin I, Njamkepo E, Rougeon F: Selective processing of submandibular rat 1 protein at dibasic cleavage sites. Salivary and bloodstream secretion products. Eur J Biochem 1994;219:765.
59 Rougeot C, Messaoudi M, Hermitte V, Rigault AG, Blisnick T, Dugave C, Desor D, Rougeon F: Sialorphin, a natural inhibitor of rat membrane-bound neutral endopeptidase that displays analgesic activity. Proc Natl Acad Sci USA 2003;100:8549.
60 Rougeot C, Vienet R, Cardona A, Le Doledec L, Grognet JM, Rougeon F: Targets for SMR1-pentapeptide suggest a link between the circulating peptide and mineral transport. Am J Physiol 1997;273:R1309.
61 Messaoudi M, Desor D, Nejdi A, Rougeot C: The endogenous androgen-regulated sialorphin modulates male rat sexual behavior. Horm Behav 2004;46:684.
62 Davies KP, Tar M, Rougeot C, Melman A: Sialorphin (the mature peptide product of Vcsa1) relaxes corporal smooth muscle tissue and increases erectile function in the ageing rat. BJU Int 2007;99:431.
63 Tong Y, Tar M, Davelman F, Christ G, Melman A, Davies KP: Variable coding sequence protein A1 as a marker for erectile dysfunction. BJU Int 2006;98:396.
64 Calenda G, Tong Y, Kanika ND, Tar MT, Suadicani SO, Xhang X, Melman, A Rougeot C, Davies KP: Reversal of diabetic vasculopathy in a rat model of type 1 diabetes by opiorphin-related peptides. Am J Physiol Heart Circ Physiol 2011;in press.
65 Tong Y, Tiplitsky SI, Tar M, Melman A, Davies KP: Transcription of G-protein coupled receptors in corporeal smooth muscle is regulated by the endogenous neutral endopeptidase inhibitor sialorphin. J Urol 2008;180:760.
66 Wisner A, Dufour E, Messaoudi M, Nejdi A, Marcel A, Ungeheuer MN, Rougeot C: Human opiorphin, a natural antinociceptive modulator of opioid-dependent pathways. Proc Natl Acad Sci USA 2006;103:17979.
67 Rougeot C, Robert F, Menz L, Bisson JF, Messaoudi M: Systemically active human opiorphin is a potent yet non-addictive analgesic without drug tolerance effects. J Physiol Pharmacol 2010;61:483.
68 Popik P, Kamysz E, Kreczko J, Wrobel M: Human opiorphin: the lack of physiological dependence, tolerance to antinociceptive effects and abuse liability in laboratory mice. Behav Brain Res 2010;213:88.
69 Javelot H, Messaoudi M, Garnier S, Rougeot C: Human opiorphin is a naturally occurring antidepressant acting selectively on enkephalin-dependent delta-opioid pathways. J Physiol Pharmacol 2010;61:355.
70 Yang QZ, Lu SS, Tian XZ, Yang AM, Ge WW, Chen Q: The antidepressant-like effect of human opiorphin via opioid-dependent pathways in mice. Neurosci Lett 2011;489:131.
71 Tong Y, Tar M, Melman A, Davies K: The opiorphin gene (ProL1) and its homologues function in erectile physiology. BJU Int 2008;102:736.

72 Kanika ND, Melman A, Davies KP: Experimental priapism is associated with increased oxidative stress and activation of protein degradation pathways in corporal tissue. Int J Impot Res 2010;22:363.

73 Kanika ND, Tar M, Tong Y, Kuppam DS, Melman A, Davies KP: The mechanism of opiorphin-induced experimental priapism in rats involves activation of the polyamine synthetic pathway. Am J Physiol Cell Physiol 2009;297:C916.

74 Kawashima A, Osman BA, Takashima M, Kikuchi A, Kohchi S, Satoh E, Tamba M, Matsuda M, Okamura N: CABS1 is a novel calcium-binding protein specifically expressed in elongate spermatids of mice. Biol Reprod 2009;80:1293.

75 Bernards A: GAPs galore! A survey of putative Ras superfamily GTPase activating proteins in man and *Drosophila*. Biochim Biophys Acta 2003;1603:47.

76 Pellinen T, Ivaska J: Integrin traffic. J Cell Sci 2006; 119:3723.

77 Thurman AC: Expression and purification of the central domain from vitronectin; University of Tennessee Honors Thesis Project, University of Tennessee – Knoxville, 2008.

78 Malerba M, Radaeli A, Mancuso S, Polosa R: The potential therapeutic role of potassium channel modulators in asthma and chronic obstructive pulmonary disease. J Biol Regul Homeost Agents 2010; 24:123.

79 Colsoul B, Nilius B, Vennekens R: On the putative role of transient receptor potential cation channels in asthma. Clin Exp Allergy 2009;39:1456.

80 Q9BX84:Q9BX84(TRPM6_HUMAN).UniProtKB/Swiss-Prot 2011.

81 Scanlan MJ, Gordan JD, Williamson B, et al: Antigens recognized by autologous antibody in patients with renal-cell carcinoma. Int J Cancer 1999;83:456–464.

82 Mathison RD, Davison JS: The tripeptide feG regulates the production of intracellular reactive oxygen species by neutrophils. J Inflamm 2006;3:9.

83 Mathison RD, Davison JS, Metwally E: Identification of a binding site for the anti-inflammatory tripeptide feG. Peptides 2003;24:1221.

84 Lautrette C, Loum-Ribot E, Petit D, Vermot-Desroches C, Wijdenes J, Jauberteau MO: Increase of Fas-induced apoptosis by inhibition of extracellular phosphorylation of Fas receptor in Jurkat cell line. Apoptosis 2006;11:1195.

85 Solstad T, Bjorgo E, Koehler CJ, Strozynski M, Torgersen KM, Tasken K, Thiede B: Quantitative proteome analysis of detergent-resistant membranes identifies the differential regulation of protein kinase C isoforms in apoptotic T cells. Proteomics 2010;10:2758.

86 Babinska A, Hogan MV, Sobocki T, Sobocka MB, Ehrlich YH, Kornecki E: Identification of ecto-PKC on surface of human platelets: role in maintenance of latent fibrinogen receptors. Am J Physiol Heart Circ Physiol 2000;278:H2008.

87 Crane JK, Vezina CM: Externalization of host cell protein kinase C during enteropathogenic *Escherichia coli* infection. Cell Death Differ 2005;12:115.

88 Yeong SS, Zhu Y, Smith D, Verma C, Lim WG, Tan BJ, Li QT, Cheung NS, Cai M, Zhu YZ, Zhou SF, Tan SL, Duan W: The last 10 amino acid residues beyond the hydrophobic motif are critical for the catalytic competence and function of protein kinase C alpha. J Biol Chem 2006;281:30768.

89 Tenovuo J: Antimicrobial function of human saliva – how important is it for oral health? Acta Odontol Scand 1998;56:250.

90 Madsen HO, Hjorth JP: Molecular cloning of mouse PSP mRNA. Nucleic Acids Res 1985;13:1.

91 Geetha C, Venkatesh SG, Bingle L, Bingle CD, Gorr SU: Design and validation of anti-inflammatory peptides from human parotid secretory protein. J Dent Res 2005;84:149.

92 Venkatesh SG, Tan J, Gorr SU, Darling DS: Isoproterenol increases sorting of parotid gland cargo proteins to the basolateral pathway. Am J Physiol Cell Physiol 2007;293:C558.

93 Declue AE, Schooley EK, Reinero CR: FEG-COOH tripeptide attenuates allergen-induced eosinophilic airway inflammation in a model of feline asthma. J Vet Intern Med 2007;21:457.

94 Mathison R, Lo P, Moore G, Scott B, Davison JS: Attenuation of intestinal and cardiovascular anaphylaxis by the salivary gland tripeptide FEG and its D-isomeric analog feG. Peptides 1998;19:1037.

95 Mathison RD, Befus AD, Davison JS, Woodman RC: Modulation of neutrophil function by the tripeptide feG. BMC Immunol 2003;4:3.

96 Rifai Y, Elder AS, Carati CJ, Hussey DJ, Li X, Woods CM, Schloithe AC, Thomas AC, Mathison RD, Davison JS, Toouli J, Saccone GT: The tripeptide analog feG ameliorates severity of acute pancreatitis in a caerulein mouse model. Am J Physiol Gastrointest Liver Physiol 2008;294:G1094.

97 Dery RE, Ulanova M, Puttagunta L, Stenton GR, James D, Marani S, Mathison R, Davison, J, Befus AD: Frontline: inhibition of allergen-induced pulmonary inflammation by the tripeptide feG. A mimetic of a neuro-endocrine pathway. Eur J Immunol 2004;34:3315.

98 Mathison R, Davison JS, Befus AD, Abraham WM: The tripeptide feG inhibits asthmatic reactions in sheep; in Monduzzi E (ed): Immunology 2004. Montreal, Medimond International Proceedings, 2004, pp 515–519.

99 Mathison R, Lo P, Tan D, Scott B, Davison JS: The tripeptide feG reduces endotoxin-provoked perturbation of intestinal motility and inflammation. Neurogastroenterol Motil 2001;13:599.
100 Bao F, John SM, Chen Y, Mathison RD, Weaver LC: The tripeptide phenylalanine-(D) glutamate-(D) glycine modulates leukocyte infiltration and oxidative damage in rat injured spinal cord. Neuroscience 2006;140:1011.
101 John SM, Bao F, Chen Y, Mathison RD, Weaver LC: Effects of a novel tripeptide on neurological outcomes after spinal cord injury. Neuroreport 2006; 17:1793.
102 Mathison R, Woodman R, Davison JS: Regulation of leukocyte adhesion to heart by the tripeptides feG and feG(NH2). Can J Physiol Pharmacol 2001; 79:785.
103 Nkemdirim M, Kubera M, Mathison R: Modulation of neutrophil activity by submandibular gland peptide-T (SGP-T). Pol J Pharmacol 1998;50:417.
104 Mathison RD, Sank C, Davison JS: Inhibition of leukocyte rolling by submandibular gland peptide-T (SGP-T). Proc West Pharmacol Soc 1999;42:39.
105 Mathison RD, Christie E, Davison JS: The tripeptide feG inhibits leukocyte adhesion. J Inflamm 2008;5:6.
106 Turesin F, Sadr A, Davison JS, Mathison R: The tripeptide FEG ameliorates systemic inflammatory responses to rat intestinal anaphylaxis. BMC Physiol 2002;2:13.
107 Rosinski-Chupin I, Kuramoto T, Courty Y, Rougeon F, Serikawa T: Assignment of the rat variable coding sequence (VCS) gene family to chromosome 14. Mamm Genome 1995;6:153.
108 Morris K, Kuo B, Wilkinson MD, Davison JS, Befus AD, Mathison RD: Vcsa1 gene peptides for the treatment of inflammatory and allergic reactions. Recent Pat Inflamm Allergy Drug Discov 2007;1: 124.
109 Rosinski-Chupin I, Rougeon F: The gene encoding SMR1, a precursor-like polypeptide of the male rat submaxillary gland, has the same organization as the preprothyrotropin-releasing hormone gene. DNA Cell Biol 1990;9:553.
110 Rougeot C, Rosinski-Chupin I, Rougeon F: Novel genes and hormones in salivary glands: from the gene for the submandibular rat1 protein (SMR1) precursor to receptor sites for SMR1 mature peptides. Biomed Rev 1998;9:17.
111 Dickinson DP, Thiesse M: cDNA cloning of an abundant human lacrimal gland mRNA encoding a novel tear protein. Curr Eye Res 1996;15:377.
112 Isemura S: Nucleotide sequence of gene PBII encoding salivary proline-rich protein P-B. J Biochem (Tokyo) 2000;127:393.
113 Isemura S, Saitoh E: Nucleotide sequence of gene PBI encoding a protein homologous to salivary proline-rich protein P-B. J Biochem (Tokyo) 1997; 121:1025.
114 Tong Y, Tar M, Monrose V, Disanto, M Melman A, Davies KP: hSMR3A as a marker for patients with erectile dysfunction. J Urol 2007;178:338.
115 Rosinski-Chupin I, Huaulme JF, Rougeot C, Rougeon F: The transcriptional response to androgens of the rat VCSA1 gene is amplified by both binary and graded mechanisms. Endocrinology 2001;142:4550.
116 Berg T, Johansen L, Nustad K: Enzymatic activity of rat submandibular gland kallikrein released into blood. Am J Physiol 1985;249:H1134.
117 Orstavik TB, Carretero OA, Scicli AG: Kallikrein-kinin system in regulation of submandibular gland blood flow. Am J Physiol 1982;242:H1010.
118 Berg T, Johansen L, Poulsen K: Exocrine and endocrine release of kallikrein after reflex-induced salivary secretion. Acta Physiol Scand 1990;139:29.
119 Aloe L, Alleva E, Bohm A, Levi-Montalcini R: Aggressive behavior induces release of nerve growth factor from mouse salivary gland into the bloodstream. Proc Natl Acad Sci USA 1986;83:6184.
120 Lakshmanan J: Aggressive behavior in adult male mice elevates serum nerve growth factor levels. Am J Physiol 1986;250:E386.
121 Tsukinoki K, Saruta J, Muto N, et al: Submandibular glands contribute to increases in plasma BDNF levels. J Dent Res 2007;86:260.
122 Gorr SU, Venkatesh SG, Darling DS: Parotid secretory granules: crossroads of secretory pathways and protein storage. J Dent Res 2005;84:500.
123 Proctor GB, Asking B, Garrett JR: Effects of secretory nerve stimulation on the movement of rat parotid amylase into the circulation. Arch Oral Biol 1989;34:609.
124 Shannon IL, Feller RP, Wescott WB: Environmental lighting and human salivary gland function. Proc Soc Exp Biol Med 1975;148:758.
125 Schmidt RE: Age-related sympathetic ganglionic neuropathology: human pathology and animal models. Auton Neurosci 2002;96:63.
126 de Pablo P, Chapple IL, Buckley CD, Dietrich T: Periodontitis in systemic rheumatic diseases. Nat Rev Rheumatol 2009;5:218.
127 Scannapieco FA, Dasanayake AP, Chhun N: Does periodontal therapy reduce the risk for systemic diseases? Dent Clin North Am 2010;54:163.

128 von Bultzingslowen I, Sollecito TP, Fox PC, Daniels T, Jonsson R, Lockhart PB, Wray D, Brennan MT, Carrozzo M, Gandera B, Fujibayashi T, Navazesh M, Rhodus NL, Schiodt M: Salivary dysfunction associated with systemic diseases: systematic review and clinical management recommendations. Oral Surg Oral Med Oral Pathol Oral Radiol Endod 2007;103(suppl):S57:e51.
129 Ladizesky MG, Cutrera RA, Boggio V, Mautalen C, Cardinali DP: Effect of unilateral superior cervical ganglionectomy on bone mineral content and density of rat's mandible. J Auton Nerv Syst 2000;78: 113.
130 Sandhu HS, Herskovits MS, Singh IJ: Effect of surgical sympathectomy on bone remodeling at rat incisor and molar root sockets. Anat Rec 1987;219:32.
131 Kim Y, Hamada N, Takahashi Y, Sasaquri K, Tsukinoki K, Onozuka M, Sato S: Cervical sympathectomy causes alveolar bone loss in an experimental rat model. J Periodontal Res 2009;44:695.
132 Haug SR, Heyeraas KJ: Effects of sympathectomy on experimentally induced pulpal inflammation and periapical lesions in rats. Neuroscience 2003; 120:827–836.
133 Aps JK, Martens LC: Review: the physiology of saliva and transfer of drugs into saliva. Forensic Sci Int 2005;150:119.
134 Jellema AP, Slotman BJ, Doornaert P, Leemans CR, Langendijk JA: Impact of radiation-induced xerostomia on quality of life after primary radiotherapy among patients with head and neck cancer. Int J Radiat Oncol Biol Phys 2007;69:751.
135 Meijer JM, Meiners PM, Huddleston Slater JJ, Spijkervet FK, Kallenberg CG, Vissink A, Bootsma H: Health-related quality of life, employment and disability in patients with Sjogren's syndrome. Rheumatology 2009;48:1077.
136 Olsen PS, Poulsen SS, Kirkegaard P, Nexo E: Role of submandibular saliva and epidermal growth factor in gastric cytoprotection. Gastroenterology 1984;87: 103.
137 Gray MR, Donnelly RJ, Kingsnorth AN: Role of salivary epidermal growth factor in the pathogenesis of Barrett's columnar lined oesophagus. Br J Surg 1991;78:1461.
138 Marcinkiewicz M, Grabowska SZ, Czyzewska E: Role of epidermal growth factor (EGF) in oesophageal mucosal integrity. Curr Med Res Opin 1998;14: 145.
139 Noto Y, Kudo M, Hirota K: Back massage therapy promotes psychological relaxation and an increase in salivary chromogranin A release. J Anesth 2010; 24:955.
140 Groer M, Mozingo J, Droppleman P, Davis M, Jolly ML, Boynton M, Davis K, Kay S: Measures of salivary secretory immunoglobulin A and state anxiety after a nursing back rub. App Nurs Res 1994;7:2.

Dr. Ronald D. Mathison
Faculty of Medicine, University of Calgary
3330 Hospital Drive NW
Calgary, AB T2N 4N1 (Canada)
Tel. +1 403 286 2731, E-Mail Ronald.Mathison@ucalgary.ca

Bienenstock J (ed): Allergy and the Nervous System.
Chem Immunol Allergy. Basel, Karger, 2012, vol 98, pp 196–221

The Mast Cell-Nerve Functional Unit: A Key Component of Physiologic and Pathophysiologic Responses

Paul Forsythe · John Bienenstock

The Brain-Body Institute, St. Joseph's Healthcare, Department of Medicine, McMaster University, Hamilton, Ont., Canada

Abstract

A key characteristic of mast cells appears to be an ability to span the division between nervous and immune system. Indeed, much of our understanding of the bi-directional relationship between the nervous and immune systems has come from the study of mast cell-nerve interaction. Although differences in species have been reported, morphologic as well as functional associations between mast cell and nerves are found in most tissues in many mammalian species, including humans. These interactions are involved in the regulation of physiologic homeostatic processes as well as in disease mechanisms. Here we discuss the influence of cholinergic and sensory neurons on mast cells as well as the importance of mast cell nerve interactions at specific tissue sites, including the brain.

Mast Cells

Mast cells are immunocytes with secretory functions that act locally to maintain tissue integrity, local hemodynamics and tissue homeostatic mechanisms. Mast cells are heterogeneous and exhibit site-specific adaptations induced by micro-environmental signals that lead to selective expression of potential mast cell characteristics. This flexibility of phenotype has important functional implications and allows these cells to adapt to organ or tissue specific roles [1].

While best known for their role in allergic inflammation through the ability of allergens to cross-link antigen-specific IgE bound to the high affinity IgE receptor (FceRI) expressed on the cell surface [2] mast cells have been identified as having diverse physiologic roles. These roles range from providing innate defense against bacteria [3] and protection from the venom of bees and snakes [4] to participating multiple aspects of adaptive immune responses such as antigen presentation [5] and lymphocyte recruitment to draining lymph nodes [6], as well as downregulation of immune responses [7]. In recent years, the pathogenic roles of mast cells have been extended to include not only allergic diseases and helminth infection, but also autoimmune diseases such as experimental allergic encephalomyelitis [8], rheumatoid arthritis [9], allograft tolerance [7], angiogenesis in tissue repair [10], and carcinogenesis [11].

A key characteristic of mast cells appears to be an ability to span the division between nervous and immune system with the cells exhibiting variably functional aspects of both systems [12]. Indeed, much of our understanding of the bi-directional relationship between the nervous and immune systems has come from the study of mast cell-nerve interaction, often considered as the archetype of neuroimmune communication. Mast cells can be activated by a range of neurotransmitters and reciprocally a variety of molecules, including histamine and serotonin, are synthesized and released by mast cells can influence neuronal activity [13] while mast cell-derived cytokines, including TNF, and growth factors, such as NGF, lower the threshold for activation of local neurons and promote nerve fiber growth [14–16].

While mast cells are distributed widely throughout the body in connective tissue and at mucosal surfaces they are concentrated at interfaces with the external environment, near blood vessels, lymphatic vessels, and nerve fibers [1]. Positioned at these strategic locations, mast cells act as sentinels of the immune system, protecting against invading microbes and signaling environmental changes or immune challenges to other cells involved in physiological and immunological responses.

There is anatomical evidence for mast cell associations with peripheral myelinated and unmyelinated nerves [17–19]. Close apposition of mast cells and neurons containing substance P, CGRP or both have been described in the rat and human gastrointestinal tract, the rat trachea and peripheral lung, the urinary bladder and several other tissues [20–22]. These interactions underlie the classical inflammatory axon reflex where antigen or noxious stimuli causes stimulation of sensory c-fibers that in turn, through collateral axons, provide an efferent route for the lateral spread of inflammatory signals [23].

While exocytosis is the most obvious event associated with secretion of the mediator molecules contained in granules the function of mast cells in health and disease often involves more subtle activities and these cells have been increasingly implicated in inflammatory processes in which degranulation is generally not observed. Mast cells can undergo ultrastructural alterations of their electron-dense granular core that are indicative of secretion but without degranulation, a process termed piecemeal degranulation, in which even molecules stored within the same granule can be secreted in a discriminatory pattern [24].

Mast cells in close proximity to unmyelinated nerve fibers have been observed to contain granules showing ultrastructural features of activation or piecemeal degranulation that have been associated with differential secretion. Histamine content of intestinal tissue increased flowing vagal stimulation without notable degranulation of mast cells [25, 26]. Selective secretion of IL-6 from mast cells appears to be distinct from degranulation and may contribute to the development of inflammation [27]. Serotonin can be released independently from histamine [28] and differential synthesis and release of arachidonic acid metabolites prostaglandins and leukotrienes have also been reported [29].

Mast cells are derived from progenitor cells that translocate from the bone marrow to tissue sites where they locally undergo differentiation into mature forms [30]. Studies have identified the remarkable facility of mast cell populations to respond to changes in the environment by significant alterations in multiple aspects of their phenotype, including morphology, mediator content, degranulation pattern and proliferative potential [1]. Consequently, mast cells can be divided into various subpopulations with distinct phenotypes. In rodents, mast cells are often classified broadly, based on tissue location, as mucosal mast cells (MMC) or connective-tissue type mast cells (CTMC) [31, 32]. However, mast cells possess a remarkable degree of plasticity and even apparently fully differentiated CTMC will transform their phenotype to that of MMC if transplanted into a mucosal environment [33]. Alternatively, and most often in human tissue, mast cells can be classified based on the protease content of secretory granules that differ between tissues, i.e. MCt for cells containing only tryptases and MCtc for those containing tryptase and chymase [30]. Tryptase is present in all mast cell subtypes and can activate cells through cleavage of protease-activated receptors (PAR) [34]. Proteases regulate neurons and glia in the central nervous system by cleaving PAR [35]. Furthermore, tryptase has been shown to cleave PAR2 on primary spinal afferent neurons, which causes the release of substance P, and CGRP and sensitization of co-expressed TRP channels that together cause plasma extravasation, amplification of inflammation and thermal and mechanical hyperalgesia [36]. Purified tryptase stimulates calcium mobilization in myenteric neurons [37] presumably through PAR2 because activation of PAR2 with trypsin or peptide agonists strongly desensitizes the response to tryptase. Mast cell proteases have also been demonstrated to degrade nerve products by enzymatic cleavage and thus may act to limit the effects of neurogenic signals [38]. It is proposed that IgE-mediated mast cell activation results in the release of tryptase from intracellular secretory granules, and the tryptase activates PAR2 on sensory neurons to stimulate the release of substance P and CGRP [39]. These neuropeptides induce the further activation of mast cells as well as inflammatory response such as arteriolar vasodilation and increased blood flow.

Molecules Involved in Mast Cell Nerve Attachments

Co-culture systems of mast cells and neurons have been particularly informative regarding the molecules involved in the formation of a neuroimmune synapse.

The adhesion molecule, cell adhesion molecule 1 (CADM1) is localized on both sides of most synapses in the brain and functions as a homophilic adhesion molecule spanning the synaptic cleft in the nervous system. CADM1 was also found to mediate mast cell/fibroblasts adhesion [40] and was subsequently demonstrated to be critical to mast cell-nerve interactions [41].

CADM1 is highly localized at the contact site between mast cells and neurites and the attachment of mast cells is dose-dependently reduced in the presence of an anti-CADM1 blocking antibody. Mast cells lacking CADM1 attach poorly to neurites, while attachment is significantly enhanced with ectopic expression of this adhesion molecule [41, 42].

The neuron-induced activation of CADM1-deficient mast cells is also markedly reduced while the response rate of CADM1+ mast cells is decreased dose-dependently in the presence of an anti-CADM1 blocking antibody. Furthermore antagonism of the substance P receptor, NK-1, attenuated the CADM-1 deficient mast cell response to neurite activation at much lower concentrations than in wild type mast cells [41, 42].

These studies indicate that CADM1 is involved not only in the physical association between mast cells and nerves but also contributes to the functional relationship enhancing mast cells sensitivity to neuronal signals. Thus, it appears that CADM1 is involved not only in the physical association between mast cells and nerves but it also contributes to the functional relationship and to the development of a microenvironment that enhances mast cells sensitivity to neuronal signals.

Indeed, variable splicing of CADM1 in neurons may be one of the molecular mechanisms that fine tune the nerve-mast cell interaction. Recently, BMMC were found to adhere to neurites expressing CADM1d splice variant more firmly than those expressing the CADM1b variant [43]. Furthermore, neuritis attached to CADM1c expressing mast cells via CADM1d were more responsive to stimulation by histamine than neurites binding with other CADM1 isoforms [43]. Therefore, it appears that CADM1d is a specific neuronal isoform that enhances nerve-mast cell interaction. Interestingly CNS neurons increase expression of CADM1d during maturation and this may influence the changes in mast cell distribution and perhaps function during CNS development.

Neurons and bone marrow-derived mast cells also express N- and E-cadherins. When in monoculture these adhesion molecules are concentrated primarily in the cytoplasm of BMMC [44, 45], but in the presence of neurons N-cadherin but not E-cadherin localizes to sites of interaction at the plasma membrane [45]. Similarly, β-catenin, a protein that associates with cadherins in the cytoplasm, also accumulates at the plasma membrane of neurite attached BMMC suggesting that N-cadherin is also involved in the contact formation between nerves and mast cells.

Nerve Growth Factor

Nerve growth factor (NGF) receptors are found on mast cells and act as autoreceptors regulating NGF synthesis and release by the cell [15, 46]. The NGF produced by mast cells can act on neurons to induce the expression of neuropeptides and lower the threshold of firing [47]. NGF has also been shown to induce degranulation and histamine release from mast cells [48], while in vivo administration of NGF in neonatal rats causes a marked increase in size and number of mast cells in peripheral tissue [49]. Indeed, mast cell proliferation in response to NGF is partially mediated by mast cell degranulation [49].

Interestingly, NGF can have anti-inflammatory as well as proinflammatory effects depending on the situation and the concentration of the growth factor. Nasal treatment of mice with NGF was shown to induce airway hyperresponsiveness as measured by electrical field stimulation [50] and nasal treatment with anti-NGF prevented the development of allergen induced airway inflammation and hyperresponsiveness [51]. Conversely, there is evidence that the increased production of NGF in the central nervous system during brain disease such as multiple sclerosis can suppress inflammation by switching to an anti-inflammatory immune response [51]. Significantly, the injection of CD4+ lymphocytes transfected with the NGF gene, either before or after the induction of allergic encephalomyelitis, inhibited the onset of demyelination [52]. Furthermore, studies support a role for interaction between nerves and NGF secreted by mast cells in the intestinal lamina propria or epithelium. NGF is enhanced in IBD [53] as is the expression of the high-affinity NGF receptor, TrkA, gene [53] and overall it appears that NGF has a protective role in colitis [54].

Sensory Neuropeptides

Peripheral sensory nerves that are involved in pain, touch and temperature perception regulate inflammation locally through the release of neuropeptides. Peripheral neuropeptides that are known to regulate inflammation include substance P, calcitonin gene-related peptide (CGRP) and vasoactive intestinal peptide (VIP). The stimulation of peripheral nerves results in the characteristic features of local inflammation, including vasodilation, vascular leakiness, edema and pain.

In clinical dermatology and gastroenterology, it is acknowledged that peptide mediators released from cutaneous c-fibers and the enteric nervous system respectively give rise to neurogenic inflammation and underlie a range of conditions, including dermatitis, psoriasis, eczema, Crohn's disease and colitis [55–58]. In asthma research there is also great interest in the role these peptides play in airway inflammation, mast cell activation, cytokine secretion, bronchial hyperresponsiveness, and mucoid secretion [59, 60]. In particular, great attention has been paid to the role of tachykinins such as substance P.

Substance P and the Functional Relationship between Neurons and Mast Cells

Substance P is an 11 amino acid peptide that acts principally at the neurokinin-1 (NK-1) G-protein coupled receptor. Substance P is generally regarded as pro-inflammatory, stimulates secretion of TNF, IL-1, IL-2 and IL-6 from macrophages and T lymphocytes in vitro [61].

Substance P is perhaps the best-known and most studied neurotransmitter in relation to mast cell activation. In vitro, high (micromolar) concentrations of substance P induce mast cell degranulation while in co-culture system substance P from activated neurites induces Ca^{2+} mobilization and degranulation of mast cells [62]. In addition to degranulation substance P also promotes production of lipid mediators such as prostaglandin D_2 and leukotriene C_4 and proinflammatory cytokines including TNF and IL-6 [63, 64].

Interestingly, low (picomolar or nanomolar) concentrations of substance P, that do not induce mediator release can increase cellular responsiveness to subsequent stimulus and so 'prime' the cell to degranulate with reapplication of a subthreshold dose [65]. This effect has great physiological significance as it likely underlies the ability substance P to activate mast cells at concentrations occurring in situ.

As described previously, the heterogeneity of mast cells is well reported and studies have described large variations in the susceptibility of mast cells to activation on challenge with neuropeptides in different tissues as well as within the same tissues in different species. Indeed, not all mast cells are activated by substance P and expression of functional NK-1 receptors appears to be dependent on microenviromental factor. Bone marrow derived mast cells BMMC co-cultured with fibroblasts for several weeks can respond to substance P [66] and BMMCs cultured in the presence of IL-4 and stem cell factor gain sensitivity to substance P by expression of functional NK-1 receptors [67]. Bischoff and colleagues determined that human intestinal mast cells do not constitutively express NK1, NK2 or NK3 receptors [68]. However, when stimulated by IgE receptor crosslinking these mast cells expressed NK1 but not NK2 or NK3 receptors, again suggesting that specific tissue conditions such as allergic inflammation may lead to mast cell expression of NK1 [68].

Electron-microscopic studies of the rat basophilic/mast cell line, RBL-2H3, cultured with SCG neurons have indicated that bradykinin-induced activation of the neurons leads to marked morphological changes in the mast cells, including membrane ruffling, associated with cell activation and exocytosis of intracellular granules and are similar to that seen following antigen stimulation of these cells [69]. Membrane ruffling and concentration of CD63, a protein located on the granule and plasma membranes of basophils and mast cells, was observed on pseudopodial extensions of the mast cell in contact with activated neurites, but not on noncontacting pseudopodia [69]. Importantly, these morphological changes were dependent on NK-1 receptor activation indicating that neuron-derived substance P induces degranulation in associated mast cells. Furthermore, association of mast cells to neurons for several days can change phenotypic and functional characteristics of the mast cell, increasing granule contents and FcεRI expression [70, 71]. This functional relationship between mast cells and substance P containing sensory nerves is thought to play a critical role in the stress induced exacerbation of a number of inflammatory conditions [72, 73].

In rats, acute immobilization stress triggered mast cell activation and degranulation via substance P released from primary afferent sensory nerve fibers in the skin [72] and the bladder [21]. Joachim et al. [73–75] utilized a mouse model of allergic airway inflammation in a series of studies which provide compelling evidence that SP is key to stress-induced enhancement of antigen-induced airway inflammation. In this model, acoustic stress increased SP expression in lung tissue and mouse airway nerves as well as increased airway inflammation in an NK-1 receptor-dependent manner [75]. In addition, many of the immunological effects of stress in this model could be mimicked by the addition of exogenous SP [76].

This pro-inflammatory neuroimmunomodulatory role for substance P is also apparent in stress-induced exacerbation of atopic dermatitis. Acoustic stress was demonstrated to enhance the number of SP-positive nerve fibers in the skin of mice [77]. These nerve fibers were more frequently in contact with mast cells and this was associated with a significant increase in the number of degranulated mast cells [77]. Correspondingly, in a mouse model of atopic dermatitis stress enhanced eosinophil infiltration, epidermal thickness accompanied by increased neurogenic inflammation which included mast cell degranulation [78]. As with the model of stress-induced asthma, the exacerbation was significantly reduced in mice deficient in the NK1 receptor [78].

CGRP

CGRP is a 37 amino acid neuropeptide that mediates its effects through G-protein coupled receptors and is expressed predominantly in sensory nerve fibers [68]. There appears to be great heterogeneity in the response of mast cells to CGRP. The LAD2 human mast cell line does not degranulate in response to CGRP [79] and BMMC expresses functional CGRP1 receptors and even though their activation does not induce degranulation of these cells, it does cause mobilization of Ca^{2+} from intracellular stores and piecemeal release of mMCP-1 [24]. In the rat, peritoneal mast cells are unresponsive to CGRP but the neuropeptide does induce histamine release from dura mater mast cells [80]. CGRP-induced activation of meningeal mast cells may be involved in the pathogenesis of headaches as the histamine released induces direct vasodilatation and activates a subset of nonmechanically sensitive neurons in the rat meninges [81]. Furthermore, CGRP induces greater histamine release from mast cells in bronchoalveolar lavage from patients with airway inflammation associated with chronic cough and cough variant asthma than from control subjects [82]. Parasite infection with schistosomiasis in the mouse ileum is accompanied by mastocytosis and a corresponding increase in the density of CGRP-immunoreactive extrinsic primary afferent nerve fibers in the lamina propria [83]. In this model, mucosal mast cells were found in close apposition to the dense network of extrinsic primary afferent nerve fibers that contained CGRP but not substance P [83]. This anatomical evidence taken together with evidence that CGRP can directly activate mast cells suggests that this neuropeptide has a role in the functional relationship between mast cells and neuronal networks. One such example of this interaction may be in the repair of intestinal mucosa injury. CGRP is released from neuroeffector junctions of extrinsic afferents as early as 4 h after the induction of intestinal mucosal injury and aids protection and repair through induction of vasodilatation and modulation of mucosal blood flow [84]. In addition, it appears that CGRP may induce additional protective responses through its action on mast cells. In an in vitro model of intestinal epithelial damage, the media of CGRP-conditioned mast cells induced a significant TGFβ-dependent increase in epithelial restitution as assessed by cell proliferation and migration [85].

Vasoactive Intestinal Peptide

Vasoactive intestinal peptide (VIP) is a 28 amino acid peptide that exerts its action on cells through two G-protein-coupled receptors, VPAC1 and VPAC2 [86]. VIPergic signaling is involved in regulating intestinal motility, induces cardiac vasodilation and, centrally, plays an essential role in the maintenance of circadian rhythm [87]. VIP is expressed widely in the nervous system, the endocrine system and the immune system and can be considered a true neuroimmunoendocrine mediator.

The interactions between VIP and mast cells appear complex and knowledge of the functional significance is limited. Mast cells can produce VIP [88], express VIP receptors [89] and degranulate in response to the peptide [79]. However, there is also evidence that VIP can stabilize mast cells in vivo [90, 91]. Furthermore, mast cell-derived proteases degrade VIP [92, 93] and have been demonstrated to limit the toxicity associated with high concentrations of VIP [92].

Systemically administered VIP can attenuate the motor response changes, neuronal cell death, and myelin sheet loss characteristic of a rat model of Parkinson's disease by 6-OHDA administration into the corpus striatum [94]. Evidence suggests that the protective effect of VIP in this model could, at least in part, be mediated by brain mast cells. Electron-microscopic studies of mast cells in the corpus stratum demonstrated that VIP treatment changes the ultrastructural morphology of mast cells in a manner characteristic of piecemeal degranulation [94].

Human airway smooth muscle cells secrete the mast cell-chemoattracting chemokine, fractalkine (FKN) [95]. Pretreatment of mast cells with VIP increases the chemoattractant effect of FKN on mast cells [95]. Interestingly, in asthmatic patients, there is an increase in both FKN and VIP expression in airway smooth muscle [96] and a positive correlation between VIP staining and mast cell infiltration of the smooth muscle layer [95]; thus, it has been suggested that airway smooth muscle-derived FKN may contribute to mast cell recruitment in asthma.

Cholinergic Neurons

In recent years, the immunoregulatory role of the parasympathetic nervous system has come into focus with the cholinergic anti-inflammatory pathway. The anti-inflammatory function of the vagus nerve was first highlighted in studies conducted by Tracey and colleagues demonstrating that electrical stimulation of the peripheral vagus nerve in vivo during lethal endotoxemia in rats prevented the development of shock through inhibition of TNF synthesis [97].

The vagus nerve also plays a counter-inflammatory role in experimental colitis [98]. Macrophages have been identified as the major source of TNF during endotoxemia, and are suggested to be the main target of the anti-inflammatory function of the vagus nerve in a murine model of inflammatory bowel disease [98]. This immunomodulatory effect of the vagus is mediated by the action of acetylcholine (Ach) on nicotinic receptors. Nicotine is as efficient as Ach in inhibiting pro-inflammatory cytokine release from human macrophages in vitro [99] while the increased disease severity observed in animal models of IBD following vagotomy can be counteracted by nicotine [98].

Nicotinic acetylcholine receptors (nAChR) are pentameric ligand-gated ion channels that can be made up of a number of different subunits (identified neuronal subtypes include α2–α10, β2–β4) and it has been reported that the homo pentameric α7 subtype of nAChR maybe essential in mediating the anti-inflammatory effect of acetylcholine [99]. However, it is clear that additional nAChR are involved in the immunomodulatory actions of the vagus [100].

Given the potential importance of the vagus nerve-mediated anti-inflammatory response in a number of inflammatory conditions including food allergy there is limited knowledge regarding the vagal regulation of mast cells. There is anatomical evidence for vagal nerves in contact with intestinal mucosal mast cells although the percentage of mucosal mast cells demonstrated to be in direct contact with vagal nerves was low (10–15%) [101]. However, removal of vagal input into the intestine of rats through vagotomy led to a 25% reduction in the number of jejunal mast cells, suggesting that the vagus does support mast cell survival [25]. Vagal stimulation has also been demonstrated to increase the histamine content of intestinal mucosal mast cells but it is not known whether this is due to increased synthesis of histamine or stabilization of the cell and decreased mediator release [26]. Interestingly, the cholinergic anti-inflammatory pathway can be activated by the administration of lipid-rich nutrition and subsequent activation of CCK receptors [102, 103]. When postoperative ileus, a mast cell-mediated process, was induced in rats, administration of lipid-rich nutrition reduced the release of rat mast cell protease II (RMCPII) indicating suggesting an inhibition of manipulation induced degranulation. Similarly, high lipid feeding was demonstrated to reduce intestinal mast cell degranulation in a model of shock.

While there is no direct evidence that the vagus acts to inhibit mast cell activation, studies have demonstrated that nictotinic receptor agonists do attenuate certain responses of the cell and this may explain reported therapeutic effects of nicotine on models of food allergy [104]. Mouse BMMC express mRNA of α3, α7 and β2 nAChR. Agonists of nicotinic receptors including the α7-specific agonist GTS-21 inhibited antigen-induced degranulation of these cells in a dose-dependent manner, an effect prevented by an α7 antagonist. More recently, a study utilizing the rat mast/basophil cell line RBL-2H3 demonstrated that these cells express the nicotinic acetylcholine receptors (nAChRs) α7, α9, and α10 [105]. Exposure to nanomolar levels of nicotine suppressed late-phase leukotriene/cytokine production but did not inhibit degranulation. The suppressive effect of nicotine on the late-phase response was blocked by the α7/α9-nAChR antagonists methyllycaconitine and α-bungarotoxin, as well as by small interfering RNA knockdowns of α7-, α9-, or α10-nAChRs [105]. These data suggest that at least three nAChRs interact functionally to mediate the effects of nicotine on the late-phase response of mast cells. From these studies, it is also clear that mast cells in different tissue sites may have distinct responses to vagal input based on AchR receptor expression. Furthermore, receptor expression may change in allergic disease. A study of human skin mast cells found that mast cells from lesions of atopic dermatitis lesions but not in healthy skin showed α3 and α5 subunit immunoreactivity [106].

It is interesting to note that the earliest description of potential cholinerergic regulation of mast cells was not an inhibitory action at the nicotinic receptors but an activation and induction of degranulation by acetylcholine acting at the muscarinic receptors [107, 108]. Mannaioni and colleagues [107] reported that histamine secretion from rat mast cells occurs in the presence of nanomolar concentrations of acetylcholine, an effect that was competitively blocked by atropine. However, other studies failed to show any effect of acetylcholine on rat mast cell degranulation [109, 110]. Masini et al. [108] went on to identify heterogeneity in response to acetylcholine with the virtual lack of sensitivity or by the full reaction to nanomolar concentrations of acetylcholine, observed in samples of serosal mast cells isolated from rats. The incubation with isolated rat mast cells with IgE induced a homogenous 'responder' population, with acetylcholine-induced histamine release proportional to the IgE concentration. Again this suggests that parasympathetic regulation of mast cells may vary significantly depending on the local tissue environment and allergic status.

Mast Cell-Nerve Interaction in the Physiology and Pathophysiology of Specific Tissues

Skin

The dermis of all mammals is innervated heavily by primary sensory afferent nerves, postganglionic cholinergic parasympathetic nerves and postganglionic adrenergic and cholinergic sympathetic nerves [111]. These nerve fibers form close contacts with mast cells and neuropeptides released by cutaneous nerves have been shown to activate a number of target cells including Langerhans cells endothelial cells and mast cells [112].

Neuropeptides such as substance P and CGRP exhibit a variety of pro-inflammatory effects in the skin where their release following nociceptive stimulation by pain, mechanical or chemical irritants mediates skin responses to infection and injury. Furthermore, skin mast cells can respond to trauma by releasing a variety of inflammatory mediators through an immediate sensory nerve stimulated response via the axon reflex inducing the release of substance P, recognized to be one of the main neuropeptides responsible for erythema pain and swelling in the skin, from peripheral nerve endings in turn leading to more mast cell degranulation with the release of histamine and TNF release from skin mast cells which in turn leads to vasodilation [113]. Mast cell-dependent passive cutaneous anaphylaxis is significantly impaired in the absence of sensory nerves [114]. This does not appear to be due to changes in mast cell numbers in denervated skin but to a decreased IgE-mediated activation of mast cells. Furthermore, pretreatment of mice with selective antagonists of substance P or CGRP also leads to reduced inflammatory responses following mast cell activation [114].

Mast cells play a crucial role in the downregulation of immune responses and the induction of tolerance after exposure of skin to ultraviolet B radiation (UVB). Hart et al. [115] reported the involvement of mast cell-derived histamine in UVB-induced immune suppression in mice. Furthermore, this UVB-mediated immune suppression appears to involve interactions between mast cells and the nervous system. Evidence indicates that CGRP released from UVB-damaged cutaneous nerve endings triggers mast cells to release TNF and that this mast cell derived TNF together with histamine is a major mediator in signaling the immunosuppressive effects of UVB [116].

There are also changes in mast cell nerve interaction in the skin during allergic disease.

In a study by Jarvikallio et al. [117], nerve-mast cell contacts were observed in the basement membrane only in biopsies from the lesional regions of patients with nummular eczema. Furthermore, SP and CGRP fibers were prominently increased in lesional samples when compared to their nonlesional controls both in atopic dermatitis and nummular eczema in the epidermis and in the papillary dermis. Since mast cells are also increased in a number in lesions of atopic dermatitis and nummular eczema, they are able to maintain neurogenic inflammation through activation by SP and CGRP. Interestingly, skin mast cells also release vascular endothelial growth factor (VEGF) and overexpression of VEGF in mouse skin causes a psoriasiform skin inflammation [118], and thus mast cells may be a key component of intracutaneous events that lead to psoriasis [119]. Recently, it was demonstrated that substance P induces VEGF production and secretion from human mast cells and that this response was significantly enhanced by co-administration of the pro-inflammatory cytokine IL-33 [120]. Such interaction between neurotransmitters and cytokines is likely an important physiological paradigm, tailoring a microenvironment-specific immune cell response to neuronal signals and likely contributes to changes in mast cell responsiveness observed in disease states.

Skin mast cells also act as transducers of the peripheral response to stress. Growth, survival and activation of skin mast cells are regulated by stress mediators. CRH, adrenocorticotropin (ACTH), SP, NGF promote proliferation and activation, whereas catecholamines and corticosteroids inhibit mast cell function [119].

It is CRH, produced following stimulation of the HPA axis, which is largely responsible for the stress-induced activation of mast cells. Theoharides et al. [121] were the first to show that CRH could act as a mast cell degranulating agent. Skin mast cells degranulate in response to acute stress or administration of CRH in vivo and in vitro [72], CRH administration induces neurogenic inflammation in rat skin while neutralizing antibodies to CRH abrogate stress-induced degranulation of skin mast cells [72]. Substance P also appears to be involved in the activation of skin mast cells following stress and stress induced exacerbation of atopic dermatitis was significantly reduced in mice deficient in the NK1 receptor [78]. A recent study provided evidence that CRH and substance P may in fact act reciprocally to modulate mast cells during stress [122]. The human LAD2 mast cell line has weak expression of corticotropin-releasing hormone receptor-1 (CRHR-1). However, treatment of these cells with SP significantly increased CRHR-1 mRNA and protein expression. These substance P 'primed' mast cells responded to CRH stimulation, synthesizing and releasing IL-8, TNF, VEGF. This upregulation of the response to CRH was blocked by pretreatment with an NK-1 receptor antagonist. Conversely, treatment of LAD2 cells with CRH induced gene expression of NK-1 compared with controls [122]. Overall there is good evidence that the mast cell nerve functional unit influences the development of inflammatory diseases of the skin and in particular stress-induced exacerbations of these disorders.

The Gastrointestinal Tract

The lamina propria of the gastrointestinal tract is densely innervated and mast cells are often observed in close proximity to these neurons. Analysis has indicated that 50–75% of mast cells are found close to nerves in the rodent and human [19, 123]. In the rat ileum, nerve terminals containing predominantly small clear neurosecretory vesicles have been observed in direct contact with the plasma membrane of mucosal mast cells [124].

Mast cell-nerve association appears to function as a homeostatic unit in the regulation of gut physiology and in response to antigens. Mast cell degranulation can directly cause nerve stimulation in the intestine. Electrical stimulation of the vagus has been shown to variably cause mast cell degranulation or an increase in mast cell histamine content [26]. Shanahan et al. [125] initially demonstrated that substance P caused mediator release from intestinal mucosal mast cells. Subsequently, substance P and CGRP fibers were reported to activate mast cells in the intestinal mucosa of healthy and infected rats as well as in patients with inflammatory bowel disease [126, 127]. However, Bischoff et al. [68] determined that human intestinal mast cells do not constitutively express any of the NK receptors and did not respond to activation with substance P. However, when stimulated by IgE receptor crosslinking these mast cells expressed the substance P receptor NK1 receptors [68], suggesting that specific tissue conditions such as allergic inflammation alter the responsiveness of intestinal mast cells to neuropeptides.

Mast cell mediators also affect nerves in the intestine. A study by Jiang et al. [128], using an intestinal model for anaphylaxis, showed that serotonin and histamine, released from the mast cells after intestinal anaphylaxis, stimulate mesenteric afferents via the 5-HT3 and histamine H1 receptors. Mesenteric afferent-nerve discharge increased approximately 1 min after luminal antigen challenge and was attenuated by serotonin and histamine receptor antagonists.

Clostridium difficile is a leading cause of infectious colitis and produces watery diarrhea and a necrotizing inflammatory colitis through the action of two exotoxins, toxin A and toxin B. Toxin A has indirect actions in the mucosa after internalization into enterocytes. Studies of toxin A have provided important insight to neuroimmune-epithelial interactions involved in the elaboration of neurogenic inflammation in the intestine.

Several mediators are released from enterocytes after toxin A has been internalized including leukotriene B4, PGE_2 and TNF from enterocytes, and IL-1β and IL-6 from monocytes. These proinflammatory mediators in turn activate primary afferent nerves. This neuroimmune interaction appears to an important component of the inflammatory cascade initiated by toxin A, as rats pretreated with capsaicin to ablate primary afferent nerves of the gut, have little response to toxin A [129]. Activation of primary afferent nerves leads to the release of neurotensin from enteroendocrine cells of the epithelium [130, 131]. Neurotensin is a potent activator of mast cells degranulation and can itself elicit fluid secretion [132, 133]. While mast cell degranulation is a major contributor to the neurogenic inflammatory effects of toxin A, it is not essential because mast cell deficient mice have a reduced, but not abolished, inflammatory and secretory response to the toxin [134].

Mast cell activation not only leads to secretory responses, but also to changes in intestinal motility and blood flow, through neuroimmune mechanisms. In vivo, degranulation of intestinal mast cells in sensitized animals leads to alterations in motility that are mediated by the ENS and other autonomic pathways [135].

Perdue and colleagues identified an integral nerve-to-mast cell and mast cell-to-nerve connection during intestinal anaphylaxis [136]. A role for the mast cell-to-nerve connection was established by increases in the short circuit current after antigen challenge was reduced in mast cell-deficient W/Wv mice as compared to their +/+ litter mates and was inhibited by different mast cell antagonists in +/+ mice but not in mast cell deficient W/Wv mice, pointing to a mast cell-to-nerve connection. Furthermore, reconstitution of the mast cell deficiency was followed by a restoration of the neural response [136]. In sensitized guinea pig intestine, the short-circuit-current secretory response to antigen occurred simultaneously with acetylcholine release and could be blocked by atropine [137]. This showed conclusively that nerve excitation and the secretion of the main cholinergic neurotransmitter could be induced by antigen via mast cells through an immune-mediated response.

Similarly, stress-induced changes in intestinal motility, mucus hypersecretion and intestinal chloride secretion as judged by increased short circuit current was mediated by CRH. This could be inhibited by intracerebral or systemic injection of CRH inhibitors. Furthermore, mast cells and multiple neural pathways in this response as mast cell stabilizers and NK-1 antagonists inhibited these effects as did ganglionic blockers and inhibition of cholinergic as well as sympathetic activity [138]. More recently, CRH has also been demonstrated to modulate intestinal permeability in human colonic mucosa acting via CRH receptor subtypes R1 and R2 on subepithelial mast cells [139].

Irritable bowel syndrome (IBS) is one of the most common gastrointestinal disorders and causes considerable morbidity. Given that mast cells are found in close apposition to nerves in the intestine and that mediators released from mast cells can induce sensorimotor dysfunction, it has been suggested that mast cell nerve interactions may play an important role in the pathophysiology of IBS [140]. Indeed, there is evidence to support this concept; in many biopsy studies of patients with IBS the number of mast cells are invariably in the small or large bowel or both [141–143]. Furthermore, there have been observations that the number of mast cells in close apposition to nerves in the colonic mucosa is increased in comparison with controls [144, 145]. Perhaps most significantly the severity and the frequency of abdominal pain have also significantly correlated with the number of mast cells closely apposed to colonic nerves [144, 146]. Moreover, the increased mast cell density in IBS colonic mucosa has been found to be associated with an increase in mucosal content of tryptase and a greater ability of mast cells to release tryptase and histamine spontaneously, as compared with controls [144, 147]. However, the observed relationship between mast cell density and disease symptoms is inconsistent and despite experimental evidence in for a prominent role of mast cells as transducers of neuroimmune signaling in IBS, the clinical relationship between mast cells and symptoms of IBS has not been conclusively established. One of the reasons for this may be the focus of many studies on correlating mast cell numbers with disease symptoms. Activated mast cells can be difficult to detect due to loss of their characteristic granules and thus standard histological techniques may underestimate mast cell numbers. Furthermore, the overall density of mast cells may not be as important to pathophysiology as changes in responsiveness and mediator release following stimulation with neuron-derived mediators.

Lung

Autonomic nerves regulate many aspects of airway function. The parasympathetic nervous system is the dominant neuronal pathway for airway smooth muscle tone. Stimulation of cholinergic nerves causes bronchoconstriction mucus secretion and bronchial vasodilation. Mast cells are located throughout the airways, including the trachea, bronchus, and sparsely in the parenchyma [17, 148]. A role for the mast cell interaction with the autonomic nervous system in the lung is supported by the fact that mast cells have been shown to be closely associated with airway nerves [20].

The NANC nervous system plays an important role in the lung. Inhibitory NANC nerves contain potent relaxants of the airway, VIP and nitric oxide that counteract bronchoconstriction. Although dysfunction of the inhibitory NANC nerves has also been proposed in asthma no difference in inhibitory NANC responses has been found between asthmatics and healthy subjects. The tachykinins and CGRP are the major excitatory NANC neuropeptides in the airways. For example, it has been reported that substance P-containing nerves in the rat trachea interact with mast cells to cause Ag-specific and Ag-dependent changes in lung solute clearance and epithelial chloride ion secretion [149, 150]. Furthermore substance P and NKA induce histamine release from human airway mast cells [82]. However, ablation of sensory C-fibers with capsaicin in either adults or neonatal mice failed to alter airway function after antigen challenge in passively sensitized mice [151], indicating that capsaicin-sensitive C-fibers do not play a primary role in allergic airway constriction. This is interesting given that depletion of C-fibers does attenuate allergic airway inflammation in mice [152] and suggests that distinct mast cell-nerve interactions regulate antigen-induced airway inflammation and bronchoconstriction.

Antigen-induced contraction of mouse trachea requires both serotonin release from airway mast cells and acetylcholine release from parasympathetic neurons [151]. However, there have been a number of mechanisms proposed for how nerves and mast cell co-operate to bring about bronchoconstriction (Fig. 1). There may be direct activation of 5-HT2 receptors on pre- or postganglionic terminals of parasympathetic cholinergic neurons that then leads to enhanced acetylcholine release that in turn stimulates smooth muscle contraction via activation of muscarinic receptors. This is supported by the location of mast cells in the mouse trachea, situated in the smooth muscle portion of the tissue well beneath the epithelium, and adjacent to postganglionic parasympathetic nerves [153, 154] and by ex vivo studies that have measured an increase in acetylcholine levels after stimulation with antigen in both mouse and canine tracheal rings [155, 156]. A second proposed mechanism involves activation of serotonin receptors on airway smooth muscle leading to smooth muscle contraction only when acetylcholine, which is released at low levels constitutively by the parasympathetic fibers, occupies muscarinic M3 receptors present on airway smooth muscle. This concept is supported by findings that only a receptor antagonist of 5-HT2A, a receptor localized to airway smooth muscle and not cholinergic fibers, can attenuate antigen-induced bronchoconstriction [151]. It is proposed that a model requiring the action of both acetylcholine and serotonin on airway smooth muscle may provide a safeguard, separating the pro-inflammatory and bronchoconstrictor roles of the mast cell nerve interactions, limiting the activity of smooth muscle modulators stored by mast cells, while at the same time allowing mast cells to protect the airway against infectious agents through rapid release of inflammatory mediators. It should be noted that compared to rodents, human mast cells make small amounts of serotonin [157] and while serotonin can activate human airway smooth muscle ex vivo

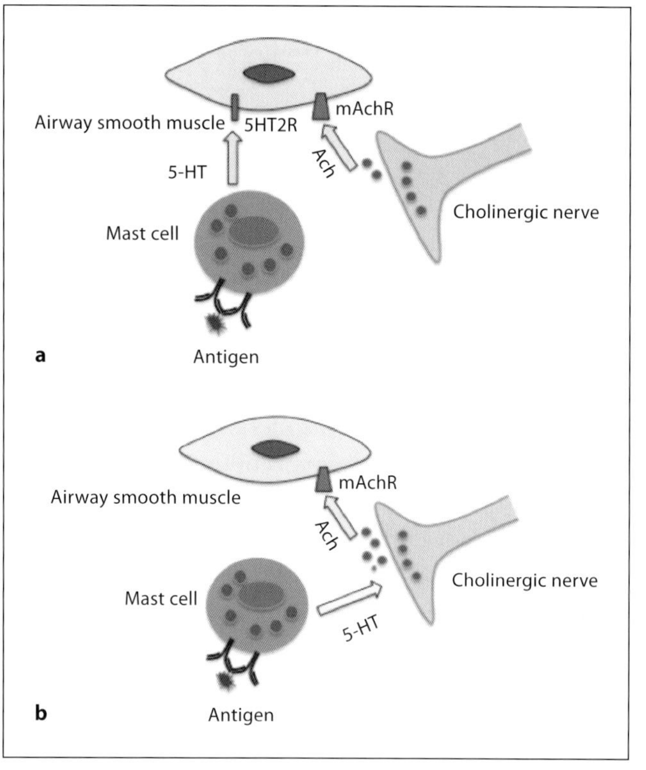

Fig. 1. The mast cell nerve unit in allergen-induced bronchoconstriction: Alternative models can be proposed: mast cell mediators, specifically serotonin, enhance the release of acetylcholine from nerve terminals that activates airway smooth muscle cells (**a**) or mast cell-derived serotonin directly activates airway smooth muscle cell contraction only when acetylcholine, constitutively released from parasympathetic fibers is bound to muscarinic receptors (**b**). Based on the work of Cyphert et al. [186]. 5-HT = Serotonin; Ach = acetylcholine; 5HT2R = type 2 5HT receptor; mAchR = muscarinic acetylcholine receptor.

[158] the relevance of this mediator to human antigen induced bronchoconstriction is far from certain.

Urinary Tract

There is an intimate relationship between mast cells and peptidergic sensory nerves in the urinary bladder. Mucosal and connective tissue type mast cells have been demonstrated in close apposition to substance P and CGRP immunoreactive nerves fibres while mast cells undergoing piecemeal degranulation have been detected in close proximity to intrinsic nerves in the bladder wall [159, 160].

As with other disorders characterized by hyperalgesia and neurogenic inflammation a putative role has been proposed for MC in Interstitial cystitis [160]. NK-1 receptor deficient mice fail to present bladder inflammatory cell infiltrate or edema in response to antigen challenge supporting a role for substance P in the development of interstitial cystitis [161]. Furthermore, CNS-induced neurogenic cystitis following pseudorabies virus infection was also associated with bladder mast cell degranulation in the rat [162]. Mast cell migration has been described and increased mast cell numbers have been reported in a subset of IC patients [163–165]. Substance P-reactive nerves have been observed close to mast cells in the bladder [141] while increased concentrations of histamine are consistent findings in the bladder biopsies from IC patients [141, 163]. Overall, there is good evidence to support a role for mast cell nerve interaction in the pathophysiology of interstitial cystitis in humans.

The Brain

Mast cells are found not only in association with nerves in the periphery but are also resident in the brain of all mammalian species [166]. In general, brain mast cells, considered a third less-common subtype, display the staining characteristics of connective tissue mast cells but the ultrastructural appearance and secretory pattern of mucosal mast cells [167]. Given the functional plasticity of mast cells, the unique microenvironment of the brain may induce the cells to express a phenotype that adapts them to roles quite distinct from their counterparts in other organs. Their role in the brain likely involves many of the mediators synthesized, stored and secreted by mast cells such as serotonin, dopamine, histamine that are important neuroregulators of the CNS. Indeed, histamine secretion from brain mast cells in response to local neurotrophic factors and neuropeptides may contribute to the etiology of neuroinflammatory conditions such as multiple sclerosis and Alzheimer's disease [168, 169]. Mast cells generate and release several mediators that have significant neuroprotective properties. The neuroprotective and tropic actions of NGF and TGFβ are well known [170–172]. More recently, proteoglycans, especially heparin and chondroitin sulfate, are receiving more attention for their role in neuronal protection and neurotransmission [173]. Thus, it is reasonable to suggest that brain mast cells may participate in neuroprotection. Furthermore, mast cells can produce the tryptophan metabolite kynurenic acid [174], which is the only known endogenous antagonist of NMDA receptors. NMDA receptors are activated by glutamate and are the major regulator of synaptic plasticity and memory function.

Mast cells have been described primarily around the third ventricle, in the thalamus, hypothalamus and hippocampal regions and appear to be strategically situated to initiate neural and vascular responses, being localized to the meninges and perivascular areas on the brain side of the blood-brain barrier in mammals [175, 176] including humans [177]. However, the physiologic significance of mast cells in brain function and/or metabolism is unclear. However, they can modulate neuroendocrine control systems [178] and may play a role in the regulation of meningeal blood flow and vessel permeability [179].

In the mammalian brain, mast cells are most prevalent in the dorsal thalamus. Here they are concentrated in some but not all dorsal thalamic nuclei, suggesting that there are chemotactic factors controlling MC migration to select regions [166]. The localization of mast cells in the developing brain differs from that of the adult animal [167, 175]. Moreover, even in adult animals the brain MC population is not static but alters with changes in the behavior and physiological state of the animal [180, 181].

The medial habenula is a major attracting nucleus for brain MC following a range of physiological, psychosocial and pharmacological stimuli that are associated with changes in behavior [182, 183]. The habenular complex has a role in mediating neurochemical and behavioral responses to stress and provides both excitatory and inhibitory inputs to the dorsal raphe nucleus (DRN), a major source of serotonergic transmission to the forebrain. Activity of the habenula is increased in several animal models of depression [184, 185] and in humans activity of the habenula/DRN pathway as assessed by fMRI is correlated with the Hamilton depression score [186]. It has been suggested that disruption of the normal balance of excitatory and inhibitory control in the habenula/DRN pathway results in aberrant serotonin release throughout the brain leading to the abnormalities of mood and cognition that characterize depression [186]. Therefore, MC have the potential to regulate neuroimmune interactions in the habenula by providing targeted delivery of neuromodulators in response to a number of local stimuli.

The particular topographical distribution of mast cells the area postrema and their relationship with the specialized ependyma and vessels without a blood-brain barrier, indicates that the cells play a critical role in the physiology of this brain region [187].

In the human area postrema mast cells are distributed perivascularly [187], suggesting that release of mast cell derived vasoactive molecules such as histamine, serotonin, prostaglandins, leukotrienes, play a role in the regulation of blood flow in this region. A subependymal location of mast cells has also been described in the thalamus of ring doves after courtship [188], and it has been suggested that mast cells play a part in controlling the ependyma in exchanges between cerebrospinal fluid and nervous tissue.

Mast cells in the central nervous system may also participate in the regulation of inflammatory responses through interactions with the HPA axis. Matsumoto et al. [189] demonstrated in dogs that degranulation of brain mast cells evokes hypothalamic-pituitary-adrenal responses via histamine and CRH release. When intracranial mast cells were passively sensitized with immunoglobulin E either via the intracerebroventricular or intravenous route, there was a marked increase in the adrenal cortisol secretion elicited by a subsequent antigenic challenge delivered via the central or peripheral route suggesting a link between intracranial mast cells and neuroendocrine networks [189].

Given that physiologic adrenal corticosteroids and pharmacologic glucocorticoids can attenuate severity allergic responses and suppress the subsequent immune-mediated inflammation [190], it has been suggested that activation of cortisol secretion after degranulation of intracranial mast cells could induce a host defense response against severe type I allergic reaction and thus provide a negative feedback mechanism to modulate peripheral inflammatory responses [189].

There is also mounting evidence that brain mast cells can influence behavior. One of the earliest indications of brain mast cell may be related to behavioral changes came from studies of courting doves. Silverman et al. [188] demonstrated that a population of mast cells is present in the medial habenula of the ring dove after a brief period of courtship. There were fewer mast cells in the medial habenula of birds housed in isolation and mast cell numbers were further reduced in long-term castrates. Mast cell-deficient mice were demonstrated to have a greater anxiety like behavior and blockade of brain but not peripheral mast cells increased anxiety like behavior [191].

Conclusions

It is clear that extensive crosstalk exists between nerves and mast cells. Although differences in species have been reported, morphologic as well as functional associations are found in most tissues in many mammalian species including humans.

The bidirectional communication between mast cells and nerves appears to serve multiple functions. Mast cells play a role in resistance to infection and are extensively involved in inflammation and subsequent tissue repair. The relationship between mast cells and neurons enables the involvement of peripheral and central nervous systems in the regulation of defense mechanisms, inflammation and response to infection.

The interaction between mast cells and nerves is involved in the regulation of physiologic homeostatic processes as well as in disease mechanisms, something that must be borne in mind when considering mast cell nerve communication as a therapeutic target. Interference in the cross-communication between mast cells and nerves also increases the risk of changing the healthy balance essential for maintaining tissue homeostasis.

More studies are required for a better understanding of how the activation of mast cells and nerves is modulated, how nerves control mast cell functions and how mast cells influence neural participation in host defense, wound repair, inflammation and associated pain responses. New findings will continue to increase our understanding of mast cell-nerve associations and their function in health and disease and will likely facilitate new therapeutic and diagnostic approaches.

References

1 Moon TC, St Laurent CD, Morris KE, et al: Advances in mast cell biology: new understanding of heterogeneity and function. Mucosal Immunol 2010;3:111–128.

2 Rivera J, Olivera A: A current understanding of Fc epsilon RI-dependent mast cell activation. Curr Allergy Asthma Rep 2008;8:14–20.

3 Marshall JS, Jawdat DM: Mast cells in innate immunity. J Allergy Clin Immunol 2004;114:21–27.

4 Metz M, Piliponsky AM, Chen CC, et al: Mast cells can enhance resistance to snake and honeybee venoms. Science 2006;313:526–530.

5 Malaviya R, Twesten NJ, Ross EA, Abraham SN, Pfeifer JD: Mast cells process bacterial Ags through a phagocytic route for class I MHC presentation to T cells. J Immunol 1996;156:1490–1496.

6 Wang HW, Tedla N, Lloyd AR, Wakefield D, McNeil PH: Mast cell activation and migration to lymph nodes during induction of an immune response in mice. J Clin Invest 1998;102:1617–1626.

7 de Vries VC, Pino-Lagos K, Elgueta R, Noelle RJ: The enigmatic role of mast cells in dominant tolerance. Curr Opin Organ Transplant 2009;14:332–337.

8 Sayed BA, Walker ME, Brown MA: Cutting edge: mast cells regulate disease severity in a relapsing-remitting model of multiple sclerosis. J Immunol 2011;186:3294–3298.

9 Hueber AJ, Asquith DL, Miller AM, et al: Mast cells express IL-17A in rheumatoid arthritis synovium. J Immunol 2010;184:3336–3340.

10 Nienartowicz A, Sobaniec-Lotowska ME, Jarocka-Cyrta E, Lemancewicz D: Mast cells in neoangiogenesis. Med Sci Monit 2006;12:RA53–56.

11 Ribatti D, Crivellato E: Mast cells, angiogenesis and cancer. Adv Exp Med Biol 2011;716:270–288.

12 Theoharides TC: The mast cell: a neuroimmunoendocrine master player. Int J Tissue React 1996;18: 1–21.

13 Frieling T, Cooke HJ, Wood JD: Histamine receptors on submucous neurons in guinea pig colon. Am J Physiol 1993;264:G74–80.

14 van Houwelingen AH, Kool M, de Jager SCA, et al: Mast cell-derived TNF-α primes sensory nerve endings in a pulmonary hypersensitivity reaction. J Immunol 2002;168:5297–5302.

15 Leon A, Buriani A, Dal Toso R, et al: Mast cells synthesize, store, and release nerve growth factor. Proc Natl Acad Sci USA 1994;91:3739–3743.

16 Kakurai M, Monteforte R, Suto H, Tsai M, Nakae S, Galli SJ: Mast cell-derived tumor necrosis factor can promote nerve fiber elongation in the skin during contact hypersensitivity in mice. Am J Pathol 2006; 169:1713–1721.

17 Andersson RG, Grundstrom N: Innervation of airway smooth muscle. Efferent mechanisms. Pharmacol Ther 1987;32:107–130.

18 Bienenstock J, Tomioka M, Matsuda H, et al: The role of mast cells in inflammatory processes: evidence for nerve/mast cell interactions. Int Arch Allergy Appl Immunol 1987;82:238–243.

19 Stead RH, Tomioka M, Quinonez G, Simon GT, Felten SY, Bienenstock J: Intestinal mucosal mast cells in normal and nematode-infected rat intestines are in intimate contact with peptidergic nerves. Proc Natl Acad Sci USA 1987;84:2975–2979.

20 Undem BJ, Riccio MM, Weinreich D, Ellis JL, Myers AC: Neurophysiology of mast cell-nerve interactions in the airways. Int Arch Allergy Immunol 1995;107:199–201.

21 Spanos C, Pang X, Ligris K, et al: Stress-induced bladder mast cell activation: implications for interstitial cystitis. J Urol 1997;157:669–672.

22 Bienenstock J, Denburg J, Scicchitano R, Stead R, Perdue M, Stanisz A: Role of neuropeptides, nerves and mast cells in intestinal immunity and physiology. Monogr Allergy 1988;24:134–143.

23 Barnes PJ: Airway inflammation and autonomic control. Eur J Respir Dis Suppl 1986;147:80–87.

24 Rychter JW, Van Nassauw L, Timmermans JP, Akkermans LM, Westerink RH, Kroese AB: CGRP1 receptor activation induces piecemeal release of protease-1 from mouse bone marrow-derived mucosal mast cells. Neurogastroenterol Motil 2011; 23:e57–68.

25 Gottwald T, Lhotak S, Stead RH: Effect of truncal vagotomy and capsaicin on mast cells and IgA-positive plasma cells in rat jejunal mucosa. Neurogastroenterol Motil 1997;9:25–32.

26 Gottwald TP, Hewlett BR, Lhotak S, Stead RH: Electrical stimulation of the vagus nerve modulates the histamine content of mast cells in the rat jejunal mucosa. Neuroreport 1995;7:313–317.

27 Kandere-Grzybowska K, Letourneau R, Kempuraj D, et al: IL-1 induces vesicular secretion of IL-6 without degranulation from human mast cells. J Immunol 2003;171:4830–4836.

28 Vliagoftis H, Dimitriadou V, Theoharides TC: Progesterone triggers selective mast cell secretion of 5-hydroxytryptamine. Int Arch Allergy Appl Immunol 1990;93:113–119.

29 Eggleston PA, Kagey-Sobotka A, Proud D, Adkinson NFJ, Lichtenstein LM: Disassociation of the release of histamine and arachidonic acid metabolites from osmotically activated basophils and human lung mast cells. Am Rev Respir Dis 1990;141:960–964.

30 Krishnaswamy G, Ajitawi O, Chi DS: The human mast cell: an overview. Methods Mol Biol 2006;315: 13–34.

31 Ruitenberg EJ, Gustowska L, Elgersma A, Ruitenberg HM: Effect of fixation on the light microscopical visualization of mast cells in the mucosa and connective tissue of the human duodenum. Int Arch Allergy Appl Immunol 1982;67:233–238.

32 Wingren U, Enerback L: Turnover of histamine in mucosal and connective tissue mast cells of the rat. Agents Actions 1984;14:358–360.

33 Kitamura Y, Kanakura Y, Sonoda S, Asai H, Nakano T: Mutual phenotypic changes between connective tissue type and mucosal mast cells. Int Arch Allergy Appl Immunol 1987;82:244–248.

34 Reed DE, Barajas-Lopez C, Cottrell G, et al: Mast cell tryptase and proteinase-activated receptor 2 induce hyperexcitability of guinea-pig submucosal neurons. J Physiol 2003;547:531–542.

35 Yuan H, Zhu X, Zhou S, et al: Role of mast cell activation in inducing microglial cells to release neurotrophin. J Neurosci Res 2010;88:1348–1354.

36 Amadesi S, Nie J, Vergnolle N, et al: Protease-activated receptor 2 sensitizes the capsaicin receptor transient receptor potential vanilloid receptor 1 to induce hyperalgesia. J Neurosci 2004;24:4300–4312.

37 Linden DR, Manning BP, Bunnett NW, Mawe GM: Agonists of proteinase-activated receptor 2 excite guinea pig ileal myenteric neurons. Eur J Pharmacol 2001;431:311–314.

38 Caughey GH, Leidig F, Viro NF, Nadel JA: Substance P and vasoactive intestinal peptide degradation by mast cell tryptase and chymase. J Pharmacol Exp Ther 1988;244:133–137.

39 Steinhoff M, Vergnolle N, Young SH, et al: Agonists of proteinase-activated receptor 2 induce inflammation by a neurogenic mechanism. Nat Med 2000;6: 151–158.

40 Adcock IM, Caramori G, Ito K: New insights into the molecular mechanisms of corticosteroids actions. Curr Drug Targets 2006;7:649–660.

41 Furuno T, Ito A, Koma Y, et al: The spermatogenic Ig superfamily/synaptic cell adhesion molecule mast-cell adhesion molecule promotes interaction with nerves. J Immunol 2005;174:6934–6942.

42 Ito A, Oonuma J: Direct interaction between nerves and mast cells mediated by the SgIGSF/SynCAM adhesion molecule. J Pharmacol Sci 2006;102:1–5.

43 Hagiyama M, Furuno T, Hosokawa Y, et al: Enhanced nerve-mast cell interaction by a neuronal short isoform of cell adhesion molecule-1. J Immunol. 2011;186:5983–5992.

44 Tegoshi T, Nishida M, Arizono N: Expression and role of E-cadherin and CD103beta7 (alphaEbeta7 integrin) on cultured mucosal-type mast cells. APMIS 2005;113:91–98.

45 Suzuki A, Suzuki R, Furuno T, Teshima R, Nakanishi M: N-cadherin plays a role in the synapse-like structures between mast cells and neurites. Biol Pharm Bull 2004;27:1891–1894.

46 Marshall JS, Gomi K, Blennerhassett MG, Bienenstock J: Nerve growth factor modifies the expression of inflammatory cytokines by mast cells via a prostanoid-dependent mechanism. J Immunol 1999;162:4271–4276.

47 Woolf CJ, Ma QP, Allchorne A, Poole S: Peripheral cell types contributing to the hyperalgesic action of nerve growth factor in inflammation. J Neurosci 1996;16:2716–2723.

48 Mazurek N, Weskamp G, Erne P, Otten U: Nerve growth factor induces mast cell degranulation without changing intracellular calcium levels. FEBS Lett 1986;198:315–320.

49 Marshall JS, Stead RH, McSharry C, Nielsen L, Bienenstock J: The role of mast cell degranulation products in mast cell hyperplasia. I. Mechanism of action of nerve growth factor. J Immunol 1990;144: 1886–1892.

50 Braun A, Quarcoo D, Schulte-Herbruggen O, Lommatzsch M, Hoyle G, Renz H: Nerve growth factor induces airway hyperresponsiveness in mice. Int Arch Allergy Immunol 2001;124:205–207.

51 Braun A, Appel E, Baruch R, et al: Role of nerve growth factor in a mouse model of allergic airway inflammation and asthma. Eur J Immunol 1998; 28:3240–3251.

52 Flugel A, Matsumuro K, Neumann H, et al: Anti-inflammatory activity of nerve growth factor in experimental autoimmune encephalomyelitis: inhibition of monocyte transendothelial migration. Eur J Immunol 2001;31:11–22.

53 di Mola FF, Friess H, Zhu ZW, et al: Nerve growth factor and Trk high affinity receptor (TrkA) gene expression in inflammatory bowel disease. Gut 2000;46:670–679.

54 Reinshagen M, Rohm H, Steinkamp M, et al: Protective role of neurotrophins in experimental inflammation of the rat gut. Gastroenterology 2000; 119:368–376.

55 Sann H, Dux M, Schemann M, Jancso G: Neurogenic inflammation in the gastrointestinal tract of the rat. Neurosci Lett 1996;219:147–150.

56 Shanahan F, Anton P: Neuroendocrine modulation of the immune system. Possible implications for inflammatory bowel disease. Dig Dis Sci 1988;33: 41S-49S.

57 Baluk P: Neurogenic inflammation in skin and airways. J Invest Dermatol Symp Proc 1997;2:76–81.

58 Mayer EA, Raybould H, Koelbel C: Neuropeptides, inflammation, and motility. Dig Dis Sci 1988;33: 71S-77S.

59 Jessop DS, Renshaw D, Larsen PJ, Chowdrey HS, Harbuz MS: Substance P is involved in terminating the hypothalamo-pituitary-adrenal axis response to acute stress through centrally located neurokinin-1 receptors. Stress 2000;3:209–220.

60 Joos GF, De Swert KO, Pauwels RA: Airway inflammation and tachykinins: prospects for the development of tachykinin receptor antagonists. Eur J Pharmacol 2001;429:239–250.

61 Lee HR, Ho WZ, Douglas SD: Substance P augments tumor necrosis factor release in human monocyte-derived macrophages. Clin Diagn Lab Immunol 1994;1:419–423.

62 Suzuki R, Furuno T, McKay DM, et al: Direct neurite-mast cell communication in vitro occurs via the neuropeptide substance P. J Immunol 1999;163: 2410–2415.

63 Anzai R, Seki S, Ogasawara K, et al: Interleukin-12 induces cytotoxic NK1+ alpha beta T cells in the lungs of euthymic and athymic mice. Immunology 1996;88:82–89.

64 Azzolina A, Bongiovanni A, Lampiasi N: Substance P induces TNF-alpha and IL-6 production through NF kappa B in peritoneal mast cells. Biochim Biophys Acta 2003;1643:75–83.

65 Janiszewski J, Bienenstock J, Blennerhassett MG: Picomolar doses of substance P trigger electrical responses in mast cells without degranulation. Am J Physiol 1994;267:C138–45.

66 Okabe T, Hide M, Hiragun T, Morita E, Koro O, Yamamoto S: Bone marrow derived mast cell acquire responsiveness to substance P with Ca(2+) signals and release of leukotriene B(4) via mitogen-activated protein kinase. J Neuroimmunol 2006;181:1–12.

67 Karimi K, Redegeld FA, Blom R, Nijkamp FP: Stem cell factor and interleukin-4 increase responsiveness of mast cells to substance P. Exp Hematol 2000;28:626–634.

68 Bischoff SC, Schwengberg S, Lorentz A, et al: Substance P and other neuropeptides do not induce mediator release in isolated human intestinal mast cells. Neurogastroenterol Motil 2004;16:185–193.

69 Mori N, Suzuki R, Furuno T, et al: Nerve-mast cell (RBL) interaction: RBL membrane ruffling occurs at the contact site with an activated neurite. Am J Physiol Cell Physiol 2002;283:C1738–C1744.

70 Blennerhassett MG, Bienenstock J: Sympathetic nerve contact causes maturation of mast cells in vitro. J Neurobiol 1998;35:173–182.

71 Suzuki A, Suzuki R, Furuno T, Teshima R, Nakanishi M: Calcium response and FcepsilonRI expression in bone marrow-derived mast cells co-cultured with SCG neurites. Biol Pharm Bull 2005;28:1963–1965.

72 Singh LK, Pang X, Alexacos N, Letourneau R, Theoharides TC: Acute immobilization stress triggers skin mast cell degranulation via corticotropin releasing hormone, neurotensin, and substance P: a link to neurogenic skin disorders. Brain Behav Immun 1999;13:225–239.

73 Joachim RA, Cifuentes LB, Sagach V, et al: Stress induces substance P in vagal sensory neurons innervating the mouse airways. Clin Exp Allergy 2006;36:1001–1010.

74 Joachim RA, Quarcoo D, Arck PC, Herz U, Renz H, Klapp BF: Stress enhances airway reactivity and airway inflammation in an animal model of allergic bronchial asthma. Psychosom Med 2003;65:811–815.

75 Joachim RA, Sagach V, Quarcoo D, Dinh QT, Arck PC, Klapp BF: Neurokinin-1 receptor mediates stress-exacerbated allergic airway inflammation and airway hyperresponsiveness in mice. Psychosom Med 2004;66:564–571.

76 Fest S, Zenclussen AC, Joachim R, Hagen E, Demuth HU, Hoffmann T: Stress and substance P but not the substance P-metabolite SP5–11 trigger murine abortion by augmenting TNF-alpha levels at the feto-maternal interface. Scand J Immunol 2006;63:42–49.

77 Peters EM, Kuhlmei A, Tobin DJ, Muller-Rover S, Klapp BF, Arck PC: Stress exposure modulates peptidergic innervation and degranulates mast cells in murine skin. Brain Behav Immun 2005;19:252–262.

78 Pavlovic S, Daniltchenko M, Tobin DJ, et al: Further exploring the brain-skin connection: stress worsens dermatitis via substance P-dependent neurogenic inflammation in mice. J Invest Dermatol 2008;128:434–446.

79 Kulka M, Sheen CH, Tancowny BP, Grammer LC, Schleimer RP: Neuropeptides activate human mast cell degranulation and chemokine production. Immunology 2008;123:398–410.

80 Ottosson A, Edvinsson L: Release of histamine from dural mast cells by substance P and calcitonin gene-related peptide. Cephalalgia 1997;17:166–174.

81 Schwenger N, Dux M, de Col R, Carr R, Messlinger K: Interaction of calcitonin gene-related peptide, nitric oxide and histamine release in neurogenic blood flow and afferent activation in the rat cranial dura mater. Cephalalgia 2007;27:481–491.

82 Forsythe P, McGarvey LP, Heaney LG, MacMahon J, Ennis M: Sensory neuropeptides induce histamine release from bronchoalveolar lavage cells in both nonasthmatic coughers and cough variant asthmatics. Clin Exp Allergy 2000;30:225–232.

83 De Jonge F, Van Nassauw L, Adriaensen D, et al: Effect of intestinal inflammation on capsaicin-sensitive afferents in the ileum of *Schistosoma mansoni*-infected mice. Histochem Cell Biol 2003;119:477–484.

84 Reinshagen M, Flamig G, Ernst S, et al: Calcitonin gene-related peptide mediates the protective effect of sensory nerves in a model of colonic injury. J Pharmacol Exp Ther 1998;286:657–661.

85 Bulut K, Felderbauer P, Deters S, et al: Sensory neuropeptides and epithelial cell restitution: the relevance of SP- and CGRP-stimulated mast cells. Int J Colorectal Dis 2008;23:535–541.

86 Abad C, Gomariz RP, Waschek JA: Neuropeptide mimetics and antagonists in the treatment of inflammatory disease: focus on VIP and PACAP. Curr Top Med Chem 2006;6:151–163.

87 Sherwood NM, Krueckl SL, McRory JE: The origin and function of the pituitary adenylate cyclase-activating polypeptide (PACAP)/glucagon superfamily. Endocr Rev 2000;21:619–670.

88 Goetzl EJ, Sreedharan SP, Turck CW: Structurally distinctive vasoactive intestinal peptides from rat basophilic leukemia cells. J Biol Chem 1988;263:9083–9086.
89 Goetzl EJ, Pankhaniya RR, Gaufo GO, Mu Y, Xia M, Sreedharan SP: Selectivity of effects of vasoactive intestinal peptide on macrophages and lymphocytes in compartmental immune responses. Ann NY Acad Sci 1998;840:540–550.
90 Undem BJ, Dick EC, Buckner CK: Inhibition by vasoactive intestinal peptide of antigen-induced histamine release from guinea-pig minced lung. Eur J Pharmacol 1983;88:247–250.
91 Tuncel N, Tore F, Sahinturk V, Ak D, Tuncel M:. Vasoactive intestinal peptide inhibits degranulation and changes granular content of mast cells: a potential therapeutic strategy in controlling septic shock. Peptides 2000;21:81–89.
92 Akahoshi M, Song CH, Piliponsky AM, et al: Mast cell chymase reduces the toxicity of Gila monster venom, scorpion venom, and vasoactive intestinal polypeptide in mice. J Clin Invest 2011;121:4180–4191.
93 Tam EK, Caughey GH: Degradation of airway neuropeptides by human lung tryptase. Am J Respir Cell Mol Biol 1990;3:27–32.
94 Tuncel N, Sener E, Cerit C, et al: Brain mast cells and therapeutic potential of vasoactive intestinal peptide in a Parkinson's disease model in rats: brain microdialysis, behavior, and microscopy. Peptides 2005;26:827–836.
95 El-Shazly A, Berger P, Girodet PO, et al: Fraktalkine produced by airway smooth muscle cells contributes to mast cell recruitment in asthma. J Immunol 2006;176:1860–1868.
96 Rimaniol AC, Till SJ, Garcia G, et al: The CX3C chemokine fractalkine in allergic asthma and rhinitis. J Allergy Clin Immunol 2003;112:1139–1146.
97 Borovikova LV, Ivanova S, Zhang M, et al: Vagus nerve stimulation attenuates the systemic inflammatory response to endotoxin. Nature 2000;405:458–462.
98 Ghia JE, Blennerhassett P, Kumar-Ondiveeran H, Verdu EF, Collins SM: The vagus nerve: a tonic inhibitory influence associated with inflammatory bowel disease in a murine model. Gastroenterology 2006;131:1122–1130.
99 Wang H, Yu M, Ochani M, et al: Nicotinic acetylcholine receptor alpha7 subunit is an essential regulator of inflammation. Nature 2003;421:384–388.
100 Karimi K, Bienenstock J, Wang L, Forsythe P: The vagus nerve modulates CD4+ T cell activity. Brain Behav Immun 2010;24:316–323.
101 Williams RM, Berthoud HR, Stead RH: Vagal afferent nerve fibres contact mast cells in rat small intestinal mucosa. Neuroimmunomodulation 1997;4:266–270.
102 Luyer MD, Greve JW, Hadfoune M, Jacobs JA, Dejong CH, Buurman WA: Nutritional stimulation of cholecystokinin receptors inhibits inflammation via the vagus nerve. J Exp Med 2005;202:1023–1029.
103 Tracey KJ: Fat meets the cholinergic antiinflammatory pathway. J Exp Med 2005;202:1017–1021.
104 Kageyama-Yahara N, Suehiro Y, Yamamoto T, Kadowaki M: IgE-induced degranulation of mucosal mast cells is negatively regulated via nicotinic acetylcholine receptors. Biochem Biophys Res Commun 2008;377:321–325.
105 Mishra NC, Rir-sima-ah J, Boyd RT, et al: Nicotine inhibits Fc epsilon RI-induced cysteinyl leukotrienes and cytokine production without affecting mast cell degranulation through alpha 7/alpha 9/alpha 10-nicotinic receptors. J Immunol 2010;185:588–596.
106 Kindt F, Wiegand S, Niemeier V, et al: Reduced expression of nicotinic alpha subunits 3, 7, 9 and 10 in lesional and nonlesional atopic dermatitis skin but enhanced expression of alpha subunits 3 and 5 in mast cells. Br J Dermatol 2008;159:847–857.
107 Fantozzi R, Masini E, Blandina P, Mannaioni PF, Bani-Sacchi T: Release of histamine from rat mast cells by acetylcholine. Nature 1978;273:473–474.
108 Masini E, Fantozzi R, Conti A, Blandina P, Brunelleschi S, Mannaioni PF: Mast cell heterogeneity in response to cholinergic stimulation. Int Arch Allergy Appl Immunol 1985;77:184–185.
109 Leung KB, Pearce FL: A comparison of histamine secretion from peritoneal mast cells of the rat and hamster. Br J Pharmacol 1984;81:693–701.
110 Kazimierczak W, Adamas B, Maslinski C: Failure of acetylcholine to release histamine from rat mast cells. Agents Actions 1980;10:1–3.
111 Rossi R, Johansson O: Cutaneous innervation and the role of neuronal peptides in cutaneous inflammation: a minireview. Eur J Dermatol 1998;8:299–306.
112 Ansel JC, Armstrong CA, Song I, et al: Interactions of the skin and nervous system. J Investig Dermatol Symp Proc 1997;2:23–26.
113 Church MK, el-Lati S, Caulfield JP: Neuropeptide-induced secretion from human skin mast cells. Int Arch Allergy Appl Immunol 1991;94:310–318.
114 Siebenhaar F, Magerl M, Peters EM, Hendrix S, Metz M, Maurer M: Mast cell-driven skin inflammation is impaired in the absence of sensory nerves. J Allergy Clin Immunol 2008;121:955–961.

115 Hart PH, Grimbaldeston MA, Swift GJ, Jaksic A, Noonan FP, Finlay-Jones JJ: Dermal mast cells determine susceptibility to ultraviolet B-induced systemic suppression of contact hypersensitivity responses in mice. J Exp Med 1998;187:2045–2053.

116 Hart PH, Townley SL, Grimbaldeston MA, Khalil Z, Finlay-Jones JJ: Mast cells, neuropeptides, histamine, and prostaglandins in UV-induced systemic immunosuppression. Methods 2002;28:79–89.

117 Jarvikallio A, Harvima IT, Naukkarinen A: Mast cells, nerves and neuropeptides in atopic dermatitis and nummular eczema. Arch Dermatol Res 2003; 295:2–7.

118 Detmar M, Brown LF, Schon MP, et al: Increased microvascular density and enhanced leukocyte rolling and adhesion in the skin of VEGF transgenic mice. J Invest Dermatol 1998;111:1–6.

119 Arck P, Paus R: From the brain-skin connection: the neuroendocrine-immune misalliance of stress and itch. Neuroimmunomodulation 2006;13:347–356.

120 Theoharides TC, Zhang B, Kempuraj D, et al: IL-33 augments substance P-induced VEGF secretion from human mast cells and is increased in psoriatic skin. Proc Natl Acad Sci USA 2010;107:4448–4453.

121 Theoharides TC, Spanos C, Pang X, et al: Stress-induced intracranial mast cell degranulation: a corticotropin-releasing hormone-mediated effect. Endocrinology 1995;136:5745–5750.

122 Asadi S, Alysandratos KD, Angelidou A, et al: Substance P (SP) induces expression of functional corticotropin-releasing hormone receptor-1 (CRHR-1) in human mast cells. J Invest Dermatol 2012;132:324–329.

123 Stead RH: Nerve remodelling during intestinal inflammation. Ann NY Acad Sci 1992;664:443–455.

124 Newson B, Dahlstrom A, Enerback L, Ahlman H: Suggestive evidence for a direct innervation of mucosal mast cells. Neuroscience 1983;10:565–570.

125 Shanahan F, Denburg JA, Fox J, Bienenstock J, Befus D: Mast cell heterogeneity: effects of neuroenteric peptides on histamine release. J Immunol 1985;135: 1331–1337.

126 Raithel M, Schneider HT, Hahn EG: Effect of substance P on histamine secretion from gut mucosa in inflammatory bowel disease. Scand J Gastroenterol 1999;34:496–503.

127 Koon HW, Pothoulakis C: Immunomodulatory properties of substance P: the gastrointestinal system as a model. Ann NY Acad Sci 2006;1088: 23–40.

128 Jiang W, Kreis ME, Eastwood C, Kirkup AJ, Humphrey PP, Grundy D: 5-HT(3) and histamine H(1) receptors mediate afferent nerve sensitivity to intestinal anaphylaxis in rats. Gastroenterology 2000;119:1267–1275.

129 Castagliuolo I, Riegler M, Pasha A, et al: Neurokinin-1 (NK-1) receptor is required in *Clostridium difficile*-induced enteritis. J Clin Invest 1998;101:1547–1550.

130 Linard C, Marquette C, Strup C, Aigueperse J, Mathe D: Involvement of primary afferent nerves after abdominal irradiation: consequences on ileal contractile activity and inflammatory mediator release in the rat. Dig Dis Sci 2003;48:688–697.

131 Margolis KG, Gershon MD: Neuropeptides and inflammatory bowel disease. Curr Opin Gastroenterol 2009;25:503–511.

132 Carraway R, Cochrane DE, Lansman JB, Leeman SE, Paterson BM, Welch HJ: Neurotensin stimulates exocytotic histamine secretion from rat mast cells and elevates plasma histamine levels. J Physiol 1982; 323:403–414.

133 Cochrane DE, Carraway RE, Harrington K, Laudano M, Rawlings S, Feldberg RS: HMC-1 human mast cells synthesize neurotensin (NT) precursor, secrete bioactive NT-like peptide(s) and express NT receptor NTS1. Inflamm Res 2011;60:1139–1151.

134 Wershil BK, Castagliuolo I, Pothoulakis C: Direct evidence of mast cell involvement in *Clostridium difficile* toxin A-induced enteritis in mice. Gastroenterology 1998;114:956–964.

135 Wood JD: Neuropathophysiology of functional gastrointestinal disorders. World J Gastroenterol 2007; 13:1313–1332.

136 Wang L, Stanisz AM, Wershil BK, Galli SJ, Perdue MH: Substance P induces ion secretion in mouse small intestine through effects on enteric nerves and mast cells. Am J Physiol 1995;269:G85–92.

137 Wang YZ, Palmer JM, Cooke HJ: Neuroimmune regulation of colonic secretion in guinea pigs. Am J Physiol 1991;260:G307–314.

138 Santos J, Saunders PR, Hanssen NP, et al: Corticotropin-releasing hormone mimics stress-induced colonic epithelial pathophysiology in the rat. Am J Physiol 1999;277:G391–399.

139 Wallon C, Yang PC, Keita AV, et al: Corticotropin-releasing hormone (CRH) regulates macromolecular permeability via mast cells in normal human colonic biopsies in vitro. Gut 2008;57:50–58.

140 Wood JD: Neuropathophysiology of irritable bowel syndrome. J Clin Gastroenterol 2002;35:S11–22.

141 Pang X, Boucher W, Triadafilopoulos G, Sant GR, Theoharides TC: Mast cell and substance P-positive nerve involvement in a patient with both irritable bowel syndrome and interstitial cystitis. Urology 1996;47:436–438.

142 Tunc B, Filik L, Altintas E, Turhan N, Ulker A, Dagli U: Mucosal mast cells in irritable bowel syndrome and inflammatory bowel disease. Acta Medica (Hradec Kralove) 2005;48:163–164.

143 Cremon C, Gargano L, Morselli-Labate AM, et al: Mucosal immune activation in irritable bowel syndrome: gender-dependence and association with digestive symptoms. Am J Gastroenterol 2009; 104:392–400.

144 Barbara G, Stanghellini V, De Giorgio R, et al: Activated mast cells in proximity to colonic nerves correlate with abdominal pain in irritable bowel syndrome. Gastroenterology 2004;126:693–702.

145 Park CH, Joo YE, Choi SK, Rew JS, Kim SJ, Lee MC: Activated mast cells infiltrate in close proximity to enteric nerves in diarrhea-predominant irritable bowel syndrome. J Korean Med Sci 2003;18:204–210.

146 Park JH, Rhee PL, Kim HS, et al: Mucosal mast cell counts correlate with visceral hypersensitivity in patients with diarrhea predominant irritable bowel syndrome. J Gastroenterol Hepatol 2006;21:71–78.

147 O'Sullivan M, Clayton N, Breslin NP, et al: Increased mast cells in the irritable bowel syndrome. Neurogastroenterol Motil 2000;12:449–457.

148 Carr MJ, Undem BJ: Bronchopulmonary afferent nerves. Respirology 2003;8:291–301.

149 Akiyama H, Amano H, Bienenstock J: Rat tracheal epithelial responses to water avoidance stress. J Allergy Clin Immunol 2005;116:318–324.

150 Sestini P, Bienenstock J, Crowe SE, et al: Ion transport in rat tracheal epithelium in vitro. Role of capsaicin-sensitive nerves in allergic reactions. Am Rev Respir Dis. 1990;141:393–397.

151 Cyphert JM, Kovarova M, Allen IC, et al: Cooperation between mast cells and neurons is essential for antigen-mediated bronchoconstriction. J Immunol 2009;182:7430–7439.

152 Rogerio AP, Andrade EL, Calixto JB: C-fibers, but not the transient potential receptor vanilloid 1 (TRPV1), play a role in experimental allergic airway inflammation. Eur J Pharmacol 2011;662:55–62.

153 Myers AC, Undem BJ, Weinreich D: Influence of antigen on membrane properties of guinea pig bronchial ganglion neurons. J Appl Physiol 1991;71: 970–976.

154 Kajekar R, Undem BJ, Myers AC: Role of cyclooxygenase activation and prostaglandins in antigen-induced excitability changes of bronchial parasympathetic ganglia neurons. Am J Physiol Lung Cell Mol Physiol 2003;284:L581–587.

155 Mitchell RW, Ndukuw IM, Ikeda K, Arbetter K, Leff AR: Effect of immune sensitization on stimulated ACh release from trachealis muscle in vitro. Am J Physiol 1993;265:L13–18.

156 Weigand LA, Myers AC, Meeker S, Undem BJ: Mast cell-cholinergic nerve interaction in mouse airways. J Physiol 2009;587:3355–3362.

157 Kushnir-Sukhov NM, Brown JM, Wu Y, Kirshenbaum A, Metcalfe DD: Human mast cells are capable of serotonin synthesis and release. J Allergy Clin Immunol 2007;119:498–499.

158 Davis C, Kannan MS, Jones TR, Daniel EE: Control of human airway smooth muscle: in vitro studies. J Appl Physiol 1982;53:1080–1087.

159 Keith IM, Jin J, Saban R: Nerve-mast cell interaction in normal guinea pig urinary bladder. J Comp Neurol 1995;363:28–36.

160 Theoharides TC, Pang X, Letourneau R, Sant GR: Interstitial cystitis: a neuroimmunoendocrine disorder. Ann NY Acad Sci 1998;840:619–634.

161 Saban R, Saban MR, Nguyen NB, et al: Neurokinin-1 (NK-1) receptor is required in antigen-induced cystitis. Am J Pathol 2000;156:775–780.

162 Jasmin L, Janni G, Ohara PT, Rabkin SD: CNS induced neurogenic cystitis is associated with bladder mast cell degranulation in the rat. J Urol 2000;164:852–855.

163 Kastrup J, Hald T, Larsen S, Nielsen VG: Histamine content and mast cell count of detrusor muscle in patients with interstitial cystitis and other types of chronic cystitis. Br J Urol 1983;55:495–500.

164 Larsen MS, Mortensen S, Nordling J, Horn T: Quantifying mast cells in bladder pain syndrome by immunohistochemical analysis. BJU Int 2008;102: 204–207.

165 Letourneau R, Sant GR, el-Mansoury M, Theoharides TC: Activation of bladder mast cells in interstitial cystitis. Int J Tissue React 1992;14:307–312.

166 Silver R, Silverman AJ, Vitkovic L, Lederhendler II: Mast cells in the brain: evidence and functional significance. Trends Neurosci 1996;19:25–31.

167 Zhuang X, Silverman AJ, Silver R: Distribution and local differentiation of mast cells in the parenchyma of the forebrain. J Comp Neurol 1999;408:477–488.

168 Rozniecki JJ, Hauser SL, Stein M, Lincoln R, Theoharides TC: Elevated mast cell tryptase in cerebrospinal fluid of multiple sclerosis patients. Ann Neurol 1995;37:63–66.

169 Dines KC, Powell HC: Mast cell interactions with the nervous system: relationship to mechanisms of disease. J Neuropathol Exp Neurol 1997;56:627–640.

170 Lin B, Pirrung MC, Deng L, Li Z, Liu Y, Webster NJ: Neuroprotection by small molecule activators of the nerve growth factor receptor. J Pharmacol Exp Ther 2007;322:59–69.

171 Nguyen N, Lee SB, Lee YS, Lee KH, Ahn JY: Neuroprotection by NGF and BDNF against neurotoxin-exerted apoptotic death in neural stem cells are mediated through Trk receptors, activating PI3-kinase and MAPK pathways. Neurochem Res 2009;34:942–951.

172 Zhu Y, Yang GY, Ahlemeyer B, et al: Transforming growth factor-beta 1 increases bad phosphorylation and protects neurons against damage. J Neurosci 2002;22:3898–3909.
173 Zhang ZG, Lu TS, Yuan HY: Neuroprotective effects of ultra-low-molecular-weight heparin in vitro and vivo models of ischemic injury. Fundam Clin Pharmacol 2011;25:300–303.
174 Knyihar-Csillik E, Chadaide Z, Okuno E, et al: Kynurenine aminotransferase in the supratentorial dura mater of the rat: effect of stimulation of the trigeminal ganglion. Exp Neurol 2004;186:242–247.
175 Ibrahim MZ: The mast cells of the mammalian central nervous system. IX. Development of the mast cells in the brain of the young rat. Acta Anat (Basel) 1985;124:149–158.
176 Florenzano F, Bentivoglio M: Degranulation, density, and distribution of mast cells in the rat thalamus: a light and electron microscopic study in basal conditions and after intracerebroventricular administration of nerve growth factor. J Comp Neurol 2000;424:651–669.
177 Dropp JJ: Mast cells in the human brain. Acta Anat (Basel) 1979;105:505–513.
178 Theoharides TC: Mast cells: the immune gate to the brain. Life Sci 1990;46:607–617.
179 Zhuang X, Silverman AJ, Silver R: Brain mast cell degranulation regulates blood-brain barrier. J Neurobiol 1996;31:393–403.
180 Cirulli F, Pistillo L, de Acetis L, Alleva E, Aloe L: Increased number of mast cells in the central nervous system of adult male mice following chronic subordination stress. Brain Behav Immun 1998;12: 123–133.
181 Kriegsfeld LJ, Hotchkiss AK, Demas GE, Silverman AJ, Silver R, Nelson RJ: Brain mast cells are influenced by chemosensory cues associated with estrus induction in female prairie voles (*Microtus ochrogaster*). Horm Behav 2003;44:377–384.
182 Cirulli F, Pistillo L, de Acetis L, Alleva E, Aloe L: Increased number of mast cells in the central nervous system of adult male mice following chronic subordination stress. Brain Behav Immun 1998;12: 123–133.
183 Serviere J, Dubayle D, Menetrey D: Increase of rat medial habenular mast cell numbers by systemic administration of cyclophosphamide. Toxicol Lett 2003;145:143–152.
184 Amat J, Sparks PD, Matus-Amat P, Griggs J, Watkins LR, Maier SF: The role of the habenular complex in the elevation of dorsal raphe nucleus serotonin and the changes in the behavioral responses produced by uncontrollable stress. Brain Res 2001;917:118–126.
185 Shumake J, Gonzalez-Lima F: Brain systems underlying susceptibility to helplessness and depression. Behav Cogn Neurosci Rev 2003;2:198–221.
186 Morris JS, Smith KA, Cowen PJ, Friston KJ, Dolan RJ: Covariation of activity in habenula and dorsal raphe nuclei following tryptophan depletion. Neuroimage 1999;10:163–172.
187 Porzionato A, Macchi V, Parenti A, De Caro R: The distribution of mast cells in the human area postrema. J Anat 2004;204:141–147.
188 Silverman AJ, Millar RP, King JA, Zhuang X, Silver R: Mast cells with gonadotropin-releasing hormone-like immunoreactivity in the brain of doves. Proc Natl Acad Sci USA 1994;91:3695–3699.
189 Matsumoto I, Inoue Y, Shimada T, Aikawa T: Brain mast cells act as an immune gate to the hypothalamic-pituitary-adrenal axis in dogs. J Exp Med 2001;194: 71–78.
190 Barnes PJ: Corticosteroid effects on cell signalling. Eur Respir J 2006;27:413–426.
191 Nautiyal KM, Ribeiro AC, Pfaff DW, Silver R: Brain mast cells link the immune system to anxiety-like behavior. Proc Natl Acad Sci USA 2008;105:18053–18057.

Dr. Paul Forsythe
The Brain-Body Institute, St. Joseph's Healthcare, Department of Medicine, McMaster University
50 Charlton Avenue East, T3302
Hamilton, ON L8N 4A6 (Canada)
Tel. +1 905 522 1155, Ext. 35890, E-Mail forsytp@mcmaster.ca

Bienenstock J (ed): Allergy and the Nervous System.
Chem Immunol Allergy. Basel, Karger, 2012, vol 98, pp 222–239

Neural and Behavioral Correlates of Food Allergy

Frederico Azevedo Costa-Pinto[a] · Alexandre Salgado Basso[b]

[a]Department of Pathology, School of Veterinary Medicine, University of Sao Paulo and [b]Department of Microbiology, Immunology, and Parasitology, Federal University of Sao Paulo, Sao Paulo, Brazil

Abstract

Food allergy accounts for a great number of reactions leading to diminished quality of life in western countries. There has been an abundance of reports of behavioral changes, as well as psychiatric conditions associated with food allergy over the past decades. Most of this field inspired little medical attention for its lack of a solid scientific ground. We review the literature on the association of food allergy and brain activity, leading to changes in emotion and behavior. Moreover, we describe an experimental paradigm employed to dissect the biological relevance of this association. Mice allergic to ovalbumin avoid a palatable sweet solution in order to escape contact with antigen. This choice is associated with increased levels of anxiety, compatible with a conflicting situation. These responses are associated with increased activity in brain areas associated with emotional and affective behavior, which are also important for anxiety and stress responses. Higher levels of corticosterone accompany these changes in behavior. These responses are mediated by specific antibodies and prevented by depletion or immunological tolerance. They are also partially mediated by C-sensitive afferents and mast cells. Far from anecdote, neural repercussions of food allergy should be considered when planning a therapeutic strategy in affected individuals.

Does the brain detect an ongoing allergic reaction that takes place elsewhere in the body? In such a case, what would the purpose of that be? What are the pathways that convey immune information to the brain, leading to changes in behavior? Are those changes adaptive, representing an evolutionary advantage? These are only a few questions asked by those interested in the core of the subject covered in this book.

Physiological feedback involving food tasting and the nervous system have been assessed in extremely creative experimental paradigms such as *Caenorhabitiditis elegans* that regularly feed on bacteria and learns to avoid pathogenic strains by conditioned taste aversion. Nevertheless, one of the cornerstones for understanding the repercussions of an allergic reaction on the central nervous system was the development of animal model of immunologically induced flavor aversion in mice [1]. This model has been employed ever since with the aim of solving the puzzle of food allergy-associated changes in the behavior of mice.

Food allergy alone represents a great deal of cases of allergic reactions leading to diminished quality of life in western countries. Moreover, costs of hospitalization and missed working days due to allergic reactions against ingested antigens are quite high and well reported. Although allergy has been on the rise in industrialized countries over the past decades, no definitive explanation that accounts for this increase in prevalence is widely accepted.

Strictly from a medical perspective, there is an abundance of reports of neuroimmune interactions associated with food allergy. We intend to review and compile clinical data supporting a role for the central nervous system, evident by behavioral traits and psychiatric or emotional conditions, in triggering crisis or leading to recurrence of allergy reactions. On the other hand, we will also exemplify how an ongoing allergic reaction in the gastrointestinal tract leads to an altered activity in the central nervous system and modifies animal behavior. Thus, approaching the same issues in experimental biology, we review scientific papers focusing on models of food allergy and its repercussions in the central nervous system.

Finally, our intention is to provide the reader with an overall idea of the mechanisms by which the central nervous system communicates with the immune system during an allergic reaction in the gut. We also intend to build solid ground on the possible outcomes of this crosstalk, both on the course of allergy and on neural activity and behavior.

Review of Clinical Findings

The presence of macromolecules in the gastrointestinal tract has several repercussions, both in immunity and on the activity of the central nervous system (CNS). Epidemiological data from patients admitted to hospitals show an association of allergy symptoms and emotional changes.

A short review of cases with a clinical correlation (rather than mechanistic explanation) will make it clear why this issue has puzzled attending physicians for quite some time. Adverse reactions to the contents of a meal have been drastically used as a Biblical example of all adversity in life being introduced by choosing the wrong food [2]. The concept of individual reactions triggered by the same food constituent (milk or cheese) puzzled Hippocrates, since 'cheese does not harm all alike, hence it is not bad in itself. Yet, some people are happy after eating it, while others suffer severely for being intolerant to its components' [3].

Modern medicine brought population statistics to build a case for an array of conditions ranging from plain intolerance to allergic reactions to food antigens. It became clear that (1) the frequency of such diseases was far higher (and currently rising) than expected, (2) their pathogenesis is highly variable and multifactorial in nature, and (3) clinical symptoms of such reactions are definitely not restricted to the gastrointestinal tract. It soon became also obvious that, other than the expected signs of gastrointestinal dysfunction, one could find preexisting behavioral or psychological traits associated with disease, or the emotional changes triggered by it.

A reasonable number of reports point to changes in behavioral patterns triggered by allergic reactions. Clinically, anxiety reactions have been the most common behavioral pattern or symptom associated with food allergy [4], sometimes comparable to those found in patients suffering from irritable bowel syndrome. Both groups (food allergy and irritable bowel syndrome) present higher levels of anxiety and depression compared to matched controls [5]. Others have pointed, although in far less well-controlled studies, that traits of psychosis [6], autism [7], or schizophrenia could be tracked down to an allergic basis (and responded well to changes in diet) [8, 9]. Depression has long been found in allergic patients exposed to the underlying food antigen, although this has probably also been the most controversial of all supposedly neuroimmune associations of allergy [10, 11]. Even migraine has been reported as possibly associated with food allergy [12]. In a series of letters to the *Canadian Medical Association Journal*, depression was discussed as being induced by the allergen to sensitive patients and prevented by 'allergy neutralizing techniques' [8]. Although the exact mechanism for this association still remains under investigation, the fact that removal of such antigens from the diet reversed emotional changes clearly points to an epidemiological association, at least. In cases of severe reactions to food allergens, patients admitted to emergency rooms with GI symptoms topped by emotional disturbance show clear improvement of behavior after being treated for the allergic reaction. One could argue that in humans this could be due to consciousness of sickness or life-threatening risk, but animal models, discussed here, helped to sort this out. Regardless of the nature of factor (predisposing, trigger, or actual cause of disease) much of the field has been confused by the general misunderstanding of psychosomatic influence on disease [13]. Although the term was created on a very rational and defined context [14] it has often been used to describe supernatural or unexplainable medical phenomena, but might easily support neuroimmune interactions in food allergy [13].

In the mid-1980s this association was the focus of a few good reviews of the literature. The clinical association reported by many of these reviews could be considered, at best, highly questionable. Many authors conclude that, even though in many cases there is resolution of psychological or neurological symptoms upon withdrawal of the insulting allergen from the diet, the criteria for diagnosing mental or psychological illness, and also for the diagnosis of allergy, is frequently weak and subjective. A few studies with groups of allergic patients at the same period have concluded that (1) there are many misdiagnosed cases of allergic reactions to food, (2) no evidence of psychological symptoms could be found at all in other patients, or (3) there was no association between food-related problems and emotional or neurological conditions [10]. Nonetheless, the same authors reporting a lack of association between food allergy and psychological symptoms found higher levels of immunoglobulin E (IgE) directed at food allergens in the serum of schizophrenics compared to matched mentally healthier controls [6]. One curious description of how biased the studies on neuroimmune interactions in food allergy and emotions can be refers to the uncertainty of diagnosis. In that particular case, instead of an association between hypersensitivity to ingested substances and psychological symptoms, the higher incidence of psychiatric disorders was found among the subjects that could not get a definitive confirmation as to being allergic or not [15]. Actually, anxiety and depression may masquerade as food allergy if care has not been taken for reaching a precise diagnosis [11]. Indeed, some have supported the view that failure to recognize symptoms and overcome the effects of placebo, suggestion, and observer or referral bias are major causes for reaching unsubstantiated conclusions [16, 17]. According to the most skeptical authors, patients suffering from nonallergic food avoidance may actually present an emergent variant of Munchausen's syndrome, in which the very fear of having food allergy sometimes put their lives in risk (in children, that parental influence would be comparable to Meadow's syndrome, or Munchausen by proxy) [18]. Even recent studies on the subject seem to reject the hypothesis that anxiety and depression are major predictors of severity of allergy, and that many patients self-referred to as allergic fail to be diagnosed as such [19, 20].

Nevertheless, although controversial, some reports proposed that there could be an overlap of other underlying conditions triggering both psychological and allergic symptoms (since it became obvious that allergy is influenced by a myriad of factors, from environment to genetics, and food), or even that the allergic reactions really cause or at least exacerbate symptoms of a psychological nature [21]. A comprehensive study with 7,000 primary school children showed that, after adjusting for several concurrent factors, a strong correlation of irritability and food intolerance remained [22]. Accordingly, the immune system has been proposed as a key factor for understanding psychopathology, reinforcing the role of diet on function of the central nervous system [23].

Although this literature can be quite vast (and the facts very obvious to clinicians who were willing to consider a less orthodox approach to pathogenesis of GI disease), it has been attacked by hordes of criticisms. Even very simple, apparently obvious connections between allergy and changes in behavior could fail to be confirmed by a rigid assessment [20] and this fact can be easily explained by the complexity of assessing behavior during different moments over the course of a disease that can either present in (1) controlled status, (2) crises, and (3) chronic, low level severity of symptoms, all leading to possibly diverse levels of influence over brain activity and behavior. Moreover, the argument of whether psychological disturbances are a consequence or cause of gastrointestinal disturbances has been challenging in human patients. The model for the association of emotion and allergy has to take into account the perceived concern triggered to the patient by the allergic reaction and the response formulated by their psychological status or makeup [24]. A basic point has always been the lack or historical or temporal perspective to the evolution of symptoms and escalating disease, particularly important for allergic diseases, since the initial condition and onset is rarely known. In human subjects it is not always easy to control for preexisting conditions, concurring factors, bias of a prior (referral) attending, lack of proposed mechanisms for psychoneuroimmune interactions underlying this phenomena, and so on. A general conclusion from several of these studies is that the relationship between food allergy and emotions is difficult to study from a clinical or epidemiological approach [25], and that the level of perceived distress (be it from allergic reactions or from emotional disturbances) is highly subjective and associated with educational level [26]. In some cases, the majority of self-reported cases of food allergy leading to emotional changes are false negatives (lack of diagnosed allergy), and rather reflects cognitive sensitization that, when triggered, is perceived and misinterpreted as food allergy [27, 28]. Since management of food allergy can per se be highly time consuming and stressful, it may also influence emotions on its own [29], having a psychosocial impact on the allergic individuals and their families [30]. This sort of situation clearly exemplifies the complexity of assessing neuroimmune interactions in allergy, and obviously claims for an experimental, multidisciplinary approach to diagnosis and treatment, since the history of coping with food allergy is key to cognitive development and emotional organization [31, 32]. Moreover, since food allergy obviously has a profound impact on quality of life (particularly in children) [33], a constant assessment of emotional distress and psychological support should be highly recommended [33].

Most of the issues with clinical studies, ranging from imprecision of terminology for diagnosis, through lack of consistency in methodology, to the influence of somatization or hypochondriasis, reinforced the need for an experimental approach based on animal models of disease [34]. All these variables and conclusions, heavily attacked by the skeptical, skating on thin ice, demanded the level of control and degree of confirmation made possible by experimental models of disease employing established animal systems.

Enter Experimental Neuroimmunomodulation

The experimental branch of psychoneuroimmunology opens the stage for setting controlled experiments in order to sort out conflicting and complicating factors from a very complex equation and shed light on robust evidence. As for many areas in biomedical sciences, hypothesis-driven experimental testing has long been used for the elucidation of causative phenomena. Moreover, this approach ultimately tests and sorts the determining influence of factors in a complex scenario rather than concurrent, confusing variables.

In this context, a major part of psychoneuroimmunology research over the past 40 years gathered effort describing the pathways used by the immune system and the central nervous system to communicate with and, especially relevant here, influence the functional outcome of each other. In our review, we will focus on the transmission of information from a peripheral immune response (peripheral here used as 'not inside the central nervous system') to the brain. The major signaling pathways thought to be relevant were reviewed elsewhere, and can be summarized as: (1) direct (hardwired) signaling through sensory nerves to the central nervous system, (2) immune signals signaling on peripheral nerves (such as cytokines, or more recently, immunoglobulin E [35, 36]), (3) circulating cytokines acting directly in the CNS (unlikely due to low crossing of the blood-brain barrier – BBB) or (4) through the circumventricular organs (CVOs – areas lacking the BBB, therefore prone to sensing circulating molecules), (5) induction of bridging molecules in the brain endothelium that can cross the BBB due to lipophilicity (such as the well-described mechanism of prostaglandin E_2 synthesis by brain endothelium upon stimulation by LPS or IL-1), (6) active transport of cytokines through the brain microvessels (unlikely since the saturation of such transporter does not appear to yield an effective concentration of the signal in brain tissue), and (7) combination of more than one mechanism (e.g. cytokines circulating through the blood reaching a CVO such as the area postrema, lying at the base of the fourth ventricle, on the brainstem, that can integrate and convey signals involved in autonomic, endocrine, and behavioral regulation). For a review, the reader is invited to consult the work of Wrona [37].

Analyzing the Behavior of Allergic Mice

Two-Bottle Preference Test: Allergic Mice Develop Food Aversion

Denise C. Cara and colleagues, working in Nelson Vaz's laboratory, have designed a very interesting experimental approach in an attempt to understand the importance of the immune system on a highly conserved behavior, namely food ingestion or diet selection. This experimental approach is based on a test hereafter referred to as the 'two-bottle preference test'. It consists of a choice between drinking from a bottle filled with tap water, or another one containing a sweetened solution of egg white in water. When facing this choice, nonimmunized mice would prefer drinking the sweetened solution, while ovalbumin (OVA)/alum-immunized animals would avoid the antigen-containing solution, drinking water instead [1]. It soon became clear that the immune system could drive a behavioral shift that leads to the avoidance of a potentially harmful molecule or context.

Since OVA/alum immunization leads to a Th_2-mediated immune response, we have employed this experimental model as a starting point to study behavioral changes in allergic animals. As seen in figure 1 (from Costa-Pinto et al. [38], with permission),

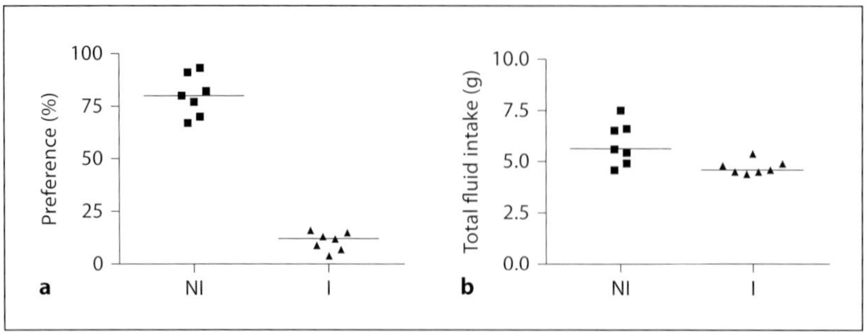

Fig. 1. Feeding behavior of allergic mice. Animals immunized with OVA or not were submitted to the two-bottle preference test, choosing between tap water and a sweetened OVA-containing solution. **a** While nonimmunized mice (NI) show a clear preference for the sweetened solution, immunized animals (I) avoid drinking the OVA-containing solution, preferring water instead. **b** Total fluid intake is not altered by prior OVA immunization. Individual values are shown as solid squares or triangles, and horizontal lines represent the medians; n = 7 per group; * $p < 0.05$; Mann-Whitney test. From Costa-Pinto et al. [38] – © 2006 New York Academy of Sciences.

we confirmed the original findings of Cara and colleagues showing that nonimmunized mice choose a 20% egg white solution in water, artificially sweetened with 0.5% saccharin, when exposed to the two-bottle preference test; OVA/alum-immunized mice drink water instead, avoiding the supposedly preferable allergen-containing solution (fig. 1a). No differences in total fluid intake were detected (fig. 1b). Allergic mice thus develop an aversion to the sweetened egg white solution, hereafter referred to as food aversion [39, 40].

In order to compare the behavior of mice challenged by the oral route (food allergy) or through the airways (asthma murine model), we adapted a passive avoidance test to analyze the behavior of allergic animals following exposure to airborne allergens. We built a transparent box consisting of two communicating compartments, one illuminated by a 60-watt bare bulb (making up one third of its total length), and another painted black (the remaining two-thirds), referred to as a light-dark box (LDB). We then replaced the classic avoidance stimulus (electric footshock) for nebulization with the allergen (OVA). Mice are placed on the training day in the lit side of the apparatus, and the delay for its first entry into the dark compartment is recorded (cutoff 5 min); the same animals are retested on the following day, without nebulization with OVA, and the delay for the first entry in the dark is recorded again (cutoff 1 min) [38, 41]. OVA/alum-immunized animals that had gone into the dark compartment and inhaled OVA on the training day avoided this compartment on the following day (test session, 24 h later). In contrast, nonimmunized mice continued to move quickly into that compartment on the following day [41].

Therefore, we were able to demonstrate that allergic mice display a shift in behavior capable of avoiding the source of the allergen that would trigger an immediate allergic reaction.

Oral Antigen Challenge Elicits Anxiety-Like Behavior in Allergic Mice

Avoidance of the antigen source, in both experimental models (challenge by the oral route or through the airways), imposes a conflict paradigm to the animals. For the two-bottle preference test, the conflict is to drink or not drink the preferable solution – due to its sweetness – that contains the antigen ultimately leading to the allergic reaction. Similarly, when placed in the light-dark box, the animals tend to prefer the dark compartment, which is exactly the one associated with the antigen source. In this setting, for allergic mice, the question is, obviously, to run or not to run into the dark compartment. Conflict and aversion are closely related to anxiety-like behavior, actually being the base of several tests utilized to experimentally evaluate anxiety and anxiolytic compounds in rodents [42]. This prompted us to ask whether or not OVA/alum-immunized mice challenged by the oral route with the allergen would display higher anxiety levels. To tackle this question, OVA/alum-immunized mice were challenged with an oral dose of OVA and observed 1 h later in an open field and, subsequently, in an elevated plus maze (EPM). The EPM is a validated behavioral model widely employed for the quantitative analysis of anxiety in mice [43]. Rodents naturally avoid open areas, and drugs or anxiogenic stimuli induce even shorter time of exploration of the open arms of this arena [43]. We found that oral OVA delivery to immunized mice induced a clear anxiogenic effect. Indeed, we observed that allergic mice challenged with the antigen spent less time exploring the open arms of the EPM than those that had received water, than nonimmunized mice receiving OVA solution, and also than naive mice [38, 40]. Furthermore, oral presentation of the antigen to immunized mice did not interfere with ambulation in the open field, which is important when interpreting data generated in the EPM.

Allergic Response Triggers Activation of Emotionality-Related Brain Areas

High levels of anxiety and development of food aversion are indicative of emotional or affective responses. We were then interested in determining which brain areas could be associated with these behavioral changes observed in our model of food allergy. We chose a relatively simple, albeit quite precise, method for assessing brain activity postmortem in rodents, i.e. the localization of Fos protein in neurons by immunohistochemistry. Fos is the product of an immediate early gene *(fos)* that plays an important role as transcription factor in many cell types, including neurons. Nuclei that had been activated over the last hour prior to euthanasia will appear dark brown after staining, allowing for the quantification of Fos-positive nuclei, directly associated with the activity of that particular brain area. We found that allergic mice had an increased c-*fos* expression mainly in the paraventricular nucleus of the hypothalamus (PVN) and in the central nucleus of the amygdala (CeA) [40]. In OVA/alum-immunized animals, we detected a high number of Fos-positive neurons 90 min after oral OVA challenge in both areas (PVN and CeA). In contrast, Fos-positive neurons were virtually absent in OVA/alum-immunized animals that received water, in nonimmunized mice that received OVA, and also in naive animals [40]. It is important to mention that we reported a very similar pattern of brain area activation when allergic mice were challenged through the airways [41]. Interestingly, these brain areas are known to be linked with emotional- and affective-related behavioral patterns. Both the PVN and the CeA are among the main areas of the CNS containing corticotropin-releasing factor (CRF)-expressing neurons. CRF is considered one of the major regulators of adaptive stress responses [44–46]. It has been shown that socially defeated rats placed on the EPM spent less time exploring the open arms and that this response was reversed by a CRF antagonist (α-helical CRF_{9-41}) injected bilaterally into the CeA [47]. Likewise, studies in which the CRF neurons of the CeA and PVN were immunotargeted and eliminated provide clear evidence for their relevance in the expression of emotionality-related behavior in stressed rats exposed to the EPM [48]. Activation of the CeA and PVN has also been detected in animals submitted to a model of conditioned taste aversion. In this model, intraperitoneal injection of lithium chloride, which is used as an unconditioned stimulus, paired with saccharin (the conditioned stimulus) causes an increased expression of c-*fos* in the CeA [49] and the PVN [50]. The importance of CeA activation in this particular experimental setting was established when microinjection of oligonucleotide antisense to c-*fos* into this area resulted in a deficient acquisition of conditioned taste aversion [51]. It is also important to mention that other immunological stimuli were also reported as capable of inducing activation of the PVN and the CeA. For instance, stimulation of T lymphocytes with staphylococcal enterotoxin B results in an increase in CRF mRNA transcripts in these areas (PVN and CeA) [52], c-*fos* expression in the PVN [53], and the expression of emotionality-related behavioral patterns [52]. Early immune events elicited by peripheral immunization with the T cell-dependent antigen Keyhole limpet hemocyanin have also been shown to induce increased c-*fos* expression in the PVN and CeA [54]. We conclude that the activation of the specific brain areas observed following an allergic reaction is compatible with the behavioral pattern displayed by allergic mice, which includes avoidance and anxiety.

We finally asked whether increased Fos expression in the PVN and the CeA in allergic mice would result in activation of the hypothalamus-pituitary-adrenal (HPA) axis, which is a well-known endocrine response occurring during stress and emotional-related behaviors. We measured corticosterone secretion following OVA challenge in allergic mice and found that animals previously immunized with OVA/alum presented higher levels of serum corticosterone than naive animals, nonimmunized mice receiving OVA by gavage, or immunized animals given water [38]. Another piece of data corroborating HPA activation in allergic animals came from experiments in which we performed in situ hybridization double labeling with Fos immunohistochemistry. As seen in figure 2, we found that Fos-positive nuclei in the PVN and CeA of allergic animals challenged orally with the antigen also express transcripts for CRF.

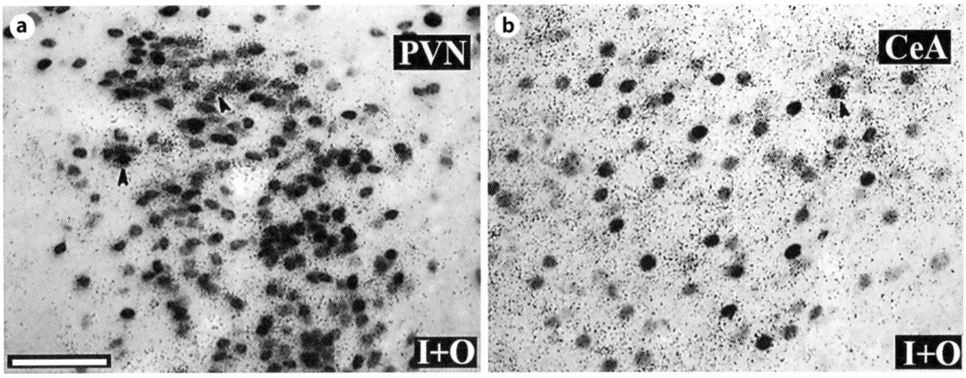

Fig. 2. Neurons in the paraventricular nucleus of the hypothalamus (**a**) and central nucleus of the amygdala (**b**) activated during food allergy display mRNA for CRF. Coronal sections of brains harvested after 90 min of ovalbumin ingestion by allergic mice (I+O) show colocalization of Fos protein (dark nuclei, around 10 micrometers in diameter) and fine, silver granules resulting from ISH for CRF mRNA. Scale bar = 50 μm.

Signaling Allergy to the Mouse Brain

Role of Antibodies and Mast Cells

As already mentioned, OVA/alum immunization leads to a Th2 (T helper type 2)-driven immune response, characterized by increased secretion of type 2 cytokines, mainly IL-4, IL-5 and IL-13. Upon challenge with the antigen, the allergic response develops into two distinct but related phases. Many of the early consequences of the first phase, named immediate phase of the allergic reaction, are triggered by mast cell contents released following cross-linking of anaphylactic antibodies bound to their high-affinity receptors expressed in the membranes of these cells. The other one is the late phase of allergic reactions that usually leads to an inflammatory milieu in which CD4+ T lymphocytes, eosinophils and type 2 cytokines play an important role. Since behavioral changes and CNS activity were mostly observed shortly after oral allergen challenge in OVA/alum immunized animals, it seemed logical to us investigating the potential role played by anaphylactic antibodies in food allergy-induced brain activation and aversion.

The role of anaphylactic antibodies (IgE and IgG1 in mice) was assessed by means of two different approaches. We used an anti-IgE antibody to completely deplete IgE in mice previously immunized with OVA and, alternatively, we precluded its production using a protocol of immunological tolerance. Immunological tolerance is accomplished by offering a solution of OVA in tap water prior to, or along with, the primary OVA immunization. The main difference between each protocol is that animals receiving oral OVA from days –7 to –2 (prior to OVA immunization) would not produce either class of antibody, while mice offered oral OVA from days 0 to +5 would generate anti-OVA IgG1, but not IgE. We found that removal of IgE, either by anti-IgE treatment or oral tolerance, was effective in preventing the development of food aversion (measured in the two-bottle preference test) [38, 40], and avoidance of the dark compartment previously associated with OVA nebulization (light-dark box) [38, 41]. Activation of the PVN and the CeA was also prevented when anti-OVA IgE was inhibited, strongly suggesting that signaling allergy to the brain uses an IgE-dependent mechanism [38, 40, 41]. Since treatment with anti-IgE antibody, or the development of oral tolerance that only precludes IgE, totally prevented the increase in Fos staining following allergic reactions, and the establishment of avoidance responses, we assumed that these phenomena are IgE mediated, and IgG1 independent. More recent data from the group led by Cara corroborate the importance of antigen-specific IgE on the development of food aversion in allergic mice. They reported that IL-4-deficient mice produce very low titers of antigen-specific IgE upon OVA/alum immunization and this was associated with failure in developing aversion to the solution containing the allergen. Passive transference of serum from allergic wild-type mice to IL-4-deficient recipients restored development of food aversion in these animals [55].

It follows that IgE-induced mast cell degranulation is likely to be the major mechanism for food allergy signaling to the brain. Since mast cells are distributed along blood vessels of the intestinal mucosa in intimate contact with substance P-positive nerve fibers (C-type fibers) [56, 57], we hypothesized that mediators released by mast cell degranulation could stimulate the nerve endings of the C-fibers that, in turn, would transmit the sensory information to the CNS. Indeed, it has already been demonstrated that when in coculture, neurons can depolarize following mast cell activation with anaphylactic anti-IgE antibody or compound 48/80 [58]. Despite the fact that the literature is full of good reasons to believe that mast cells play an important role signaling food allergy to the brain, we do not have any direct experimental evidence supporting this idea. However, we did perform studies addressing the participation of mast cells signaling allergy to the CNS in the murine model of asthma. In this series of experiments, we aimed at the pharmacological inhibition of mast cell degranulation using dissodium cromoglycate (cromolyn), a mast cell membrane stabilizer commonly used in humans to prevent allergic reactions in the airways. Mice in this model of experimental allergic asthma were treated with cromolyn prior to OVA challenge and used for the evaluation of PVN and CeA activity. Inhibition of mast cell degranulation by cromolyn totally precluded the increase in neuronal activity assessed in these two areas, as measured by Fos expression [59]. Moreover, OVA/alum-immunized mice treated with cromolyn no longer developed the aversion to the dark compartment previously associated with OVA nebulization [59]. Altogether, our data support the notion that allergy-induced changes on behavior and brain activity are dependent on IgE and mast cells.

An alternate mechanism that would exclude the participation of mast cells in signaling allergy to the CNS was recently brought up by interesting findings describing the expression of fully functional high-affinity Fc-receptors (FcεRI) for IgE in neurons. The group led by John Bienenstock has found that mouse neurons from the superior cervical ganglion (SCG) do express the tetrameric form of the high-affinity IgE receptor and that in neurons sensitized with dinitrophenylated (DNP)-specific IgE, in vitro challenge with the antigen, but not with an unrelated protein, led to a rapid rise in intracellular Ca^{2+} levels [35]. They also showed that Ca^{2+} signals elicited by FcεRI stimulation could be transferred to interconnected neuritis [35]. Some of their findings were also described for neurons from the myenteric plexus within the gut [35]. This clearly raises the possibility that in the gut, an allergic reaction can signal to the brain in a mast cell-independent manner. In spite of these results, experimental data confirming this hypothesis is yet to be gathered.

Another question puzzling us refers to the nature of the stimulus leading to behavioral changes and brain activity following food allergy. Mast cells release a myriad of mediators upon activation and degranulation due to antigen-induced crosslinking of IgE molecules bound to high-affinity receptors present in the membrane of these cells. Some of them, such as serotonin and histamine, signaling through H_1 and 5-HT_2 receptors, respectively, are known to play a key role in the edema formation during the immediate phase of allergic responses. Indeed, increased vascular permeability and edema were observed in allergic mice after oral challenge with the antigen [60]. However, treatment with antagonists of serotoninergic and histaminergic receptors, albeit blocking edema formation, did not preclude the development of food aversion in allergic mice [60] or rats [61]. These results suggest that avoidance of the diet containing the allergen is not directly related to the edema present during immediate allergic responses. In contrast, treatment with an antagonist of 5-HT_3 receptors, despite not completely impeding food aversion, was able to diminish its magnitude to a certain extent [61]. Interestingly, 5-HT_3 receptor signaling is not involved in mast cell-induced edema formation but rather might be involved in transmitting sensory information to the CNS following anaphylactic responses. Thus, it has already been demonstrated that vagal afferents present in the gut mucosa do express 5-HT_3 receptors [62, 63], and evidence has been provided that they are activated following antigen-induced mast cell degranulation [64, 65]. The potential role of other mast cell-released mediators – and their receptors – in food allergy-induced behavioral changes and brain activity are still to be determined.

Neural Pathways Involved in Food Allergy Signaling to the Mouse Brain: Role of Type C-Sensitive Fibers

We were also interested in studying how sensory information following an allergic reaction in the gut would be conveyed to the already mentioned emotionality-related brain areas. For that purpose, we adopted the same strategy of looking at Fos expression in brain areas known to receive afferents from the periphery. We found that food allergy, besides leading to activation of the PVN and the CeA, also induces Fos expression in the nucleus of tractus solitarii (NTS) [66]. This is not surprising, as this nucleus receives visceral sensory inputs from both spinal and vagal afferents

[67, 68]. Cell bodies of vagal and spinal primary afferents conveying visceral sensory information are located within the nodose and the dorsal root ganglia, respectively. Central projections from the nodose ganglion directly reach the NTS, whereas the fibers from the dorsal root ganglion enter the dorsal horn of the spinal cord and make synaptic connections with second-order neurons which, in turn, project to the NTS (spinosolitary tract) [69]. This makes the NTS an important relay station integrating sensory information and underlying viscero-visceral reflexes. In particular, concomitant activation of the NTS and motor alterations in the GI tract have been described after antigen challenge of an isolated intestinal segment in OVA-sensitized rats [70, 71]. Some of these studies raised the possibility of a role for the CNS in intestinal motor response while demonstrating that extrinsic neural pathways are required for full manifestation of anaphylaxis-induced alterations in GI motility and NTS activation [70]. Anatomical data showing that the efferent ascending targets of the NTS include the PVN and the CeA [72, 73] corroborates our previous experimental findings reporting the activation of the PVN and the CeA.

Once we had a more complete picture regarding the specific pattern of brain activation following food allergy, our further step was to investigate the possible afferent pathways conveying this sensory information to the NTS. Although several studies have investigated the routes involved in NTS activation following intestinal anaphylaxis, this issue is still controversial. Some authors have suggested that vagal afferent pathways are essential for brain stem activation and intestinal motor response following IgE-mediated mast cell degranulation. In fact, Castex et al. [64] reported that perivagal capsaicin treatment eliminated both Fos expression in the NTS and the alteration in fasting motility observed in OVA-sensitized rats challenged with the antigen. However, others have not confirmed these findings. Indeed, it has been shown that subdiaphragmatic vagotomy not only failed to block anaphylaxis-induced disturbances in intestinal motility but also did not modify the degree of Fos immunoreactivity in the NTS [70]. The latter investigators argued that intestinal allergic response signaling to the brain stem occurs through the spinal pathways. They have demonstrated that splanchnectomy abolished changes in jejunal motor responses and diminished the number of Fos-positive nuclei in the NTS of sensitized animals challenged with the antigen [71].

Our experimental approach did not allow any further analysis regarding the participation of spinal or vagal afferent fibers in the pattern of brain activation we have described. Employing neonatal capsaicin treatment, we evaluated the role of unmyelinated primary afferent C-fibers on food allergy signaling to the mouse brain. As already mentioned, within the mucosa of the gastrointestinal tract, mast cells and C-sensitive fibers are closely related. Capsaicin is a widely used neurotoxin known to promote a deficit in sensory modalities subserved by these fibers [74]. It is important to mention that capsaicin treatment per se did not alter antibody production, or preference for the sweetened solution in allergic mice [39]. We showed that while neonatal capsaicin only diminished the number of Fos-positive nuclei in the NTS, it completely blocked c-*fos* expression in the PVN of OVA-sensitized mice challenged orally with the antigen [66]. Thus, although there are extensive projections from the NTS to the PVN [73], it is unlikely that this pathway accounts for complete food allergy-induced PVN activation. Some studies have described that a large number of neurons in the spinal cord of rats project directly to the hypothalamus [75, 76]. Since it has been shown that this spinohypothalamic tract conveys visceral sensory information [77, 78], this could be an alternative route for food allergy signaling to the PVN. Whether the fibers composing the spinohypothalamic tract are more susceptible to the neonatal capsaicin treatment remains to be elucidated.

We also found that capsaicin treatment did not modify the degree of Fos immunoreactivity in the CeA. This could indicate that food allergy signaling to the PVN and to the CeA occurs through different pathways. Since the amygdala also receives afferent inputs from the NTS [73], this route could be involved in at least part of food allergy-induced c-*fos* expression in the CeA, even considering the lower activation seen in the NTS of capsaicin-treated animals. Despite the fact that neonatal capsaicin has been shown to destroy only 30% of the number of vagal neurons in the nodose ganglia [79] and 41–75% of unmyelinated fibers in spinal cord roots [80], these results led us to suggest that additional mechanisms, apart from the capsaicin-sensitive C-fibers, are likely to be involved in food allergy signaling to specific brain areas. This suggestion is in accordance with another piece of data we have gathered showing that, albeit diminishing the magnitude of food aversion in allergic mice, capsaicin treatment was not able to completely block its development [39]. Other studies have demonstrated that transmission of certain visceral sensory information is only partially dependent on capsaicin-sensitive C-fibers. Thus, colon distension-induced c-*fos* expression in the NTS was not completely abolished after neonatal capsaicin treatment in rats [81]. Similarly, while systemic capsaicin reduced the number of Fos-positive cells by 50% in the PVN 1 h after abdominal surgery, it did not modify Fos staining in the NTS and in the CeA [82].

In conclusion, these experimental studies provided evidence showing that unmyelinated type C-sensitive fibers are part of the neural pathways involved in food allergy-induced activation of specific brain areas, specially the PVN and to a lesser extent the NTS.

Current Approaches and Future Perspectives

There has been increasing interest in the assessment of behavioral and emotional changes associated with the onset of food allergy. From an experimental perspective, the existence and constituency of microbiota plays a major role during development of the immune system, as well as both of the enteric nervous system and central nervous system. Recently, the role of microbiota, not only on gut immunity but also on systemic disease, has gained strong support. Monocolonization of the gut with specific classes of bacteria predisposes to an array of medical conditions not restricted to the gastrointestinal tract (such as heart disease). On the other hand, motor activity, learning and anxiety have also been associated to microbiota in mouse models. The gastrointestinal tract represents the largest surface of the body exposed to the environment and deals with trillions of bacteria (mostly harmless, commensal individuals) but also several grams a day of dietary proteins. In order to accomplish the amazing task of avoiding unnecessary inflammatory reactions, yet retaining the capability of mounting immune responses and clearing pathogens, the intestine is endowed with the highest concentration of lymphoid cells in the body. Additionally, there are more neurons in the enteric nervous system than in the spinal cord, making it the largest collection of nerves outside the brain. These facts combined should support the existence of an intricate network of neuroimmune relationships in the gut. We are only beginning to understand the relevance of this crosstalk for health and disease.

References

1 Cara DC, Conde AA, Vaz NM: Immunological induction of flavor aversion in mice. Braz J Med Biol Res 1994;27:1331–1341.

2 Cohen SG, Saavedra-Delgado AM: Through the centuries with food and drink, for better or worse. Allergy Proc 1989;10:281–290.

3 Cohen SG, Saavedra-Delgado AM: Through the centuries with food and drink, for better or worse. Part II. Allergy Proc 1989;10:363–373.

4 Fand R, Hubbard RC: Acute anxiety reaction secondary to food allergy. Conn Med 1976;40:188–189.

5 Addolorato G, Marsigli L, Capristo E, Caputo F, Dall'Aglio C, Baudanza P: Anxiety and depression: a common feature of health care seeking patients with irritable bowel syndrome and food allergy. Hepatogastroenterology 1998;45:1559–1564.

6 Rix KJ, Ditchfield J, Freed DL, Goldberg DP, Hillier VF: Food antibodies in acute psychoses. Psychol Med 1985;15:347–354.

7 Lucarelli S, Frediani T, Zingoni AM, et al: Food allergy and infantile autism. Panminerva Med 1995;37:137–141.

8 Glaisher IL: Letter: allergy and psychosis. Can Med Assoc J 1974;111:1048.

9 Fields M, Fields P: The relationship between problem behavior and food allergies: one family's story. J Autism Child Schizophr 1976;6:75–91.

10 Rix KJ, Pearson DJ, Bentley SJ: A psychiatric study of patients with supposed food allergy. Br J Psychiatry 1984;145:121–126.

11 Seggev JS, Eckert RC: Psychopathology masquerading as food allergy. J Fam Pract 1988;26:161–164.

12 Stevenson DD, Dalessio DJ: Food allergies and migraine. Lancet 1979;ii:103.

13 Vatn MH: Food intolerance and psychosomatic experience. Scand J Work Environ Health 1997;23(suppl 3):75–78.

14 Halliday JL: Rising incidence of psychosomatic illness. Br Med J 1938;ii:11–14.

15 Pearson DJ, Rix KJ, Bentley SJ: Food allergy: how much in the mind? A clinical and psychiatric study of suspected food hypersensitivity. Lancet 1983;i:1259–1261.

16 Pearson DJ: Psychologic and somatic interrelationships in allergy and pseudoallergy. J Allergy Clin Immunol 1988;81:351–360.

17 Peveler R, Mayou R, Young E, Stoneham M: Psychiatric aspects of food-related physical symptoms: a community study. J Psychosom Res 1996;41:149–159.

18 Pearson DJ: Pseudo food allergy. Br Med J 1986;292:221–222.

19 Lillestol K, Berstad A, Lind R, Florvaag E, Arslan Lied G, Tangen T: Anxiety and depression in patients with self-reported food hypersensitivity. Gen Hosp Psychiatry 2010;32:42–48.

20 Lind R, Lied GA, Lillestol K, Valeur J, Berstad A: Do psychological factors predict symptom severity in patients with subjective food hypersensitivity? Scand J Gastroenterol 2010;45:835–843.

21 Gettis A: Food sensitivities and psychological disturbance: a review. Nutr Health 1989;6:135–146.

22 Price CE, Rona RJ, Chinn S: Associations of excessive irritability with common illnesses and food intolerance. Paediatr Perinat Epidemiol 1990;4:156–160.
23 Smith RS: The immune system is a key factor in the etiology of psychosocial disease. Med Hypotheses 1991;34:49–57.
24 Mandell M, Rose GJ: May emotional reactions be precipitated by allergens? Conn Med 1968;32:300–302.
25 Kelsay K: Psychological aspects of food allergy. Curr Allergy Asthma Rep 2003;3:41–46.
26 Lyons AC, Forde EM: Food allergy in young adults: perceptions and psychological effects. J Health Psychol 2004;9:497–504.
27 Berstad A, Arslan G, Lind R, Florvaag E: Food hypersensitivity-immunologic (peripheral) or cognitive (central) sensitisation? Psychoneuroendocrinology 2005;30:983–989.
28 Teufel M, Biedermann T, Rapps N, Hausteiner C, Henningsen P, Enck P, et al: Psychological burden of food allergy. World J Gastroenterol 2007;13:3456–3465.
29 Jones SM, Scurlock AM: The impact of food allergy: the real 'fear factor'. Ann Allergy Asthma Immunol 2006;96:385–386.
30 Akeson N, Worth A, Sheikh A: The psychosocial impact of anaphylaxis on young people and their parents. Clin Exp Allergy 2007;37:1213–1220.
31 Dunn GA, Gaffney A, Hourihane JO: Developmental pathways in food allergy: a new theoretical framework. Allergy 2009;64:560–568.
32 Lebovidge JS, Strauch H, Kalish LA, Schneider LC: Assessment of psychological distress among children and adolescents with food allergy. J Allergy Clin Immunol 2009;124:1282–1288.
33 Cummings AJ, Knibb RC, King RM, Lucas JS: The psychosocial impact of food allergy and food hypersensitivity in children, adolescents and their families: a review. Allergy 2010;65:933–945.
34 Crayton JW: Adverse reactions to foods: relevance to psychiatric disorders. J Allergy Clin Immunol 1986;78:243–250.
35 van der Kleij H, Charles N, Karimi K, Mao YK, Foster J, Janssen L, et al: Evidence for neuronal expression of functional Fc (epsilon and gamma) receptors. J Allergy Clin Immunol 2010;125:757–760.
36 Liang H, Xu L, Zhou C, Zhang Y, Xu M, Zhang C: Vagal activities are involved in antigen-specific immune inflammation in the intestine. J Gastroenterol Hepatol 2011;26:1065–1071.
37 Wrona D: Neural-immune interactions: an integrative view of the bidirectional relationship between the brain and immune systems. J Neuroimmunol 2006;172:38–58.
38 Costa-Pinto FA, Basso AS, De Sa-Rocha LC, Britto LR, Russo M, Palermo-Neto J: Neural correlates of IgE-mediated allergy. Ann NY Acad Sci 2006;1088:116–131.
39 Basso AS, de Sa-Rocha LC, Palermo-Neto J: Immune-induced flavor aversion in mice: modification by neonatal capsaicin treatment. Neuroimmunomodulation 2001;9:88–94.
40 Basso AS, Pinto FA, Russo M, Britto LR, de Sa-Rocha LC, Palermo Neto J: Neural correlates of IgE-mediated food allergy. J Neuroimmunol 2003;140:69–77.
41 Costa-Pinto FA, Basso AS, Britto LR, Malucelli BE, Russo M: Avoidance behavior and neural correlates of allergen exposure in a murine model of asthma. Brain Behav Immun 2005;19:52–60.
42 Bailey KR, Crawley JN: Anxiety-related behaviors in mice; in Buccafusco JJ (ed.): Methods of Behavior Analysis in Neuroscience. Boca Raton, CRC Press, 2009.
43 Lister RG: The use of a plus-maze to measure anxiety in the mouse. Psychopharmacology (Berl) 1987;92:180–185.
44 Gray TS: Amygdaloid CRF pathways. Role in autonomic, neuroendocrine, and behavioral responses to stress. Ann NY Acad Sci 1993;697:53–60.
45 Gray TS, Bingaman EW: The amygdala: corticotropin-releasing factor, steroids, and stress. Crit Rev Neurobiol 1996;10:155–168.
46 Swanson LW, Sawchenko PE, Rivier J, Vale WW: Organization of ovine corticotropin-releasing factor immunoreactive cells and fibers in the rat brain: an immunohistochemical study. Neuroendocrinology 1983;36:165–186.
47 Heinrichs SC, Pich EM, Miczek KA, Britton KT, Koob GF: Corticotropin-releasing factor antagonist reduces emotionality in socially defeated rats via direct neurotropic action. Brain Res 1992;581:190–197.
48 Menzaghi F, Heinrichs SC, Pich EM, Weiss F, Koob GF: The role of limbic and hypothalamic corticotropin-releasing factor in behavioral responses to stress. Ann NY Acad Sci 1993;697:142–154.
49 Yamamoto T, Sako N, Sakai N, Iwafune A: Gustatory and visceral inputs to the amygdala of the rat: conditioned taste aversion and induction of c-fos-like immunoreactivity. Neurosci Lett 1997;226:127–130.
50 Lamprecht R, Dudai Y: Differential modulation of brain immediate early genes by intraperitoneal LiCl. Neuroreport 1995;7:289–293.

51 Lamprecht R, Dudai Y: Transient expression of c-Fos in rat amygdala during training is required for encoding conditioned taste aversion memory. Learn Mem 1996;3:31–41.
52 Kusnecov AW, Liang R, Shurin G: T-lymphocyte activation increases hypothalamic and amygdaloid expression of CRH mRNA and emotional reactivity to novelty. J Neurosci 1999;19:4533–4543.
53 Goehler LE, Gaykema RP, Hansen MK, Kleiner JL, Maier SF, Watkins LR: Staphylococcal enterotoxin B induces fever, brain c-Fos expression, and serum corticosterone in rats. Am J Physiol Regul Integr Comp Physiol 2001;280:R1434–R1439.
54 Pacheco-Lopez G, Espinosa E, Zamorano-Rojas HM, Ramirez-Amaya V, Bermudez-Rattoni F: Peripheral protein immunization induces rapid activation of the CNS, as measured by c-Fos expression. J Neuroimmunol 2002;131:50–59.
55 Dourado LP, Saldanha JC, Gargiulo DL, et al: Role of IL-4 in aversion induced by food allergy in mice. Cell Immunol 2010;262:62–68.
56 Stead RH, Dixon MF, Bramwell NH, Riddell RH, Bienenstock J: Mast cells are closely apposed to nerves in the human gastrointestinal mucosa. Gastroenterology 1989;97:575–585.
57 Stead RH, Tomioka M, Quinonez G, Simon GT, Felten SY, Bienenstock J: Intestinal mucosal mast cells in normal and nematode-infected rat intestines are in intimate contact with peptidergic nerves. Proc Natl Acad Sci USA 1987;84:2975–2979.
58 Janiszewski J, Bienenstock J, Blennerhassett MG: Activation of rat peritoneal mast cells in coculture with sympathetic neurons alters neuronal physiology. Brain Behav Immun 1990;4:139–150.
59 Costa-Pinto FA, Basso AS, Russo M: Role of mast cell degranulation in the neural correlates of the immediate allergic reaction in a murine model of asthma. Brain Behav Immun 2007;21:783–790.
60 Cara DC, Conde AA, Vaz NM: Immunological induction of flavour aversion in mice. II. Passive/adoptive transfer and pharmacological inhibition. Scand J Immunol 1997;45:16–20.
61 Zarzana EC, Basso AS, Costa-Pinto FA, Palermo-Neto J: Pharmacological manipulation of immune-induced food aversion in rats. Neuroimmunomodulation 2009;16:19–27.
62 Castex N, Fioramonti J, Fargeas MJ, More J, Bueno L: Role of 5-HT3 receptors and afferent fibers in the effects of mast cell degranulation on colonic motility in rats. Gastroenterology 1994;107:976–984.
63 Gershon MD: 5-HT (serotonin) physiology and related drugs. Curr Opin Gastroenterol 2000;16:113–120.
64 Castex N, Fioramonti J, Fargeas MJ, Bueno L: c-fos expression in specific rat brain nuclei after intestinal anaphylaxis: involvement of 5-HT3 receptors and vagal afferent fibers. Brain Res 1995;688:149–160.
65 Kreis ME, Muller M, Zittel TT, Glatzle J, Grundy D: Mediators of neuronal activation in the rat brainstem following intestinal anaphylaxis. Neurosci Lett 2000;289:45–48.
66 Basso AS, Costa-Pinto FA, Britto LR, de Sa-Rocha LC, Palermo-Neto J: Neural pathways involved in food allergy signaling in the mouse brain: role of capsaicin-sensitive afferents. Brain Res 2004;1009:181–188.
67 Altschuler SM, Bao XM, Bieger D, Hopkins DA, Miselis RR: Viscerotopic representation of the upper alimentary tract in the rat: sensory ganglia and nuclei of the solitary and spinal trigeminal tracts. J Comp Neurol 1989;283:248–268.
68 Menetrey D, Basbaum AI: Spinal and trigeminal projections to the nucleus of the solitary tract: a possible substrate for somatovisceral and viscerovisceral reflex activation. J Comp Neurol 1987;255:439–450.
69 Grundy D: Neuroanatomy of visceral nociception: vagal and splanchnic afferent. Gut 2002;51(suppl 1):i2–i5.
70 Scott RB, Tan DT, Miampamba M, Sharkey KA: Anaphylaxis-induced alterations in intestinal motility: role of extrinsic neural pathways. Am J Physiol 1998;275:G812–G821.
71 Scott RB, Tan DT, Sharkey KA: Effect of splanchnectomy on jejunal motility and fos expression in brain stem after intestinal anaphylaxis in rat. Am J Physiol Gastrointest Liver Physiol 2000;279:G990–G997.
72 Cechetto DF: Central representation of visceral function. Fed Proc 1987;46:17–23.
73 Petrov T, Krukoff TL, Jhamandas JH: Branching projections of catecholaminergic brainstem neurons to the paraventricular hypothalamic nucleus and the central nucleus of the amygdala in the rat. Brain Res 1993;609:81–92.
74 Holzer P: Capsaicin: cellular targets, mechanisms of action, and selectivity for thin sensory neurons. Pharmacol Rev 1991;43:143–201.
75 Burstein R, Cliffer KD, Giesler GJ Jr: Cells of origin of the spinohypothalamic tract in the rat. J Comp Neurol 1990;291:329–344.
76 Cliffer KD, Burstein R, Giesler GJ Jr: Distributions of spinothalamic, spinohypothalamic, and spinotelencephalic fibers revealed by anterograde transport of PHA-L in rats. J Neurosci 1991;11:852–868.

77 Katter JT, Dado RJ, Kostarczyk E, Giesler GJ Jr: Spinothalamic and spinohypothalamic tract neurons in the sacral spinal cord of rats. II. Responses to cutaneous and visceral stimuli. J Neurophysiol 1996;75:2606–2628.
78 Zhang X, Gokin AP, Giesler GJ Jr: Responses of spinohypothalamic tract neurons in the thoracic spinal cord of rats to somatic stimuli and to graded distention of the bile duct. Somatosens Mot Res 2002;19:5–17.
79 Carobi C: A quantitative investigation of the effects of neonatal capsaicin treatment on vagal afferent neurons in the rat. Cell Tissue Res 1996;283:305–311.
80 Hiura A, Sakamoto Y: Quantitative estimation of the effects of capsaicin on the mouse primary sensory neurons. Neurosci Lett 1987;76:101–106.
81 Monnikes H, Ruter J, Konig M, et al: Differential induction of c-fos expression in brain nuclei by noxious and non-noxious colonic distension: role of afferent C-fibers and 5-HT3 receptors. Brain Res 2003;966:253–264.
82 Bonaz B, Tache Y: Corticotropin-releasing factor and systemic capsaicin-sensitive afferents are involved in abdominal surgery-induced Fos expression in the paraventricular nucleus of the hypothalamus. Brain Res 1997;748:12–20.

Dr. Frederico Azevedo Costa-Pinto
Department of Pathology, School of Veterinary Medicine, University of Sao Paulo
Av Prof Dr Orlando Marques de Paiva, 87, Cidade Universitaria
Sao Paulo, SP 05508–270 (Brazil)
Tel. +55 11 30911373, E-Mail fpinto@usp.br

Co-corresponding author: Dr. Alexandre Salgado Basso
Department of Microbiology, Immunology and Parasitology
Paulista Medical School, UNIFESP
Rua Botucatu, 862. Ed. Ciencias Biomedicas, 4 andar
Sao Paulo, SP 04023–062 (Brazil)
Tel. +55 11 55723328 ext. 29, E-Mail asbasso@unifesp.br

Bienenstock J (ed): Allergy and the Nervous System.
Chem Immunol Allergy. Basel, Karger, 2012, vol 98, pp 240–252

The Neuroendocrine-Immune Connection Regulates Chronic Inflammatory Disease in Allergy

Eva M.J. Peters

University-Medicine Charité, CharitéCenter 12 (CC12) for Internal Medicine and Dermatology, Department of Psychosomatic Medicine, Berlin, and Justus Liebig University, Department of Psychosomatic Medicine, Giessen, Germany

Abstract

Allergy is an instructive model to study neuroendocrine-immune interaction in chronic inflammation, a key research task taken on by a relatively new scientific field: psychoneuroimmunology (PNI). Itch, as the prime symptom of many chronic inflammatory diseases but especially of allergic inflammation, hints at the prominent role of neurogenic inflammation in the course of the disease. Environmental factors ranging from allergens to perceived stress can trigger the release of neuropeptides from peripheral nerve endings that than activate mast cells and induce an exaggerated alarm response in peripheral organs such as the skin. Beyond this innate immune response, neuroendocrine-immune interaction regulates specific immune balance. Depending on intensity and timing of neuroendocrine activation, especially neuropeptides and neurotrophins either enhance or suppress tissue regeneration and inflammation, the conditions of which will be discussed in detail here. Allergic inflammation thus serves to understand the clinical and therapeutic implications of neuroendocrine-immune interaction in chronic inflammatory disease and its implications for future treatment strategies.

In the 18 hundreds the term 'neurodermitis' [1] was coined to describe what we now rather label as allergic dermatitis or atopic eczema. This historical name implicated what clinicians observed: that there might be a close connection between nerves and skin and that this interaction may be intimately involved in the cause and progression of chronic inflammation and its sensitivity to environmental as well as emotional strain. Since then continuous advances in the methodology allow us not only to locate and differentiate distinct nerve fiber subsets in peripheral tissues and identify specific mediators within, but also to investigate their interaction with the local immune system [2–5]. Moreover, animal experimental set-ups and broad availability of laboratory support enable researchers today to regularly target the neuroendocrine-immune circuitry in the investigation of novel treatment options for allergic inflammation [6].

From this point in science we have a sound understanding of the 'neuro' in '-dermitis' and are able to appreciate the prominent impact of a neurotrophin/neuroepeptide stress response axis (NNA) complementing the classical stress response pathways along the hypothalamus pituitary adrenal axis (HPA) or the sympathetic axis (SA) not only centrally but also peripherally [7]. Together and regulating each other, these three axes conduct a multi-layered neuroendocrine concert in organs at the self-environment border, which controls inflammation in response to diverse challenges. Presently, the insights into the complexity of neuroendocrine-immune interactions are still marginalized in standard recommendations for allergic diseases (e.g. [8, 9]). While more and more data accumulate that proof their potent impact on the clinical course and progression of allergic inflammation, this integrative perspective will increasingly gain appreciation.

Neuroanatomy of the Skin: A Key to Understand Neuroendocrine-Immune Interactions in Peripheral Tissues

To understand the role of neuroendocrine-immune interactions in the skin and in allergy, it is important to get an idea of the neuroanatomy of the skin (fig. 1) [10, 11]. The skin is equipped with an abundant supply of mixed nerve fibers containing autonomic as well as sensory nerve fibers that get into contact with virtually all functional skin cell populations. Nerve fibers in the epidermis, dermis and subcutis are never farther away than a few cells from any keratinocyte, fibroblast, endothelial cell or Schwann cell, to name only some of the most frequent structural cell types involved in and co-directing inflammation, and they maintain close direct contacts with immunocytes residing in and invading peripheral tissues [5, 6]. One could say, the skin is hardwired with a complex neuronal alarm system ready to respond to any environmental challenge and that without it, challenges such as allergens do not become recognized (e.g. [12, 13]).

Before we became higher organized organisms, we started out as single cell entities. Most neuroendocrine mediators such as neurotrophins are highly conserved and already present in protozoa, which use them to produce a tolerant immune bias in their hosts [14]. It is thus not surprising that apart from the neuroendocrine-immune circuitry there is also in loco production of neuroendocrine mediators. To make things even more complex, for many of the mediators in question, low and high doses, single versus frequent exposure, or presence versus absence of adjuvants often appear to exert opposite effects, some of which will be discussed in detail below (fig. 1). Neuroendocrine-immune regulation of peripheral inflammatory events is thus not simply 'pro-inflammatory' but requires close scrutiny of a specific setting.

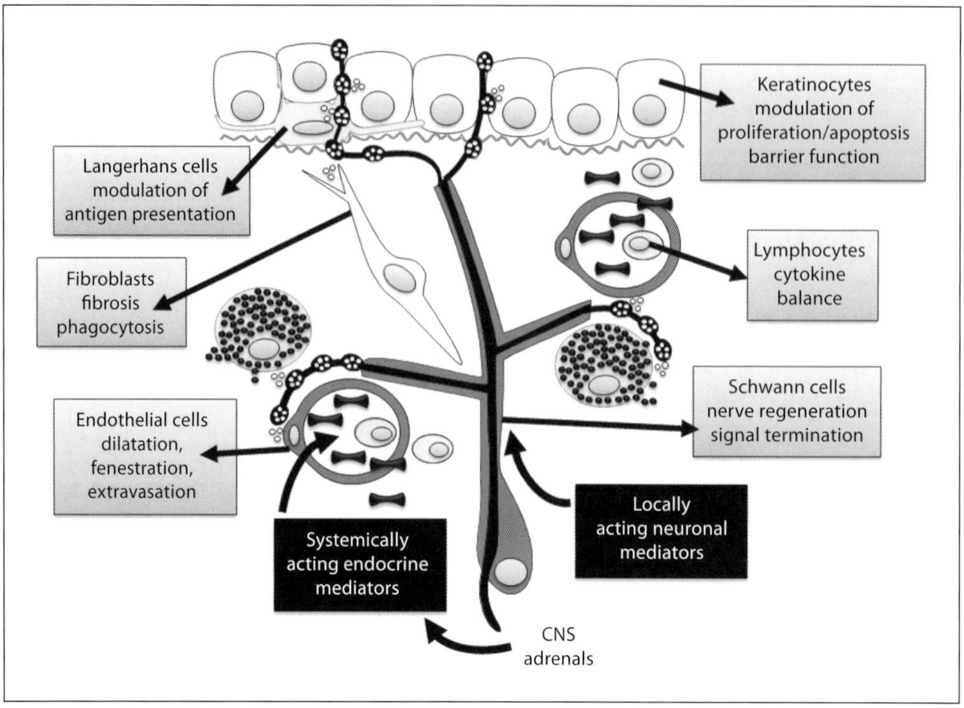

Fig. 1. Basic neuroendocrine-immune interactions in the skin. Small dots implicate mediator release.

Intriguingly, all of the above named cell populations express functional receptors for at least one neuroendocrine mediator, produce them themselves or carry enzymes that are ready to terminate, e.g. neuropeptide function [6, 15–17]. Thus, neuroendocrine-immune interaction is not a one way street but comprises afferent as well as efferent functions. Neurotrophins and release of neuropeptides can regulate a wide variety of cell functions in skin ranging from epidermal barrier via blood supply to the fine tuning of the local with the systemic immune response, all of which are affected in allergic inflammation. Accordingly, chronic inflammation is always characterized by increased neurotrophin expression and rising numbers of peptidergic nerve fibers, which are mostly found in compartments where they interact with the immune system, e.g. epidermis and dermis [6].

Neuroendocrine Immune Interaction in the Epidermis Involves Structural and Functional Cells Regulating Barrier Function and Antigen Presentation

In the epidermis mostly unmyelinated sensory nerve fibers upon local but also central stimulation release neuropeptides such as substance P (SP) or calcitonine gene-related peptide (CGRP) and many more, which we will not be able to all discuss in detail here (exemplary reviews [6, 10, 11, 16–25]). We will here discuss some key data that give a comprehensive idea on the time course and role of neuroendocrine-immune interaction in the various stages of allergy development.

The constant adaptation of the peripheral innervation to environmental changes and its interaction with the immune system is supported by locally produced neurotrophins, enabling livelong plasticity of the peripheral nervous system. Peptidergic nerve fibers are able to release their mediators along long stretches of their endings and besides keratinocytes maintain close contacts with the antigen-presenting cells of the epidermis.

In the epidermis-constituting keratinocytes, neuropeptides and neurotrophins directly promote proliferation through interaction with their high affinity receptors such as neurokinin 1 receptor (NK1) or tyrosinekinase A (TrkA) and thereby contribute to epidermal hyperplasia in inflamed skin [16, 17, 26–28]. By contrast interaction of neurotrophins such as nerve growth factor (NGF) and brain derived neurotrophic factor (BDNF) or their prohormones with the p75 neurotrophin receptor promotes keratinocyte apoptosis which plays a prominent negative role in tissue regeneration [17, 29]. Life or death decisions in neuroendocrine regulation of epithelial homeostasis thus greatly depend on receptor expression patterns and ligand availability which in allergic inflammation is shifted to a pro-proliferative profile. To understand neuroendocrine disturbances in barrier function therefor requires analysis of all involved mediators and receptors as well as the time course of their expression [6, 27].

During times of low barrier function such as in autumn, neuropeptides released by nerve fibers and their effects on keratinocytes increase [30]. In addition neuropeptides and neurotrophins are generated in loco in response to environmental challenges including allergens and noise [27, 31]. Thus physical as well as perceived stressors are suited to enhance peripheral neuroendocrine-immune circuitry and kick the skin's alarm system off.

Interestingly, acute inflammation and stress are associated with decreased numbers of SP+ nerve fibers in peripheral tissue indicating massive mediator release, while chronic inflammatory conditions and chronic stress are associated with increased numbers of SP+ nerve fibers [6]. Also, high levels of cortisol as generated by acute stressors suppress SP expression of keratinocyte and their pro-inflammatory cytokine production while low levels as observed under chronic stress conditions enhance it [32]. It therefor appears that NNA and HPA mediators complement each other in the adaptation of peripheral tissues to chronic exposure to stressors.

In analogy to the effects in the epidermis, much could be said about the neuroendocrine regulation of hair growth, as this model of epithelial tissue regeneration also shows antagonistic effects of SP and CGRP [33]. However, in atopics its only relevance appears to be in the explanation of the often sparse growing hair that may be due to a constant overactivation of neurogenic inflammation together with increased neurotrophin-p75 interaction in hair follicles in inflamed tissue.

In the initial inflammatory response to neuroendocrine activation in the epidermis, increased neuropeptides result in increased pro-inflammatory cytokine production by keratinocytes such as IL1α, IL6 and IL8 which contributes to neutrophilic inflammation [34–37]. Most prominently, however, high and acutely released nerve derived SP as well as acute perceived stress have been associated with an enhanced migration and antigen presentation by Langerhans cells which facilitates allergic sensitization [38–41]. CGRP on the contrary suppresses antigen presentation and therefore should act anti-inflammatory or sensitization protective in allergy [22, 42, 43].

Recent data from our laboratory also shows that repeated SP release by mild stress exposure or low SP levels in culture result in an increase of T regulatory functions and suppression of allergic inflammation in a mouse model for atopic-dermatitis like allergic dermatitis generated by sensitization against ovalbumin [44]. Moreover, neutrophils attracted to the site of inflammation contain CGRP [45]. Thus, neuropeptide effects on epidermal immunity appear to be biphasic with a pro-inflammatory initial phase under massive SP release and a counter-regulatory anti-inflammatory phase under low SP levels and CGRP (fig. 2).

Deeper Skin Structures Are Characterized by Prominent Innate Neuroendocrine Immune Regulation

Directly underneath the epidermis, sensory nerve fibers are intermingled with noradrenergic and actylcholinergic nerve fibers containing additional neuropeptides such as neuropeptide Y (NPY) or vasoactive intestinal peptide (VIP). Here and in the deeper regions of the dermis and subcutis they are commonly found in close contact with mast cells, blood vessels or hair follicles and their arrector pili muscles but are also seen to seemingly terminate freely between the mesenchymal cells.

The prime role of peptidergic nerve fibers in the dermis and subcutis appears to be the activation of mast cells. In mast cells, SP is known for its prominent neurogenic inflammation inducing effect meaning degranulation of mast cells and subsequent pro-inflammatory effects of mediators such as histamine or tumor necrosis factor-α [6, 16]. A large body of evidence has accumulated over the past decades that enhanced SP+ nerve fiber numbers in the dermis, a standard feature of chronic inflammation, is associated with enhanced nerve fiber-mast cell contacts.

SP-induced mast cell degranulation is clearly involved in the pathogenesis of allergic inflammation as for example IgE-induced mast cell degranulation depends on mast cell innervation [13]. Also, mast cells exposed to pro-allergic cytokines such as IL-4 further enhance their responsiveness to SP [46]. Thus a vicious cycle is created where nerve fiber-mast cell contacts not only increase in frequency but also in susceptibility for further activation. But perhaps the most interesting findings demonstrate

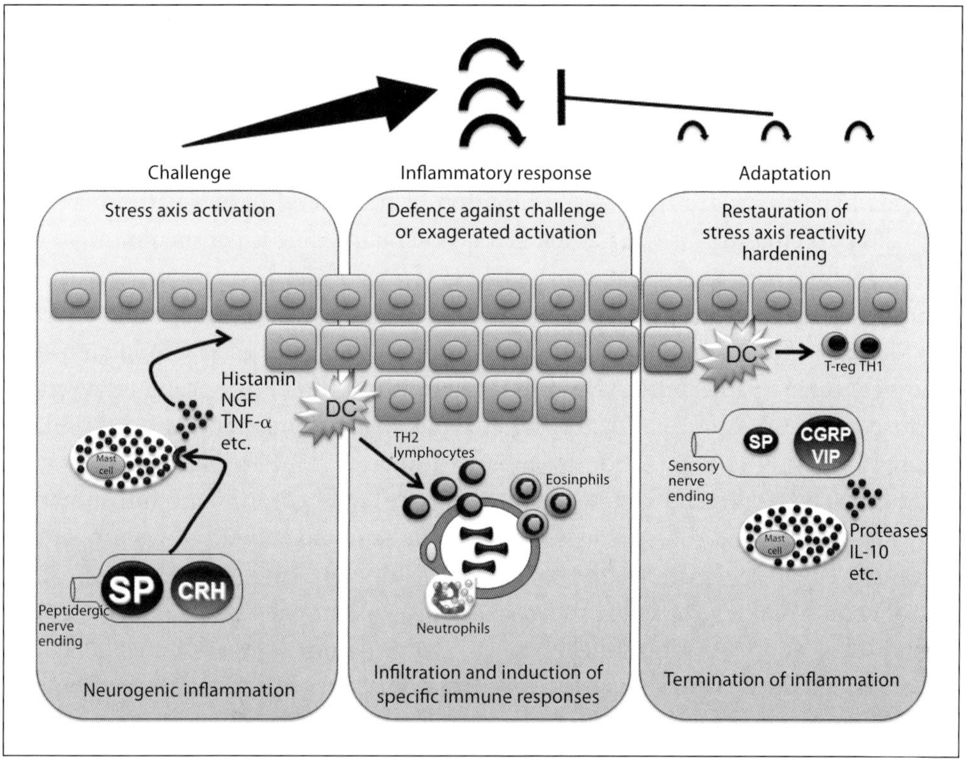

Fig. 2. Time course of neuroendocrine-immune interaction upon challenge and exacerbating effects of additional challenges contrary anti-inflammatory effects of regeneration and repeated mild challenge.

that concomitant encounter of different stressors such as for example acute noise together with allergen exposure exerts adjuvant and additive effects on neurogenic inflammation, almost doubling disease parameters [47] (fig. 2).

In contrast, NGF was shown to generate mast cell degranulation in cultured mast cells exposed to high concentrations, but in vivo it appears not to be effective [27]. Also, histamine via the H3 receptor on peripheral nerves inhibits CGRP signaling [48]. This is especially interesting in the context of therapeutic approaches that employ neuropeptide- or neurotrophin-neutralizing strategies. Here it can be expected that antagonists of the SP receptor NK1 and CGRP attenuate neurogenic inflammation and block acute exacerbation of allergic inflammation by environmental and endogenous factors while NGF-neutralization is suited to block events that contribute to chronification of allergic inflammation such as the development of peptidergic hyperinnervation or of epidermal hyperplasia.

Often underestimated, neuropeptides also potently modulate the function of endothelial cells. Release of SP increases not only plasma extravasation but also ICAM and VCAM expression on vascular epithelial cells [49]. CGRP promotes the expression of the proinflammatory cytokine IL-8 but suppresses chemokine production by endothelial cells further contributing to neutrophilic infiltration [50, 51]. Moreover, SP induces VEGF release from mast cells and slow release formulations of SP implanted into the skin increase as well as CGRP promote endothelial cell proliferation and vascularization [52–55], another stress sensitive circuit [47]. These changes facilitate hypervascularization and infiltration of peripheral tissues with inflammatory cells perpetuating disease pathology beyond neurogenic inflammation.

The many nerve fibers that can be detected in the dermis suggest neuroendocrine regulation of fibroblast function [56]. Interestingly, fibroblasts express receptors for SP, produce it and increase receptor expression as well as SP production after exposure to SP or interferon-γ [57, 58]. Interestingly, this response is followed by increased expression of a SP degrading enzyme, neutral endopeptidase. Fibroblasts also respond to NK1 stimulation by enhanced migration and proliferation [59, 60]. In addition NGF directly promotes collagen production in allergic inflammation [61, 62], while skin fibroblast elastase appears to be identical with the neuropeptide degrading enzyme neprilysin and its enhanced function in aging cells [63]. Thus, neuropeptides and neurotrophins act as acute pro-inflammatory signaling molecules in fibroblasts and may contribute to exaggerated inflammatory responses in acutely stressed skin which overexpresses SP, NGF and interferon-γ and later contribute to fibrosis in chronified allergic inflammation.

Disease Pathology in Allergic Inflammation Is an Instructive Model for Misguided Neuroendocrine Stress Responses

From the data collected above it is evident that the NNA regulates inflammatory responses and that this may have a prominent impact on chronic inflammatory disease for example in allergy. However, the diversity of individual responses makes it difficult to draw a comprehensive picture which depicts what is happening when and where in neuroendocrine-immune control of chronic inflammation (fig. 2). In addition to the neuroanatomy and observations made in individual cell populations exposed to neuroendocrine mediators, analysis of the development of neuroendocrine-immune interaction over time and in response to environmental challenges during allergic inflammatory disease progression may lead the way to our understanding of its pathogenetic relevance in the clinical context of complex disease pathologies.

A good example for the diverse effects of neuroendocrine-immune activation was given by a study collecting data on patients with atopic diseases after an earthquake in Japan, were 38% showed deterioration while 9% showed improvement of the disease in response to the stressor [64]. Likewise, animal experiments employing acute versus chronic or repeated stress conditions often show exacerbating versus attenuating effects of neuroendocrine activation [65]. Therefore, especially additive or counter-regulatory effects of different triggers of neuroendocrine-immune interaction in a specific situation have to be considered to understand the clinical outcome and therapeutic options.

Neurogenic inflammation as a prime pathogenetic element in neuroendocrine-immune exacerbation of allergic inflammation can be confirmed. Neuropeptide release and subsequent mast cell activation in skin produces itch and scratching behavior within minutes and for up to a week following itch induction as was demonstrated in mice [66]. This classical clinical sign of atopic dermatitis is therefore generated acutely and locally [23].

Flare and wheal are additional witnesses of NNA activation and the difficulties with sweating together with the maladaptation of the vasculature to pressure – the so-called white dermographism – illustrate that the enhanced susceptibility of the NNA goes hand in hand with an enhanced excitability of the SA in noradrenergic innervated structures and a decreased excitability of the SA in cholinergic innervated structures.

As discussed above this hyperactive NNA promoting neurogenic inflammation is relevant for exacerbation of allergic inflammation under conditions of acute challenge both in allergen encounter and in additional stress exposure. In chronified allergic inflammation a higher sensitivity to acutely itch inducing agents may result from enhanced SP expression but also from the downregulated expression of opiod receptors and a shift in pain perception as seen, e.g., in atopic dermatitis skin [32, 67]. This is further promoted by signaling molecules and inflammatory mediators released by activated mast cells that desensitize nerve fibers as they express the anti-nociceptive histamine 3 receptor [68]. At the same time, mast cell-derived enzymes such as tryptase activate PAR-2 on nerve fibers and sensitize them for itch perception [23, 69, 70].

Similar observations have been made in models of chronic infection such as leishmaniasis or in TH1 driven inflammatory disease such as psoriasis, where acute stress also enhances SP signaling and worsens the disease [71, 72]. Neurogenic inflammation thus appears to be a common feature of any chronic inflammatory disease in which itch can be observed as a symptom. Accordingly, a wide variety of chronic inflammatory diseases are characterized by increased neuropeptides in the chronically inflamed tissue together with further increased itch perception and other signs of neurogenic inflammation upon acute stress exposure [73, 74].

Besides neurogenic inflammation, the skins' immune system in allergic inflammation is initially characterized by prominent so-called T helper cell type 2 (TH2) immunity. Concerning the bias of immune responses towards the production of TH2 cytokines such as IL4 and IL5, which initiate humoral immune responses and eosinophilia, the NNA appears to play a less prominent role. Here a misconducted altered reactivity of the HPA and SA may facilitate TH2 bias development as a prerequisite for allergic disease development [7, 75]. In addition, NGF was shown to enhance TH2 cytokine production, and the NNA may therefor contribute to the TH2 bias through neurotrophin signaling [27].

In long-standing disease, however, enhanced NNA signaling may travel different roads as indicated by clinical improvement occasionally observed under stress as cited above. Also, treatment with antihistamines can increase SP levels alongside with improved disease [76]. These observations indicate a shift in SP signaling away from neurogenic inflammation. Clinically, in chronified allergic inflammation additional TH1 cytokine activity is added to the TH2-driven inflammation and T regulatory mechanisms are affected. Both can be conducted by SP and counterbalance TH2 driven inflammation [6, 44]. An anti-inflammatory role for SP in inflammation can also be concluded from the observation that capsaicin-denervated asthmatic lungs contain higher numbers of neutrophils in mice [77] and that acute stress enhances delayed type hypersensitivity as well as allergic dermatitis while chronic stress acts suppressive [44, 47, 78].

Certain bacteria are another exogenous challenge suited to shift the TH1/TH2 balance to an anti-inflammatory state and induce allergy suppressing T regulatory cells [79]. And again opposing effects of CGRP and SP in the regulation of T cell function can be observed as direct interaction of CGRP with T cells promotes cell adhesion by upregulation of integrins while SP provokes the opposite [80].

In addition to enhanced susceptibility of neurogenic inflammation to acute challenges, the anti-allergic inflammation effects of NNA activation characterize the chronification of allergic diseases. Staying within the analogy of an alarm system, the installation of enhanced neurogenic inflammation together with regulatory immunity in highly challenged peripheral tissues may be viewed as an unspecific learning effect resulting in a high security alarm system and the attempt at its counterbalance as compared to the standard equipment under physiological conditions.

Conclusion

In summary, neuroendocrine-immune interaction in chronic inflammation is complex but distinct corner stones can be defined (fig. 2). (1) Neuroendocrine generation of a TH2-dominated immune imbalance facilitates the development of allergic inflammation. (2) Neuroendocrine-immune interaction occurs following disturbance in the skins' defense mechanisms and barrier and promotes the induction of neurogenic inflammation by a wide variety of challenges including perceived stress. (3) Neurogenic inflammation exacerbates ongoing inflammation in allergy and many other chronic inflammatory conditions. (4) Under chronic or repeated challenge, neuroendocrine circuitry seems also to be involved in the attempt to counter- or downregulate the initial inflammatory response. Regular assessment of the neuroendocrine-immune interaction should provide us with the tools to understand the specific situation in a given patient affected with allergic disease and to identify individualized means to block its malfunction.

References

1 Brocq L, Jacquet l: Note pour servir á l'histoire des neurodermites. Ann Dermatol Syphiligr 1891:193.

2 Arthur RP, Shelley WB: The technology of in vitro staining of nerves in human skin with thiazin dyes. J Invest Dermatol 1959:121.

3 Allenby CF: Nerves of the skin; in Champion RH, Gillman T, Rook AJ, et al (eds): An Introduction to the Biology of the Skin. Saunders, Philadelphia, 1970, pp 1–124.

4 Ansel JC, Kaynard AH, Armstrong CA, Olerud J, Bunnett N , Payan D: Skin-nervous system interactions. J Invest Dermatol 1996;1:198.

5 Hendrix S, Picker B, Liezmann C, Peters EMJ: Skin and hair follicle innervation in experimental models: a guide for the exact and reproducible evaluation of neuronal plasticity. Exp Dermatol 2008;17: 214.

6 Liezmann C, Klapp B , Peters EM: Stress, atopy and allergy: a re-evaluation from a psychoneuroimmunologic persepective. Dermatoendocrinol 2011;1: 37.

7 Buske-Kirschbaum A, Hellhammer DH: Endocrine and immune responses to stress in chronic inflammatory skin disorders. Ann NY Acad Sci 2003;992: 231.

8 Montoro J, Mullol J, Jauregui I, Davila I, Ferrer M, Bartra J, del Cuvillo A, Sastre J , Valero A: Stress and allergy. J Investig Allergol Clin Immunol 2009; 19(suppl 1):40–47.

9 Shams K, Grindlay DJ, Williams HC: What's new in atopic eczema? An analysis of systematic reviews published in 2009–2010. Clin Exp Dermatol 2011;6: 573.

10 Roosterman D, Goerge T, Schneider SW, Bunnett NW, Steinhoff M: Neuronal control of skin function: the skin as a neuroimmunoendocrine organ. Physiol Rev 2006;4:1309.

11 Cevikbas F, Steinhoff A, Homey B, Steinhoff M: Neuroimmune interactions in allergic skin diseases. Curr Opin Allergy Clin Immunol 2007;5:365.

12 Suzuki R, Furuno T, McKay DM, Wolvers D, Teshima R, Nakanishi M , Bienenstock J: Direct neurite-mast cell communication in vitro occurs via the neuropeptide substance P. J Immunol 1999;5: 2410.

13 Siebenhaar F, Magerl M, Peters EM, Hendrix S, Metz M, Maurer M: Mast cell-driven skin inflammation is impaired in the absence of sensory nerves. J Allergy Clin Immunol 2008;4:955.

14 Akpan N, Caradonna K, Chuenkova MV, PereiraPerrin M: Chagas' disease parasite-derived neurotrophic factor activates cholinergic gene expression in neuronal PC12 cells. Brain Res 2008;1217:195.

15 Scholzen TE, Luger TA: Neuropeptides, a never-ending story? Termination of cutaneous inflammation by proteolytic peptidases. Exp Dermatol 2004; 33:573.

16 Peters EM, Ericson ME, Hosoi J, Seiffert K, Hordinsky MK, Ansel JC, Paus R, Scholzen TE: Neuropeptide control mechanisms in cutaneous biology: physiological and clinical significance. J Invest Dermatol 2006;9:1937.

17 Botchkarev VA, Yaar M, Peters EM, Raychaudhuri SP, Botchkareva NV, Marconi A, Raychaudhuri SK, Paus R , Pincelli C: Neurotrophins in skin biology and pathology. J Invest Dermatol 2006;8:1719

18 Goetzl EJ, Cheng PP, Hassner A, Adelman DC, Frick OL, Sreedharan SP: Neuropeptides, mast cells and allergy: novel mechanisms and therapeutic possibilities. Clin Exp Allergy 1990;20(suppl 4):3–7.

19 Black PH: Stress and the inflammatory response: a review of neurogenic inflammation. Brain Behav Immun 2002;6:622.

20 Frieri M: Neuroimmunology and inflammation: implications for therapy of allergic and autoimmune diseases. Ann Allergy Asthma Immunol 2003; 6(suppl 3):34.

21 Slominski A: Neuroendocrine system of the skin. Dermatology 2005;3:199.

22 Seiffert K, Granstein RD: Neuroendocrine regulation of skin dendritic cells. Ann NY Acad Sci 2006; 1088:195.

23 Steinhoff M, Bienenstock J, Schmelz M, Maurer M, Wei E, Biro T: Neurophysiological, neuroimmunological, and neuroendocrine basis of pruritus. J Invest Dermatol 2006;8:1705.

24 Ziemssen T, Kern S: Psychoneuroimmunology – cross-talk between the immune and nervous systems. J Neurol 2007;254(suppl 2):II8–II11.

25 Elenkov IJ: Neurohormonal-cytokine interactions: implications for inflammation, common human diseases and well-being. Neurochem Int 2008;1–2:40.

26 Seike M, Ikeda M, Morimoto A, Matsumoto M, Kodama H: Increased synthesis of calcitonin gene-related peptide stimulates keratinocyte proliferation in murine UVB-irradiated skin. J Dermatol Sci 2002;2:135.

27 Peters EM, Liezmann C, Spatz K, Daniltchenko M, Joachim R, Gimenez-Rivera A, Hendrix S, Botchkarev VA, Brandner JM , Klapp BF: Nerve growth factor partially recovers inflamed skin from stress-induced worsening in allergic inflammation. J Invest Dermatol 2011;3:735.

28 Yu XJ, Li CY, Xu YH, Chen LM, Zhou CL: Calcitonin gene-related peptide increases proliferation of human HaCaT keratinocytes by activation of MAP kinases. Cell Biol Int 2009;11:1144.

29 Peters EM, Raap U, Welker P, Tanaka A, Matsuda H, Pavlovic-Masnicosa S, Hendrix S, Pincelli C: Neurotrophins act as neuroendocrine regulators of skin homeostasis in health and disease. Horm Metab Res 2007;2:110.

30 Tupker RA, Coenraads PJ, Fidler V, De Jong MC, Van der Meer JB, De Monchy JG: Irritant susceptibility and weal and flare reactions to bioactive agents in atopic dermatitis. II. Influence of season. Br J Dermatol 1995;3:365.

31 Peters EM, Kuhlmei A, Tobin DJ, Muller-Rover S, Klapp BF, Arck PC: Stress exposure modulates peptidergic innervation and degranulates mast cells in murine skin. Brain Behav Immun 2005;3:252.

32 Katayama I, Bae SJ, Hamasaki Y, Igawa K, Miyazaki Y, Yokozeki H, Nishioka K: Stress response, tachykinin, and cutaneous inflammation. J Investig Dermatol Symp Proc 2001;1:81.

33 Peters EM, Botchkarev VA, Botchkareva NV, Tobin DJ, Paus R: Hair-cycle-associated remodeling of the peptidergic innervation of murine skin, and hair growth modulation by neuropeptides. J Invest Dermatol 2001;2:236.

34 Park YM, Kim CW: The effects of substance P and vasoactive intestinal peptide on interleukin-6 synthesis in cultured human keratinocytes. J Dermatol Sci 1999;22:17.

35 Song IS, Bunnett NW, Olerud JE, Harten B, Steinhoff M, Brown JR, Sung KJ, Armstrong CA, Ansel JC: Substance P induction of murine keratinocyte PAM 212 interleukin 1 production is mediated by the neurokinin 2 receptor (NK-2R). Exp Dermatol 2000; 1:42.

36 Burbach GJ, Kim KH, Zivony AS, Kim A, Aranda J, Wright S, Naik SM, Caughman SW, Ansel JC, Armstrong CA: The neurosensory tachykinins substance P and neurokinin A directly induce keratinocyte nerve growth factor. J Invest Dermatol 2001;5: 1075.

37 Dallos A, Kiss M, Polyanka H, Dobozy A, Kemeny L, Husz S: Effects of the neuropeptides substance P, calcitonin gene-related peptide, vasoactive intestinal polypeptide and galanin on the production of nerve growth factor and inflammatory cytokines in cultured human keratinocytes. Neuropeptides 2006; 4:251.

38 Niizeki H, Kurimoto I, Streilein JW: A substance p agonist acts as an adjuvant to promote hapten-specific skin immunity. J Invest Dermatol 1999;4: 437.

39 Nakano Y: Stress-induced modulation of skin immune function: two types of antigen-presenting cells in the epidermis are differentially regulated by chronic stress. Br J Dermatol 2004;1:50.

40 Beresford L, Orange O, Bell EB, Miyan JA: Nerve fibres are required to evoke a contact sensitivity response in mice. Immunology 2004;1:118.

41 Joachim RA, Handjiski B, Blois SM, Hagen E, Paus R, Arck PC: Stress-induced neurogenic inflammation in murine skin skews dendritic cells towards maturation and migration: key role of intercellular adhesion molecule-1/leukocyte function-associated antigen interactions. Am J Pathol 2008;5:1379.

42 Hosoi J, Murphy GF, Egan CL, Lerner EA, Grabbe S, Asahina A, Granstein RD: Regulation of Langerhans cell function by nerves containing calcitonin gene-related peptide. Nature 1993;6425;159

43 Mathers AR, Tckacheva OA, Janelsins BM, Shufesky WJ, Morelli AE, Larregina AT: In vivo signaling through the neurokinin 1 receptor favors transgene expression by Langerhans cells and promotes the generation of Th1- and Tc1-biased immune responses. J Immunol 2007;11:7006.

44 Pavlovic S, Liezmann C, Blois SM, Joachim R, Kruse J, Romani N, Klapp BF, Peters EM: Substance P is a key mediator of stress-induced protection from allergic sensitization via modified antigen presentation. J Immunol 2011;2:848.

45 Kay AB: Calcitonin gene-related peptide- and vascular endothelial growth factor-positive inflammatory cells in late-phase allergic skin reactions in atopic subjects. J Allergy Clin Immunol 2011;1:232.

46 van der Kleij HP, Ma D, Redegeld FA, Kraneveld AD, Nijkamp FP , Bienenstock J: Functional expression of neurokinin 1 receptors on mast cells induced by IL-4 and stem cell factor. J Immunol 2003;4: 2074.

47 Pavlovic S, Daniltchenko M, Tobin DJ, Hagen E, Hunt SP, Klapp BF, Arck PC, Peters EM: Further exploring the brain-skin connection: stress worsens dermatitis via substance P-dependent neurogenic inflammation in mice. J Invest Dermatol 2008;2: 434.

48 Sun P, Takatori S, Jin X, Koyama T, Tangsucharit P, Li S, Zamami Y, Kitamura Y, Kawasaki H: Histamine H(3) receptor-mediated modulation of perivascular nerve transmission in rat mesenteric arteries. Eur J Pharmacol 2011;1–3:67.

49 Lindsey KQ, Caughman SW, Olerud JE, Bunnett NW, Armstrong CA , Ansel JC: Neural regulation of endothelial cell-mediated inflammation. J Investig Dermatol Symp Proc 2000;1:74.

50 Ansel JC, Armstrong CA, Song I, Quinlan KL, Olerud JE, Caughman SW, Bunnett NW: Interactions of the skin and nervous system. J Investig Dermatol Symp Proc 1997;1:23.

51 Huang J, Stohl LL, Zhou X, Ding W, Granstein RD: Calcitonin gene-related peptide inhibits chemokine production by human dermal microvascular endothelial cells. Brain Behav Immun 2011;4:787.

52 Castellani ML, Galzio RJ, Felaco P, Tripodi D, Toniato E, De Lutiis MA, Conti F, Fulcheri M, Conti C, Theoharides TC, Caraffa A, Antinolfi P, Felaco M, Tete S, Pandolfi F, Shaik-Dasthagirisaheb YB: VEGF, substance P and stress, new aspects: a revisited study. J Biol Regul Homeost Agents 2010;3:229.

53 Kohara H, Tajima S, Yamamoto M, Tabata Y: Angiogenesis induced by controlled release of neuropeptide substance P. Biomaterials 2010;33:8617.

54 Mishima T, Ito Y, Hosono K, Tamura Y, Uchida Y, Hirata M, Suzsuki T, Amano H, Kato S, Kurihara Y, Kurihara H, Hayashi I, Watanabe M, Majima M: Calcitonin gene-related peptide facilitates revascularization during hindlimb ischemia in mice. Am J Physiol Heart Circ Physiol 2011;2:H431.

55 Zhou Z, Hu CP, Wang CJ, Li TT, Peng J, Li YJ: Calcitonin gene-related peptide inhibits angiotensin II-induced endothelial progenitor cells senescence through up-regulation of klotho expression. Atherosclerosis 2010;1:92.

56 Xie L, Takahara M, Nakahara T, Oba J, Uchi H, Takeuchi S, Moroi Y, Furue M: CD10-bearing fibroblasts may inhibit skin inflammation by down-modulating substance P. Arch Dermatol Res 2011;1:49.

57 Bae SJ, Matsunaga Y, Takenaka M, Tanaka Y, Hamazaki Y, Shimizu K, Katayama I: Substance P induced preprotachykinin-a mRNA, neutral endopeptidase mRNA and substance P in cultured normal fibroblasts. Int Arch Allergy Immunol 2002;4:316.

58 Liu JY, Hu JH, Zhu QG, Li FQ, Sun HJ: Substance P receptor expression in human skin keratinocytes and fibroblasts. Br J Dermatol 2006;4:657.

59 Parenti A, Amerini S, Ledda F, Maggi CA, Ziche M: The tachykinin NK1 receptor mediates the migration-promoting effect of substance P on human skin fibroblasts in culture. Naunyn Schmiedebergs Arch Pharmacol 1996;5:475.

60 Jing C, Jia-Han W, Hong-Xing Z: Double-edged effects of neuropeptide substance P on repair of cutaneous trauma. Wound Repair Regen 2010;3:319.

61 Kilic A, Sonar SS, Yildirim AO, Fehrenbach H, Nockher WA, Renz H: Nerve growth factor induces type III collagen production in chronic allergic airway inflammation. J Allergy Clin Immunol 2011;128:1058–1066.

62 Palazzo E, Marconi A, Truzzi F, Dallaglio K, Petrachi T, Humbert P, Schnebert S, Perrier E, Dumas M, Pincelli C: Role of neurotrophins on dermal fibroblast survival and differentiation. J Cell Physiol 2011, doi: 10.1002/jcp.22811 [Epub ahead of print].

63 Morisaki N, Moriwaki S, Sugiyama-Nakagiri Y, Haketa K, Takema Y, Imokawa G: Neprilysin is identical to skin fibroblast elastase: its role in skin aging and UV responses. J Biol Chem 2010;51:39819.

64 Kodama A, Horikawa T, Suzuki T, Ajiki W, Takashima T, Harada S, Ichihashi M: Effect of stress on atopic dermatitis: investigation in patients after the great hanshin earthquake. J Allergy Clin Immunol 1999;1:173.

65 Dhabhar FS: Enhancing versus suppressive effects of stress on immune function: implications for immunoprotection and immunopathology. Neuroimmunomodulation 2009;5:300.

66 Yamaoka J, Kawana S: Rapid changes in substance P signaling and neutral endopeptidase induced by skin-scratching stimulation in mice. J Dermatol Sci 2007;2:123.

67 Bigliardi-Qi M, Lipp B, Sumanovski LT, Buechner SA, Bigliardi PL: Changes of epidermal mu-opiate receptor expression and nerve endings in chronic atopic dermatitis. Dermatology 2005;2:91.

68 Cannon KE, Chazot PL, Hann V, Shenton F, Hough LB, Rice FL: Immunohistochemical localization of histamine H3 receptors in rodent skin, dorsal root ganglia, superior cervical ganglia, and spinal cord: potential antinociceptive targets. Pain 2007;1–2:76.

69 Steinhoff M, Buddenkotte J, Shpacovitch V, Rattenholl A, Moormann C, Vergnolle N, Luger TA, Hollenberg MD: Proteinase-activated receptors: transducers of proteinase-mediated signaling in inflammation and immune response. Endocr Rev 2005;1:1.

70 Steinhoff M, Neisius U, Ikoma A, Fartasch M, Heyer G, Skov PS, Luger TA, Schmelz M: Proteinase-activated receptor-2 mediates itch: a novel pathway for pruritus in human skin. J Neurosci 2003;15:6176.

71 Ruiz MR, Quinones AG, Diaz NL, Tapia FJ: Acute immobilization stress induces clinical and neuroimmunological alterations in experimental murine cutaneous leishmaniasis. Br J Dermatol 2003;4:731.

72 Raychaudhuri SP, Raychaudhuri SK: Role of NGF and neurogenic inflammation in the pathogenesis of psoriasis. Prog Brain Res 2004;146:433.

73 Fischer A, Wussow A, Cryer A, Schmeck B, Noga O, Zweng M, Peiser C, Dinh QT, Heppt W, Groneberg DA: Neuronal plasticity in persistent perennial allergic rhinitis. J Occup Environ Med 2005;1:20.
74 Remrod C, Lonne-Rahm S, Nordlind K: Study of substance P and its receptor neurokinin-1 in psoriasis and their relation to chronic stress and pruritus. Arch Dermatol Res 2007;2:85.
75 Buske-Kirschbaum A, Ebrecht M, Hellhammer DH: Blunted HPA axis responsiveness to stress in atopic patients is associated with the acuity and severeness of allergic inflammation. Brain Behav Immun 2010; 8:1347.
76 Izu K, Tokura Y: The various effects of four H1-antagonists on serum substance P levels in patients with atopic dermatitis. J Dermatol 2005;10:776.
77 Franco-Penteado CF, De Souza IA, Camargo EA, Teixeira SA, Muscara MN, De Nucci G, Antunes E: Mechanisms involved in the enhancement of allergic airways neutrophil influx by permanent C-fiber degeneration in rats. J Pharmacol Exp Ther 2005;1: 440.
78 Dhabhar FS: Stress-induced enhancement of cell-mediated immunity. Ann NY Acad Sci 1998;840: 359.
79 Karimi K, Inman MD, Bienenstock J, Forsythe P: *Lactobacillus reuteri*-induced regulatory T cells protect against an allergic airway response in mice. Am J Respir Crit Care Med 2009;3:186.
80 Levite M: Nerve-driven immunity. The direct effects of neurotransmitters on T-cell function. Ann NY Acad Sci 2000;917:307.

Dr. Eva M.J. Peters
Department of Psychosomatic Medicine, Justus Liebig University
Ludwigstrasse 78
DE–35392 Giessen (Germany)
Tel. +49 641 99 45642, E-Mail eva.peters@eva-peters.com

Bienenstock J (ed): Allergy and the Nervous System.
Chem Immunol Allergy. Basel, Karger, 2012, vol 98, pp 253–265

Itch and the Brain

F. Pfab[a,b] · M. Valet[c] · V. Napadow[a] · T.-R. Tölle[c] · H. Behrendt[d] · J. Ring[b,d] · U. Darsow[b,c]

[a]Department of Radiology, Massachusetts General Hospital, Harvard Medical School, Boston, Mass., USA; [b]Department of Dermatology and Allergy and [c]Department of Neurology, Klinikum r.d. Isar, Technische Universität München and [d]Division of Environmental Dermatology and Allergy, Helmholtz Zentrum München/TUM, ZAUM-Center for Allergy and Environment, Munich, Germany

Abstract

The sensation of itch – defined as unpleasant sensation inducing the urge to scratch – is processed by a network of different brain regions contributing to the encoding of sensory, emotional, attention-dependent, cognitive-evaluative and motivational patterns. Patients with atopic eczema show different activation patterns and kinetics compared to healthy volunteers. This review summarizes current studies investigating itch in the brain.

Itch is the major symptom of many diseases; yet it is still difficult to measure objectively. Recent technological advances in the field of brain imaging paved the way for neuroimaging studies on central itch pathways. Positron emission tomography (PET) Scan studies and later studies using functional magnetic resonance imaging (1.5 and 3 Tesla) technology were able to show that itch is processed by a network of brain regions contributing to the encoding of sensory, emotional, attentional, evaluative and motivational aspects. This central itch matrix may be an interesting target for different therapies.

Itch is a complex and unpleasant sensory experience that induces the urge to scratch [1]. It is the most prevalent symptom of inflammatory skin diseases [2, 3] and difficult to be measured objectively. With its well-known psychophysiologic aspects, it has substantial impact on the quality of life of patients [4]. Its pathophysiology remains poorly understood in spite of numerous studies [2].

Quantity and quality of perceived itch show specific characteristics in different pruritic skin diseases. Clinical observations point to differences in the central nervous processing of pruritus. The multidimensional 'Eppendorf Itch Questionnaire' (EIQ) [5] was used in hospitalized patients suffering from atopic eczema (AE, n = 62) and chronic urticaria (CU, n = 58). Total scores (127 items), emotional and sensory ratings, reactive behavior and visual analogue scale (VAS) ratings for itch intensity were evaluated. The mean VAS ratings of itch intensity showed no significant difference between the two diseases. In contrast, the total EIQ score was significantly higher in the AE group with 231.6 ± 11.5 versus 175.2 ± 9.4. In 34 of 127 items, a significantly different rating was obtained, mostly with higher load for affective and some sensory items in AE. Significant differences were also seen in the description of the scratch response. Thus, itch perception in AE and CU differs on a qualitative level, influencing items relevant for quality of life. Similar findings were perceived in a study investigating the preventive effect of acupuncture on experimental itch – showing a preventive point-specific effect on the emotional items of the EIQ [6]. These findings accentuate the emotional component of the itch sensation; with possibly differences in CNS processing.

Itch can easily be elicited experimentally – most effectively via a histamine stimulus [7]. With its mainly subjective characteristics itch has some psychophysiological similarity to pain. Although some degree of overlap is present, recent neurophysiological studies have confirmed that itch pathways are clearly distinct from pain pathways [8–10]. In recent years, progress in central nervous system imaging technologies had substantial impact on itch research. New models to measure itch may also be useful for the development of new therapeutic strategies against pruritus.

Neuroimaging of Itch by Positron Emission Tomography

Objective covariates of itch and differences to pain processing were shown using imaging techniques for the CNS: a complex pattern of cerebral activation after experimental itch induction with histamine dihydrochloride (0.03 to 8%) at the right lower arm in healthy volunteers was observed in a $H_2{}^{15}O$ PET correlation study (n = 6) [8]. Subtraction analysis of histamine versus control condition revealed significant activation of the primary somatosensory cortex and motor-associated areas, predominantly left-sided activations of frontal, orbitofrontal and superior temporal cortex and anterior cingulate cortex. Compared to activation patterns induced by pain stimuli [11] itch did not lead to thalamus activation, but significant activation in the insula region and differences in sensory, motor and cingulate areas.

Mochizuki et al. [12] investigating the central modulation of histamine-itch by application of a contralateral cold pain stimulus, showed significant increases in regional cerebral blood flow in the anterior cingulate cortex, thalamus, parietal cortex, dorsolateral prefrontal cortex and premotor cortex.

These results give evidence for central nervous processing of itch, and clearly demonstrate differences to pain processing. Planning of a scratch response is mirrored by extensive activation of motor areas in the cortex, while other areas may be involved in emotional evaluation of pruriception.

New Methodology Enabling Itch Measurement by Functional MRI

Until recently functional magnetic resonance imaging (fMRI) studies on itch had been hampered by the lack of a phasic stimulus. In contrast to pain, no method had been described to elicit and stop the sensation of itch within seconds. In a recent study the itch sensation was investigated using a methodology with short term temperature changes for modulation of histamine-induced itch [13].

In 9 healthy right-handed male volunteers, 1% histamine dihydrochloride was used as the evaluated itch stimulus [5] on the right forearm with subsequent modulation of the target skin area temperature by a Medoc TSA thermode. The latter is capable of heating or cooling the skin and was placed exactly above the stimulus area. Using a boxcar design 14 equal cycles were applied: Each cycle started with a warm block producing a constant skin temperature of 32°C for 20 s then changing within 1.5 s (ramp 5°C/s) to a cold block of 25°C also lasting for 20 s.

Subjective scales were recorded using a computerized visual analogue scale (VAS) ranging from 0 to 100 at 4-second intervals. At one-third of the VAS (33/100) the intervention point 'scratch threshold' was installed. Above this threshold each individual felt the clear-cut desire to scratch; this, however, was not permitted nor done. Itch intensity was quantitatively expressed in percent of the maximum VAS value.

All subjects reported itch without pain within 40 s after histamine application. None of the volunteers felt pain sensation at any time during the course of the experiment.

In each individual subject as well as in the total group, significant differences between VAS rating intervals concerning itch intensity were noted. In each cycle itch intensity was generally perceived as higher during 25°C-blocks than during 32°C-blocks. Mean itch intensity was 50.6 ± 3.5% during the 25°C-block (intervals 6 to 10) and 33.8 ± 3.9% during the 32°C-block (intervals 1 to 5) with a highly significant difference ($p < 0.0001$) between the two temperature blocks (fig. 1).

Alternating changes in mean itch perception comparing warm and cold blocks were remarkably reproducible.

In spite of the common knowledge that intensive cold inhibits itch sensation, a reproducible, significant enhancement of histamine-induced itch by short-term moderate cooling was shown. This effect might be explained by peripheral and central adaptation processes triggered by abnormal afferent activity patterns.

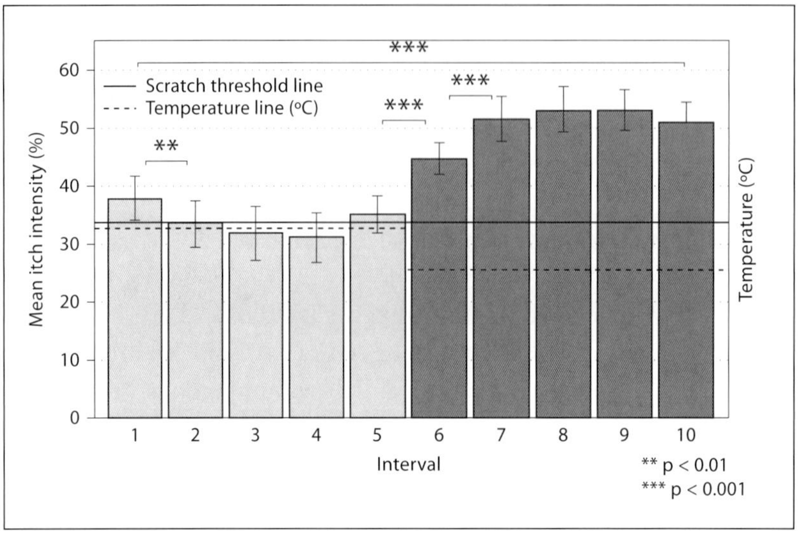

Fig. 1. Demonstrating increased itch intensity on lower temperature and in lesional compared to nonlesional skin as well as delayed onset of itch modulation in patients with atopic eczema. Mean itch intensity of both sessions at the various temperature intervals (n = 10). As indicated by the dotted line the red columns numbered 1 to 5 indicate warm temperature intervals (32°C), whereas the blue columns numbered 6 to 10 mark relatively cold temperature intervals (25°C), each lasting 4 s. Columns with horizontal line pattern represent healthy skin, columns with ascending line pattern represent nonlesional AE skin, columns with downward line pattern lesional AE skin. The yellow line represents the scratch threshold (33% itch intensity). Asterisks indicate selected significant differences between intervals. * $p < 0.05$, ** $p < 0.01$, *** $p < 0.001$. From Pfab et al. [21].

This method allows controlled and rapid modulation of itch. Short-term cooling enhances histamine-induced itch, providing the possibility of further and more detailed investigations of itch by functional imaging methods such as fMRI.

In a further study we evaluated this itch stimulus model in lesional (LS) and nonlesional (NLS) atopic eczema (AE) skin (n = 13, healthy skin (HS) of age-matched volunteers served as control (n = 9).). Thermal modulation was performed on a histamine stimulus in randomized order on LS or NLS in rapid alternating order from 32°C (warm) to 25°C (cold). Subjective itch ratings were recorded.

Mean VAS itch intensity was significantly ($p < 0.0001$) higher during the relative cold (55.2 ± 8.3% (LS); 48.6 ± 8.2% (NLS)) compared to the relative warm blocks (36.0 ± 7.3% (LS); 33.7 ± 7.6% (NLS)). Compared to HS the itch response was delayed in LS and NLS. Itch intensity was perceived highest in LS, followed by NLS and HS.

Moderate short-term temperature modulation led to a reproducible, significant enhancement of histamine-induced itch with the strongest effect in LS.

The differences in itch perception and itch kinetics between healthy volunteers and NLS in patients point towards an ongoing central inhibitory activity patients with AE, especially at the beginning of the itch provocation.

Cerebral Processing of Histamine-Induced Itch Using Short-Term Alternating Temperature Modulation – An fMRI Study

Using the previously established biphasic temperature stimulus model, we investigated the cerebral activation pattern of itch processing in 12 healthy volunteers with functional MRI [14].

Itch was provoked on the right forearm with 1% histamine-dihydrochloride. Local temperature modulation allowed reproducible itch provocation above scratch threshold (defined as 33/100 on a VAS) during 25°C whereas itch declined below scratch threshold during the 32°C stimulation period. No itch sensation was reported using 0.9% saline with temperature modulation.

The calculation of itch-specific activation maps for the first 4, 8, 12, 16 and 20 s of the 25°C stimulation period confirmed that the changes during the first 8 s are reflected by the higher brain activations during this time period than during the other time periods. Focusing on the first 8 s of 25°C stimulation, the thalamus, pre-SMA, lateral prefrontal cortex, anterior insular cortex and inferior parietal cortex were more active than during the saline condition ($p < 0.001$; fig. 2). The medial frontal cortex, orbitofrontal cortex, dorsal part of the anterior cingulate cortex (dACC) and primary motor cortex (M1) were all less active during histamine induced itch than during saline ($p < 0.001$; fig. 2).

So far this is the only imaging study on itch using a phasic supra-threshold itch model comparing itch and nonitch phases.

Further Neuroimaging Studies in Healthy Volunteers

Neuroimaging studies on itch have been performed using both PET [8, 12, 15–17] and more recently fMRI [18, 19]. Table 1 summarizes the findings of current neuroimaging studies.

Taking the results of these studies together key centers of histamine-itch perception in healthy volunteers seem to be ipsilateral pre-motor and supplementary motor area and contralateral cingulate cortex , insular cortex, thalamus and frontal inferior gyrus (inferior parietal and dorsolateral prefrontal cortex).

So far, one study [19] investigated the effect of allergen-induced itch in patients with mucosal atopy showing similarities to histamine itch (table 1). Mochizuki et al. [18] directly compared itch and pain stimuli with fMRI in healthy volunteers: Neural activity in the posterior cingulate cortex and the posterior insula associated with itch was significantly higher than that associated with pain; pain in contrast to itch, induced an activation of the thalamus correlating to pain sensation.

Leknes et al. [19] were the first to investigate the cerebral processing of allergen-induced itch, postulating a dysfunction of striato-thalamo-orbitofrontal circuits,

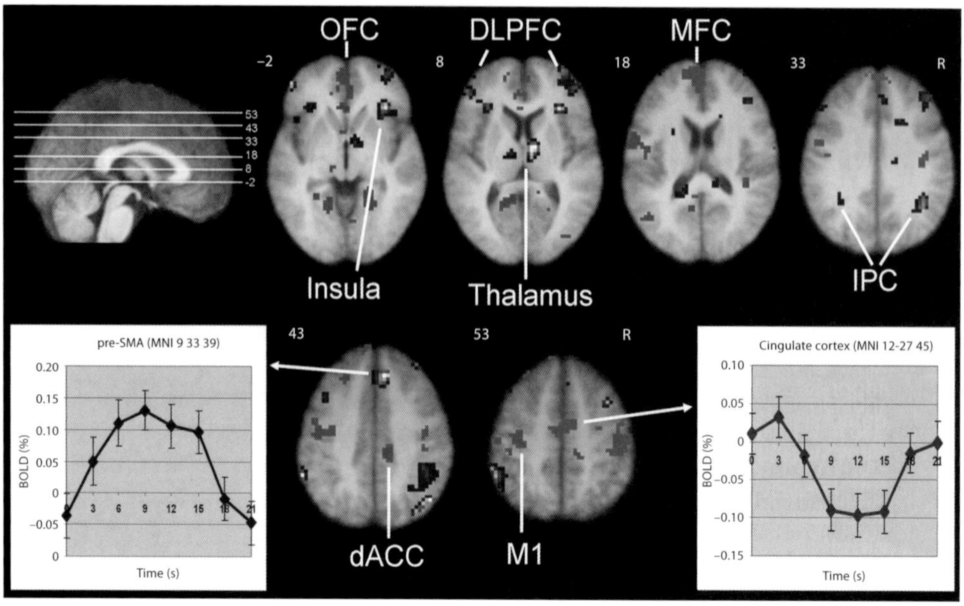

Fig. 2. Cerebral activation (red) and deactivation (blue) patterns induced by itch provocation: nonlesional skin of patients with atopic eczema, lesional skin of patients with atopic eczema, healthy control skin. Activation maps of histamine-induced itch compared to saline were calculated for the first 4, 8, 12, 16 and 20 s of the 25°C stimulation period and are superimposed on the averaged normalized T_1-weighted brain of all subjects. A dynamic process with increase and decrease of regional brain activation can be observed in the time course of the 25°C stimulation period. The statistical parametric maps were thresholded at $p < 0.005$. The right side of the image corresponds to right side of the brain (neurological convention). From Pfab et al. [21].

which are believed to underlie the failure to regulate the motivational drive in disorders associated with strong urges, e.g. addiction and obsessive compulsive disorder. Mochizuki et al. [20] investigated histamine-induced itch in 10 healthy volunteers using magnet encephalography (MEG) as well as fMRI suggesting the importance of the precuneus as well as premotor, primary motor, and anterior cingulate cortices (table 1).

Neuroimaging Studies in Patients Suffering Chronically from Itch

We characterized the cerebral responses in lesional skin (LS) and nonlesional skin (NLS) of 13 patients with atopic eczema (AE) using fMRI [21]:

Histamine-induced itch in NLS at 25°C stimulation was reflected by a deactivation of brain structures, such as the primary and secondary somatosensory, insular, cingulate and prefrontal cortex, supplementary motor area, premotor areas and basal ganglia. These deactivations were less pronounced in the later course of 25°C stimulation with a parallel activation increase in the basal ganglia.

In contrast, histamine-induced itch in LS at 25°C stimulation was associated with an activation of the basal ganglia, insular cortex, prefrontal areas and parietal cortex. Deactivations were seen in the parietal, temporal, primary and secondary somatosensory, cingulate cortex, premotor and prefrontal areas, but were less robust than for NLS.

Our study supports a peripheral as well as a central component in the pathophysiology of chronic itch in patients suffering from atopic eczema. On the one hand, pathological skin conditions such as a skin barrier abnormality and local inflammation processes in atopic eczema patients [22, 23] point to a peripherally increased sensitivity to itch stimuli. On the other hand, central filter mechanisms might counteract this pathological skin condition to a certain point when the threshold of the pruriceptive input is exceeded.

Schneider et al. [24] demonstrated significant differences in central imaging of histamine-induced itch between patients with atopic dermatitis in non lesional skin and healthy subjects in a study correlating itch intensity with cerebral activation using PET.

Ishiuji et al. [25] recently compared itch induced by histamine-iontopheresis in lesional skin of 8 patients with AE compared to 7 healthy controls, showing significant differences between patients and healthy controls (table 1).

Key Anatomic Brain Regions of Itch and Their Function

Insular Cortex

The anterior insula is assumed to subserve subjective feelings [26] and to integrate sensory and emotional experiences [27]. It has been suggested that the insular cortex is part of an interoceptive system providing the basis for a cortical image of homeostatic activity that reflects all aspects of the physiological condition [28]. In this context, itch activation of the insular cortex might indicate an interference on homeostatic balance, leading to the desire to scratch [13, 19].

Pre-Supplementary Motor Area and Primary Motor Cortex, Motor Part of the Cingulate Cortex

The pre-SMA is thought to encode motor actions prior to self-initiated voluntary movements and during imagination of motor action [29]. M1 is typically involved in motor planning and execution highlighting the definition of itch which includes the intention to scratch [1]. As the subjects were not allowed to scratch the deactivation might indicate a suppression of motor activity. The dorsal anterior cingulate cortex (dACC) is also thought to be engaged in premotor planning [30, 31] as well as in stimulus intensity encoding [32, 33]. Translating this information from pain to itch

Table 1. Summarizing findings of current neuroimaging studiesActivation in the corresponding region is marked by I (ipsilateral) or C (contralateral); the minus (–) indicates reduced activation in comparison to a saline control stimulus.

	Healthy volunteers						
	Hsieh et al. [16], 1994	Drzezga et al. [15], 2001	Mochizuki et al. [12], 2003	Schneider et al. [24], 2008	Walter et al. [17], 2005	Leknes et al. [19], 2007	Valet et al. [14], 2007
Scanner	PET	PET	PET	PET	fMRI 1.5T	fMRI 3T	fMRI 1.5T
Neuroimaging analysis	subtraction	correlation	subtraction	correlation	correlation	correlation	subtraction
Itch induction	intracutaneous injection	skin prick model	Iontophoresis	Iontophoresis	skin prick model	skin prick model	skin prick model
Itch stimulus	histamine	histamine	histamine	histamine	histamine	histamine	histamine
Number of subjects	10	6	15	6	6	14	12
Brain region							
Primary somatosensory cortex (BA 1–3)		I,C		C			C-
Somatosensory associated/ parietal cortex (BA 5, 7)		I,C	I	C			
Primary motor cortex (BA 4)		C					
Pre-motor and supplementary motor cortex (BA 6)	I,C	I,C	I	C			I
Cerebellum	I,C				C		
Insular cortex (BA 13, 14)		C				I,C	C
Cingulate cortex (BA 23, 24, 25, 29, 30, 32)	C	I,C	C	C	C	I,C	I-
Prefrontal cortex (BA 9)	I,C	C		I			
Frontopolar and orbitofrontal area (BA 8, 10–12)		C			I,C		I-,C-
Inferior parietal and dorsolateral prefrontal cortex (BA 45, 46, 47)		C	I,C				I,C
Temporal gyrus (BA 20–22)					C		
Temporal lobe/Wernicke's area (BA 38–40)			I				I,C

				Atopic patients	Patients with atopic eczema			
Mochizuki et al. [18], 2007	Herde, 2007	Ishiuji et al. [25], 2009	Mochizuki et al. [20], 2009	Leknes et al. [19], 2007	Schneider et al. [24], 2008	Ishiuji et al. [25], 2009	Pfab et al. [21], 2010	Pfab et al. [21], 2010
fMRI 3.0T	fMRI 1.5T	fMRI 1.5T	fMRI 3T and MEG	fMRI 3T	PET	fMRI 1.5T	fMRI 3T	fMRI 3T
correlation	subtraction	correlation	correlation	correlation	correlation	correlation	subtraction	subtraction
ionto-phoresis	intracuta-neous microdialysis	ionto-phoresis		skin prick model	ionto-phoresis	ionto-phoresis	skin prick model non-lesional skin	skin prick model lesional skin
histamine	histamine and codeine	histamine	electricity	histamine	histamine	histamine	histamine	histamine
14	10	8	10	14	8	8	13	13
	C	C		C			I-,C-	I-,C-
	C	C				I,C		I-,C-
		C		C			I-,C-	
I	I,C		I	C	I,C	I,C		I-,C-
	I,C		C		I,C			
C	I,C		I,C		I	I	I-,C-	I,C
C	I,C		C	I,C		I,C	I-,C-	I-,C-
	I,C				I		I-,C-	I,C
I	C			I,C	I	I,C		
	I,C		I			I,C		I,C
	I,C							I-,C-
	I,C	C	I,C	C	C			

Table 1. Continued

	Healthy volunteers						
	Hsieh et al. [16], 1994	Drzezga et al. [15], 2001	Mochizuki et al. [12], 2003	Schneider et al. [24], 2008	Walter et al. [17], 2005	Leknes et al. [19], 2007	Valet et al. [14], 2007
Thalamus			C			I,C	I,C
Basal ganglia						I	
SII (BA 40, 43)							
Precuneus (BA 7, 31)							
Putamen							
Visual association gyrus (BA 18)							
Anterior entorhinal cortex (BA 34)							

processing, we hypothesize that the dual function of the dACC, with the anatomically neighboring M1, is advantageous for the generation of an adequate motor response to the itching stimulus (planning of a scratch response).

Thalamus and Primary Somatosensory Cortex

The activation of the thalamus and S1 cortex can be attributed to sensory aspects of itch processing. The ability to localize itch (S1) plays an important role in the initiation of withdrawal behavior. These brain structures are fulfilling important functions regarding detection, localization, discrimination and intensity encoding of sensory stimuli [34].

Inferior Parietal Cortex and Dorsolateral Prefrontal Cortex

The inferior parietal cortex is known to be involved in the spatial representation of the intra- and extrapersonal space (body scheme) and regarded as polymodal association area integrating multisensory information from the thalamus, insula, anterior cingulate cortex and prefrontal cortex [35]. It is known that lesions of this region in the non-dominant hemisphere are highly associated with neglect and inattention syndromes. Activation of this region may therefore reflect a spatially directed attention to the itching stimulus.

The dorsolateral prefrontal cortex is associated with cognitive evaluative, attention-dependent, working memory and executive functions [36]. Besides input from the thalamus and cingulate cortex, it receives and processes multisensory information

				Atopic patients	Patients with atopic eczema			
Mochizuki et al. [18], 2007	Herde, 2007	Ishiuji et al. [25], 2009	Mochizuki et al. [20], 2009	Leknes et al. [19], 2007	Schneider et al. [24], 2008	Ishiuji et al. [25], 2009	Pfab et al. [21], 2010	Pfab et al. [21], 2010
	I,C		I	I,C	C			
I	I,C			I,C	I	C	I-,C-	I,C
			I,C					
		C	I			I,C		
						C		
						I,C		
						C		

mainly from the inferior parietal cortex [36]. The sensory convergence and integration is required in the preparation of motor action.

Conclusion

Itch sensation is processed by a network of brain regions contributing to the encoding of sensory, emotional, attention-dependent, cognitive-evaluative and motivational patterns. Patients with atopic eczema show different activation patterns and kinetics compared to healthy volunteers. It now seems possible to further analyze the specific effects of various therapies on these significant activation patterns.

Acknowledgement

This work was supported by the Christine Kühne Center of Allergy Research and Education (CK-CARE).

References

1 Hafenreffer S: In Kuhnen B (ed): De pruritu, in Nosodochium, in quo cutis, eique adaerentium partium, affectus omnes, singulari methodo, et cognoscendi et curandi fidelissime traduntur. Ulm, 1660, pp 98–102.

2 Charlesworth EN, Beltrani VS: Pruritic dermatoses: overview of etiology and therapy. Am J Med 2002; 113(suppl 9A):25S–33S.

3 Behrendt H, Krämer U, Schäfer T, et al: Allergotoxicology – a research concept to study the role of environmental pollutants in allergy. ACI Int 2001;13:122–128.

4 Stander S, Weisshaar E, Mettang T, et al: Clinical classification of itch: a position paper of the International Forum for the Study of Itch. Acta Dermato-venereol 2007;87:291–294.

5 Darsow U, Scharein E, Simon D, Walter G, Bromm B, Ring J: New aspects of itch pathophysiology: component analysis of atopic itch using the 'Eppendorf Itch Questionaire'. Int Arch Allergy Immunol 2001;124:326–331.

6 Pfab F, Hammes M, Backer M, et al: Preventive effect of acupuncture on histamine-induced itch: a blinded, randomized, placebo-controlled, crossover trial. J Allergy Clin Immunol 2005;116:1386–1388.

7 Darsow U, Ring J, Scharein E, Bromm B: Correlations between histamine-induced wheal, flare and itch. Arch Dermatol Res 1996;288:436–441.

8 Darsow U, Drzezga A, Frisch M, et al: Processing of histamine-induced itch in the human cerebral cortex: a correlation analysis with dermal reactions. J Invest Dermatol 2000;115:1029–1033.

9 Schmelz M, Schmidt R, Bickel A, Handwerker HO, Torebjoerk HE: Specific C-receptors for itch in human skin. J Neurosci 1997;17:8003–8008.

10 Ikoma A, Steinhoff M, Stander S, Yosipovitch G, Schmelz M: The neurobiology of itch. Nat Rev 2006;7:535–547.

11 Sprenger T, Ruether K, Boecker H, et al: Altered metabolism in frontal brain circuits in cluster headache. Cephalalgia 2007;27:1033–1042.

12 Mochizuki H, Tashiro M, Kano M, Sakurada Y, Itoh M, Yanai K: Imaging of central itch modulation in the human brain using positron emission tomography. Pain 2003;105:339–346.

13 Pfab F, Valet M, Sprenger T, et al: Short-term alternating temperature enhances histamine-induced itch: a biphasic stimulus model. J Invest Dermatol 2006;126:2673–2678.

14 Valet M, Pfab F, Sprenger T, et al: Cerebral processing of histamine-induced itch using short-term alternating temperature modulation – an fMRI study. J Invest Dermatol 2008;128:426–433.

15 Drzezga A, Darsow U, Treede RD, et al: Central activation by histamine-induced itch: analogies to pain processing: a correlational analysis of O-15 H_2O positron emission tomography studies. Pain 2001;92:295–305.

16 Hsieh JC, Hagermark O, Stahle-Backdahl M, et al: Urge to scratch represented in the human cerebral cortex during itch. J Neurophysiol 1994;72:3004–3008.

17 Walter B, Sadlo MN, Kupfer J, et al: Brain activation by histamine prick test-induced itch. J Invest Dermatol 2005;125:380–382.

18 Mochizuki H, Sadato N, Saito DN, et al: Neural correlates of perceptual difference between itching and pain: a human fMRI study. NeuroImage 2007;36: 706–717.

19 Leknes SG, Bantick S, Willis CM, Wilkinson JD, Wise RG, Tracey I: Itch and motivation to scratch: an investigation of the central and peripheral correlates of allergen- and histamine-induced itch in humans. J Neurophysiol 2007;97:415–22.

20 Mochizuki H, Inui K, Tanabe HC, et al: Time course of activity in itch-related brain regions: a combined MEG-fMRI study. J Neurophysiol 2009;102:2657–2666.

21 Pfab F, Valet M, Sprenger T, et al: Temperature modulated histamine-itch in lesional and nonlesional skin in atopic eczema – a combined psychophysical and neuroimaging study. Allergy 2010;65:84–94.

22 Elias PM, Hatano Y, Williams ML: Basis for the barrier abnormality in atopic dermatitis: outside-inside-outside pathogenic mechanisms. J Allergy Clin Immunol 2008;121:1337–1343.

23 Sicherer SH, Leung DY: Advances in allergic skin disease, anaphylaxis, and hypersensitivity reactions to foods, drugs, and insects in 2007. J Allergy Clin Immunol 2008;121:1351–1358.

24 Schneider G, Stander S, Burgmer M, Driesch G, Heuft G, Weckesser M: Significant differences in central imaging of histamine-induced itch between atopic dermatitis and healthy subjects. Eur J Pain 2008;12:834–841.

25 Ishiuji Y, Coghill RC, Patel TS, Oshiro Y, Kraft RA, Yosipovitch G: Distinct patterns of brain activity evoked by histamine-induced itch reveal an association with itch intensity and disease severity in atopic dermatitis. Br J Dermatol 2009;161:1072–1080.

26 Singer T, Seymour B, O'Doherty J, Kaube H, Dolan RJ, Frith CD: Empathy for pain involves the affective but not sensory components of pain. Science 2004;303:1157–1162.

27 Gracely RH, Geisser ME, Giesecke T, et al: Pain catastrophizing and neural responses to pain among persons with fibromyalgia. Brain 2004;127:835–843.
28 Craig AD: Interoception: the sense of the physiological condition of the body. Curr Opin Neurobiol 2003;13:500–505.
29 Cunnington R, Windischberger C, Moser E: Premovement activity of the pre-supplementary motor area and the readiness for action: studies of time-resolved event-related functional MRI. Hum Mov Sci 2005;24:644–656.
30 Vogt BA: Pain and emotion interactions in subregions of the cingulate gyrus. Nat Rev 2005;6:533–544.
31 Kwan CL, Crawley AP, Mikulis DJ, Davis KD: An fMRI study of the anterior cingulate cortex and surrounding medial wall activations evoked by noxious cutaneous heat and cold stimuli. Pain 2000;85:359–374.
32 Tölle TR, Kaufmann T, Siessmeier T, et al: Region-specific encoding of sensory and affective components of pain in the human brain: a positron emission tomography correlation analysis. Ann Neurol 1999;45:40–47.
33 Buchel C, Bornhovd K, Quante M, Glauche V, Bromm B, Weiller C: Dissociable neural responses related to pain intensity, stimulus intensity, and stimulus awareness within the anterior cingulate cortex: a parametric single-trial laser functional magnetic resonance imaging study. J Neurosci 2002;22:970–976.
34 Apkarian AV, Bushnell MC, Treede RD, Zubieta JK: Human brain mechanisms of pain perception and regulation in health and disease. Eur J Pain 2005; 9:463–484.
35 Freund HJ: The parietal lobe as a sensorimotor interface: a perspective from clinical and neuroimaging data. NeuroImage 2001;14:S142–146.
36 Fuster JM: The Prefrontal Cortex. Anatomy, Physiology and Neuropsychology of the Frontal Lobe. Philadelphia, Lippincott-Raven, 1997.

PD Dr. Florian Pfab
Department of Radiology, Massachusetts General Hospital
Harvard Medical School
Building 149, Room 2301, 13th Street
Charlestown, MA 02129 (USA)
Tel. +1 617 838 6644, E-Mail pfab@nmr.mgh.harvard.edu

Author Index

Subject Index